CASE REVIEW
Genitourinary Imaging

Series Editor

David M. Yousem, MD, MBA
Professor of Radiology
Director of Neuroradiology
Russell H. Morgan Department of Radiology and Radiological Science
The Johns Hopkins Medical Institutions
Baltimore, Maryland

Other Volumes in the CASE REVIEW Series

Brain Imaging
Breast Imaging
Cardiac Imaging
Gastrointestinal Imaging
General and Vascular Ultrasound
Head and Neck Imaging, Second Edition
Musculoskeletal Imaging
Nuclear Medicine
Obstetric and Gynecologic Ultrasound
Pediatric Imaging
Spine Imaging
Thoracic Imaging
Vascular and Interventional Imaging

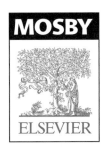

Ronald J. Zagoria, M.D.
Professor of Radiology
Section Head of Abdominal Imaging
Vice Chairman for Medical Affairs
Wake Forest University Baptist Medical Center
Winston-Salem, North Carolina

William W. Mayo-Smith, M.D.
Professor of Radiology
Brown University School of Medicine
Director of Computed Tomography
Rhode Island Hospital
Providence, Rhode Island

Julia R. Fielding, M.D.
Section Head of Abdominal Imaging
Associate Professor, Radiology
University of North Carolina, Chapel Hill
Chapel Hill, North Carolina

WITH OVER 500 ILLUSTRATIONS

CASE REVIEW

Genitourinary Imaging

SECOND EDITION

CASE REVIEW SERIES

MOSBY
ELSEVIER

1600 John F. Kennedy Blvd.
Suite 1800
Philadelphia, PA 19103-2899

GENITOURINARY IMAGING: CASE REVIEW   ISBN-13: 978-0-323-03714-3
Copyright © 2007, 2000 by Mosby, Inc., an affiliate of Elsevier Inc.   ISBN-10: 0-323-03714-3

Library of Congress Cataloging-in-Publication Data

Zagoria, Ronald J.
  Genitourinary imaging : case review / Ronald J. Zagoria, William W. Mayo-Smith, Julia R.
Fielding. — 2nd ed.
      p. ; cm. — (Case review series)
  Cross-referenced to: Genitourinary radiology / Ronald J. Zagoria. 2nd ed.
c2004.
  Includes bibliographical references and index.
  ISBN 0-323-03714-3
  1. Genitourinary organs—Imaging—Examinations, questions, etc.
  I. Zagoria, Ronald J. Genitourinary radiology. II. Fielding, Julia R.
III. Mayo-Smith, William W. IV. Title. V. Series.
  [DNLM: 1. Urogenital Diseases—diagnosis—Examination Questions.
2. Diagnostic Imaging—Examination Questions. WJ 18.2 Z18g 2007]
  RC874.Z34 2007
  616.6'0754076—dc22   2006043831

Acquisitions Editor: Meghan McAteer
Developmental Editor: Ryan Creed
Project Manager: Bryan Hayward

Printed in the United States of America

Last digit is the print number: 9 8 7 6 5 4 3 2 1

To my favorite people, Kathy, David, Michael, Sam, and Sylvia, who bring so much pleasure to my life.

RJZ

To dear Margaret and Bill, who cultivated intellectual curiosity.
To Leslie, who has supported me throughout.
And to my dogs, James, Andrew, and Chris, who keep it all in perspective.

WWM-S

To my parents, who made sure that I was prepared for anything.
To my husband and son, who make every day a delight.
And to my residents, who convince me of a bright future for radiology.

JRF

I have been very gratified by the popularity of the Case Review Series and the positive feedback the authors have received on the publication of the first edition of their volumes. Reviews in journals and word-of-mouth comments have been uniformly favorable. The authors have done an outstanding job in filling the niche of an affordable, easy-to-read, case-based learning tool that supplements the material in *THE REQUISITES* series. While some students learn best in a noninteractive study-book mode, others need the anxiety or excitement of being quizzed, being put on the hot seat. Recognizing this need, the publisher and I selected the format of the Case Review Series to simulate the Boards experience by showing a limited number of images needed to construct a differential diagnosis and asking a few clinical and imaging questions (the only difference being that the Case Review books give you the correct answer and immediate feedback!). Cases are scaled from relatively easy to very hard to test the limit of the reader's knowledge. A brief authors' commentary, a cross-reference to the companion *REQUISITES* volume, and an up-to-date literature reference are also provided for each case.

Because of the success of the series, we have begun to roll out the second editions of the volumes. The expectation is that the second editions will bring the material to the state-of-the-art, introduce new modalities and new techniques, and provide new and even more graphic examples of pathology.

Ron Zagoria, Bill Mayo-Smith, and Julia Fielding have certainly fulfilled the mission of the second editions of the Case Review Series by providing a balanced array of cases from different modalities and pathologies and of varying difficulty. There are new cases, new techniques, new insights, and new entities. The image quality and the new emphasis on differential diagnosis (as demanded by trainees across the globe) add to the value of this second edition.

I welcome the *Genitourinary Radiology* volume by Drs. Zagoria, Mayo-Smith, and Fielding to the second edition Case Review Series line-up, which also includes *Head and Neck Imaging*, second edition, by myself and Dr. Ana Carolina B. S. da Motta. First edition volumes include *Breast Imaging* by Emily F. Conant and Cecilia M. Brennecke, *Cardiac Imaging* by Gautham Reddy and Robert Steiner; *Vascular and Interventional Imaging* by Suresh Vedantham and Jennifer Gould, *Pediatric Imaging* by Rob Ward and Hans Blickman, *Nuclear Medicine* by Harvey A. Zeissman and Patricia Rehm, *General and Vascular Ultrasound* by William D. Middleton, *Musculoskeletal Imaging* by Joseph Yu, *Obstetric and Gynecologic Ultrasound* by Al Kurtz and Pam Johnson, *Spine Imaging* by rian Bowen, *Thoracic Imaging* by Phil Boiselle and Theresa McLoud, *Gastrointestinal Imaging* by Peter Feczko and Robert Halpert, and *Brain Imaging* by Laurie Loevner.

David M. Yousem, MD, MBA

When the publisher asked me to step up to lead this project, and Glen Tung declined participation, the task of revising this textbook seemed formidable. This was before Bill Mayo-Smith and I recruited Julia Fielding as the third contributor. Fortunately, Dr. Fielding enthusiastically embraced the project. Readers will quickly find that there are many new cases in the textbook and that many of the cases in the first edition have been updated. Outdated cases have been deleted and replaced with ones more relevant today. We have greatly expanded the number of MR cases as well as the number and breadth of gynecologic cases. The timeliness of these contributions could not be better. With improved techniques, the impact of imaging studies on the treatment of gynecologic diseases has increased substantially since the writing of the first edition. Because students frequently use the book to prepare for the oral examination given by the American Board of Radiology, we felt that expansion of these segments of the book would lead to better preparation for the exam, which is constantly updated to reflect practice patterns. In addition, there is an increased emphasis on cross-sectional imaging as the first test used in diagnosis of gastrourinary diseases. Since publication of the first edition, the use of multidetector CT and newer MR protocols has increased, and these new applications are reflected in this second edition.

The three of us are very proud of this new textbook. We feel it offers an engaging way to learn and review genitourinary imaging techniques. Careful reading of this textbook and assimilation of the learning points presented within should prepare the reader well for approaching even the most difficult gastrourinary imaging cases. For those readers using this in preparation for the board examination, we feel confident that this textbook, used in conjunction with other learning tools and practical experience, will prepare them well for the cases shown during the gastrourinary segment of the exam.

The three of us hope that the second edition of *Genitourinary Imaging: Case Review* helps the reader learn about this ever-changing, interesting, and challenging subspecialty of radiology.

Ronald J. Zagoria, MD

I acknowledge the wonderful contributions to this textbook provided by Drs. William Mayo-Smith and Julia Fielding. Without them it would have been impossible to complete this second edition. Glen Tung, MD, was the lead author on the first edition of this textbook. He contributed a large number of cases, and his write-ups were fantastic. Much of this material was used in the second edition, albeit updated when needed, but his contributions remain substantial. I am grateful to him for allowing us to include those cases that we felt were germane. In addition, I gratefully acknowledge the help of my colleagues and mentors in the Department of Diagnostic Radiology at the Wake Forest University School of Medicine. These include my long-time mentor Ray Dyer, MD, and the other members of the abdominal radiology section, but in particular John Leyendecker, MD, for his help with the cases focused on MR imaging. I thank David and Michael Zagoria for their help with the crucial task of organizing the cases for this edition. Many residents and fellows contributed to this textbook, and I gratefully acknowledge their contributions. These include Drs. Scott Baginski, Noel Berquist, Forrest Carson, Lance Dasher, Andy Deibler, Kathryn Olsen, Joe Pastrano, Alex Pertile, Christian Scales, Grant Thaxton, and Chris Whitlow. I also am extremely grateful for the contributions made by my administrative assistant, Maureen Crumley. Without her, chaos would reign, and it would be difficult to complete projects such as this. Finally, I want to thank my wife Kathy for her support and patience, for which I am forever thankful. Projects like this require sacrifices from one's family. Kathy's willingness to support my participation in academic efforts such as this is nothing less than noble.

RJZ

In the first edition of this text, I learned that writing a book is not an easy task. In this second edition, I learned that revising a book is easier than writing it, but not by much! I owe much to my colleagues for this edition. Drs. Baird, Beland, Dubel, Kalinsky, Khan, Lourenco Potter, Prince, Salad, and Yoo all contributed new and interesting cases to the book. Particular thanks go to Liz Lazarus, who wrote multiple "women's imaging" cases, and I wish her well in her budding career. I would also like to acknowledge my Chair, John Cronan, who has been very supportive of academics at Brown; Mark Ridlen, who somehow schedules us; and my colleagues, who have performed clinical duties during my academic absences. Also thanks to my office mate Damian Dupuy for his energy and sense of humor.

Ron Zagoria, who prepared the final edits and layout, has been an exemplary senior author for this edition. Readers will notice that the authorship has changed with the second edition. My friend and colleague Glenn Tung has shifted to a different academic arena and is thriving there. When Ron asked me who we should recruit as a new third author, my response was nearly instantaneous: Julia Fielding. Julia is smart, has a tremendous work ethic, and completes tasks in a timely manner. I know the text has been greatly strengthened by her additions.

Finally, I would like to acknowledge my wife, Leslie, and my three sons, James, Andrew, and Chris. Writing a book takes time away from family life, and they have been very supportive of this endeavor the second time around.

I hope you enjoy our new edition of *Genitourinary Imaging: Case Review*!

WWM-S

Color Plates

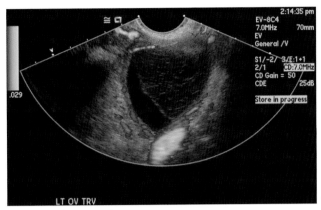

Case 37 (page 55).

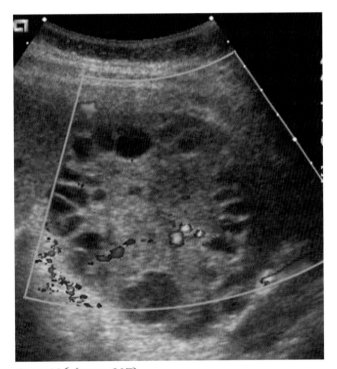

Case 126 (page 207).

Opening Round

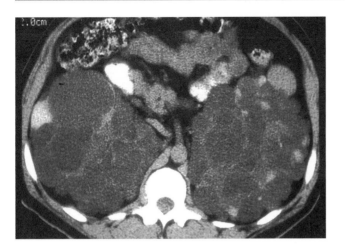
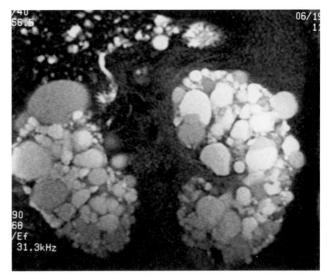

1. What causes the numerous low attenuation renal lesions seen on this patient's CT scan?

2. What is the most likely underlying diagnosis in these two patients with the same disease?

3. Why are some of the masses of lower signal intensity on the coronal T2W MRI?

4. What is the risk of renal cell carcinoma development in this group of patients?

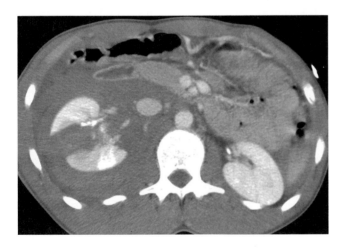

1. What type of kidney injury is shown?

2. On this 120-second delayed image, is there urine extravasation?

3. Is this type of injury usually caused by penetrating or blunt trauma?

4. How are these injuries usually treated?

Kidney: Autosomal Dominant Polycystic Kidney Disease

1. Numerous renal cysts.

2. Autosomal dominant polycystic kidney disease.

3. These represent cysts complicated by infection or hemorrhage, resulting in higher protein content in the fluid, pp 1–6.

4. The same as in the general population.

Reference

Hartman DS: An overview of renal cystic disease. In Hartman DS, ed: *Renal Cystic Disease*, Philadelphia, 1989, Saunders, pp 1–6.

Cross-Reference

Zagoria RJ, *Genitourinary Radiology: THE REQUISITES*, 2nd ed, pp 135, 152.

Comment

Autosomal dominant polycystic kidney disease (ADPKD) is a hereditary disorder that is inherited in an autosomal dominant pattern. This disease may come to light as a result of hematuria, hypertension, or renal insufficiency. Up to 15% of patients develop intracranial aneurysms that may lead to subarachnoid hemorrhage and later discovery of the underlying renal disease. Although there is no increased risk for malignancy development in these patients, the disease, which has a high degree of penetrance, nearly always progresses to complete renal failure and the need for long-term dialysis. As the patient ages, more and more renal cysts develop, leading to complete replacement of the parenchyma by cystic masses, as seen on this MRI. In addition these patients often develop cysts in other organs. Hepatic cysts, as seen on the MRI, occur in up to 75% of ADPKD patients. Cysts in other abdominal and pelvic viscera also are relatively common.

Notes

Kidney: Fractured Kidney

1. A deep laceration, also called a fracture, of the right kidney.

2. Yes. Contrast material as dense as the urine excreted by the opposite kidney is leaking between the two right kidney fragments.

3. The vast majority of these injuries result from blunt force, usually from motor vehicle collisions.

4. Renal lacerations are usually treated conservatively, with resection reserved for protracted renal bleeding, and for removal of nonviable kidneys. This patient did undergo a nephrectomy.

Reference

Kawashima A, Sandler CM, Corl FM, et al: Imaging of renal trauma: a comprehensive review, *Radiographics* 21:557–574, 2001.

Cross-Reference

Zagoria RJ, *Genitourinary Radiology: THE REQUISITES*, 2nd ed, pp 153–157.

Comment

Renal trauma is best evaluated with contrast-enhanced CT as part of an evaluation of the entire abdomen and pelvis. The most common renal injury is contusion, or a bruise. Contusions comprise about 75% of renal injuries. A contusion is a minor injury that causes nephrographic abnormalities, including focal areas of decreased contrast excretion. They generally do not require more than supportive care. Other minor renal injuries include small subcapsular hematomas and minor surface lacerations without significant hematomas. These are graded as category I injuries by the CT classification scheme referenced above. Class II injuries are major lacerations of the kidney. These include the full-thickness tears that result in separation of the kidney into two or more fragments, a fracture. Concomitant with these lacerations are perirenal hematomas and urinomas. Active bleeding can be demonstrated as vascular contrast extravasation on early-phase contrast-enhanced CT images. To diagnose urine extravasation, more delayed images are required, usually greater than 120 seconds after initiation of contrast injection. Treatment of class II injuries largely depends on the patient's stability and sequential changes demonstrated on follow-up CT scans.

Class III and IV injuries are much less common and generally require surgical repair. Class III injuries include catastrophic injuries such as renal vascular pedicle disruptions and severe multifocal renal lacerations. Class IV injuries are ureteropelvic junction disruptions, including lacerations and avulsions.

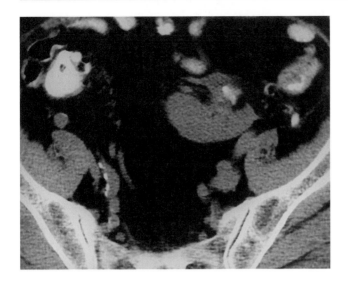 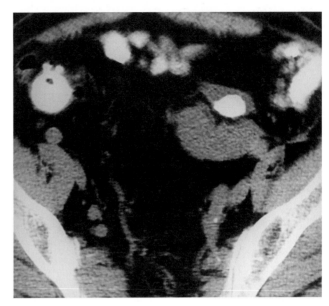

1. What findings are evident on these images?

2. What is the normal path of renal migration during development?

3. What complications are associated with this condition?

4. Which radiologic examination may be helpful before surgery is performed on patients with this condition?

C A S E   3

Kidney: Nephrolith in a Pelvic Kidney

1. Left pelvic kidney with a renal pelvis calculus.

2. Ureteral bud develops at the S1 level and migrates cranially to the L2 level.

3. Obstruction, vesicoureteral reflux, and stone formation.

4. CT or MR angiography, because the vascular supply to a pelvic kidney may be quite variable.

References

Bader AA, Tamussino KF, Winter R: Ectopic (pelvic) kidney mimicking bulky lymph nodes at pelvic lymphadenectomy, *Gynecol Oncol* 96(3):873–875, 2005.

Daneman A, Alton DJ: Radiographic manifestation of renal anomalies, *Radiol Clin North Am* 29:351, 1991.

Cross-Reference

Zagoria RJ, *Genitourinary Radiology: THE REQUISITES*, 2nd ed, pp 55–61.

Comment

Both the ureteral bud and the metanephric blastema are necessary for the normal development of a kidney. The kidneys develop from the ureteral bud and metanephric blastema between the 4th and 8th weeks of gestation. The kidney starts developing at approximately the S1 vertebral level and migrates cranially to the L2 level. Any arrest in this cranial migration results in renal ectopia. Pelvic kidney, as illustrated in this case, has an incidence of approximately 1 per 1000 live births. Most patients with a pelvic kidney have no symptoms. However, some may have symptoms resulting from vesicoureteral reflux or obstruction; ureteropelvic junction obstruction is particularly common. In this case there is a renal pelvis stone, presumably caused by urinary stasis. Pelvic kidneys are usually maloriented and are often smaller than their normal counterparts. Renal function may also be decreased.

It is important to confirm that a pelvic "mass" is a pelvic kidney to avoid unnecessary surgery. Imaging of the upper abdomen at the time a reniform pelvic mass is discovered confirms the diagnosis of ectopic kidney if the ipsilateral renal fossa is empty. If surgery is planned, CT or MR angiography may be helpful because the blood supply to ectopic kidneys is variable. The arterial supply to the embryonic kidney starts with the iliac vessels, then involves the distal aorta, and finally arises from the middle aorta at the L1–L2 level. As new vessels develop, the initial caudal vessels usually regress. However, a duplicated arterial supply is common from persistence of the embryologic vessels.

Notes

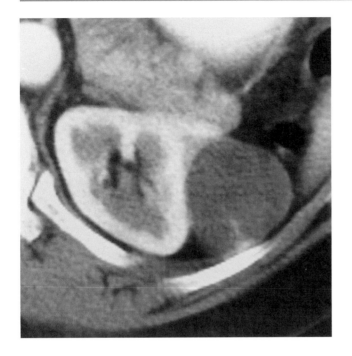 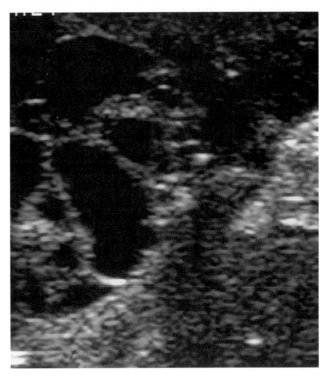

1. Would the renal mass shown be treated surgically or would it usually be treated conservatively?

2. What are the main differential diagnoses for this type of mass?

3. Using the Bosniak classification, what class is this lesion?

4. What single imaging feature is specific for the diagnosis of multilocular cystic nephroma?

Kidney: Cystic Renal Cell Carcinoma

1. Based on the multiple septations and slight thickening of the peripheral margins, this mass should be considered a surgical renal mass. This determination is further confirmed by the sonographic image showing thick septations.

2. Renal cell carcinoma, multilocular cystic nephroma, and renal cyst complicated by infection or hemorrhage.

3. Based on the CT scan, this is a Bosniak class IV lesion with some enhancing tissue in the mass. Cystic lesions with enhancing solid components are Bosniak class IV.

4. Herniation of the mass into the renal pelvis.

Reference

Hartman DS, Choyke PL, Hartman MS: From the RSNA Refresher Courses: a practical approach to the cystic renal mass, *Radiographics* 24(Suppl 1):101–115, 2004.

Cross-Reference

Zagoria RJ, *Genitourinary Radiology: THE REQUISITES*, 2nd ed, pp 87–89.

Comment

Any ball-shaped renal mass that is not a simple cyst and does not contain detectable fat should be considered a renal cell carcinoma. Lesions that are predominantly cystic can be further classified using the Bosniak classification system. This system allows for some complex cystic lesions with additional features, such as thin peripheral calcifications or one or two septa, to be classified as benign cysts. However, Bosniak class III and IV lesions are surgical renal masses, unless there are extenuating circumstances, such as metastatic disease, or features strongly suggestive of an alternative nonsurgical diagnosis, like an abscess. Renal masses that appear to be cysts must be scrutinized very carefully. As demonstrated by this case, enhancement can be very subtle; multiple septations are faintly visible within this mass. When there is doubt regarding the diagnosis, sonography can help further elucidate the internal architecture of a renal mass. Sonography clearly shows the complicated internal architecture of this mass, which was a renal cell carcinoma.

Multilocular cystic nephroma can have an appearance identical to that of renal cell carcinoma. Sometimes multilocular cystic nephromas herniate into the renal sinus. This sign is diagnostic of this entity, but it is not sensitive for this diagnosis. Most multilocular cystic nephromas do not herniate into the renal pelvis.

Notes

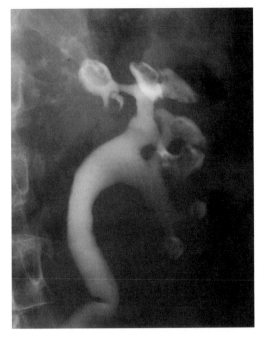

1. Are the filling defects seen in this case located within the calyx or the medulla of the kidney?

2. What is the most likely diagnosis for these filling defects?

3. What processes may cause unilateral papillary necrosis?

4. What is this radiologic appearance of filling defects surrounded by contrast material called in this location?

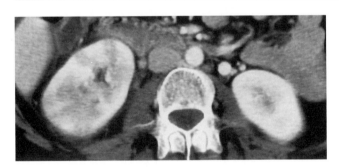

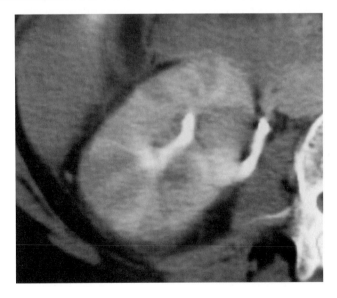

1. What is the diagnosis in this febrile patient?

2. What causes the areas of decreased enhancement in the right kidney?

3. In the setting of blunt trauma, what type of renal injury can have an identical radiographic appearance?

4. True or false: When hydronephrosis is present with this type of renal abnormality, it is the result of ureteral obstruction.

CASE 5

Kidney: Papillary Necrosis

1. Medulla.

2. Papillary necrosis.

3. Pyelonephritis, ureteral obstruction, tuberculosis, and renal vein thrombosis.

4. Signet ring.

Reference

Davidson AJ, Hartman DS, eds: In *Radiology of the Kidney and Urinary Tract*, 2nd ed, Philadelphia, 1994, Saunders, pp 177–189.

Cross-Reference

Zagoria RJ, *Genitourinary Radiology: THE REQUISITES*, 2nd ed, p 196.

Comment

Papillary necrosis is a cause of gross hematuria and a common cause of chronic renal insufficiency. It usually results from ischemia of the medulla of the kidneys. Common causes of papillary necrosis can be remembered by the mnemonic *POSTCARD*, which abbreviates the following common causes: *p*yelonephritis, *o*bstruction, *s*ickle cell disease, *t*uberculosis, *c*irrhosis/pancreatitis, *a*nalgesic abuse, *r*enal vein thrombosis, and *d*iabetes mellitus. Necrosis of the papillae may be predominantly central, causing a cavity that communicates with the nadir of the calyceal concavity. The result is the "ball on tee" pattern that is seen on contrast studies. Alternatively, papillary necrosis originating at the margins of the papilla initially causes sloughing of the edges of the papilla, resulting in apparent elongation of the fornices (angles) of the calyx and causing a "lobster claw" pattern. Further necrosis leads to complete sloughing of a large segment of the papillary tip. Contrast material can then extend from the calyx and surround this necrotic segment of the medulla. If this tissue remains in place, it causes the signet ring appearance, as seen in this case. All of these radiologic patterns are typical of papillary necrosis. The necrotic papilla may pass into the calyx and advance into the ureter, causing ureteral obstruction and a radiologic appearance similar to that seen with a ureteral stone. Clues that help diagnose a sloughed papilla include a roughly triangular filling defect and evidence of papillary necrosis in the upper tract of the kidney on the involved side.

Notes

CASE 6

Kidney: Acute Pyelonephritis

1. Acute pyelonephritis.

2. Interstitial edema of the kidney leads to urinary stasis in some tubules in the medulla. These tubules do not opacify to the degree of normal areas of kidney filled with opacified urine.

3. Renal contusion.

4. False. Some bacteria that cause acute pyelonephritis release an endotoxin, which leads to smooth muscle paralysis and nonobstructive hydronephrosis.

Reference

Gash JR, Zagoria RJ, Dyer RB: Imaging features of infiltrating renal lesions, *Crit Rev Diagn Imaging* 33:293–310, 1992.

Cross-Reference

Zagoria RJ, *Genitourinary Radiology: THE REQUISITES*, 2nd ed, pp 135–138.

Comment

Acute pyelonephritis is almost always the result of infection ascending from the bladder via reflux of infected urine or lymphatic communication with bladder infection. It usually is a unilateral process. Radiographically, acute pyelonephritis may be focal or diffuse, as in this case. On intravenous urography, 70% of patients with pyelonephritis have no abnormal findings. However, CT is much more sensitive for the detection of abnormalities caused by pyelonephritis. Typical CT findings include unilateral nephromegaly, striated nephrogram, and patchy, wedge-shaped areas of low attenuation in the otherwise enhanced kidney. The bacteria often secrete an endotoxin, which can cause hydronephrosis as a result of diminished peristalsis and flaccidity of the smooth muscle of the ureter. This finding should not be confused with ureteral obstruction. The differential diagnosis for the parenchymal abnormalities seen with pyelonephritis includes renal contusion, infarcts, and radiation therapy–induced injury.

Imaging is not usually required to diagnose pyelonephritis because this condition is easily diagnosed on a clinical basis. On occasion, imaging findings of pyelonephritis may precede detectable bacteriuria and fever by several days. Possible complicating features include emphysematous pyelonephritis, abscess formation, and xanthogranulomatous pyelonephritis, all of which may require additional treatment.

Notes

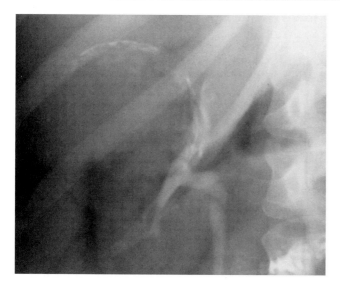

1. What is the most likely diagnosis for the calcified renal mass shown?

2. What percentage of lesions such as the one shown here are malignant?

3. Regardless of the calcification pattern, what diagnosis encompasses the majority of calcified renal masses?

4. What imaging test should be recommended for further evaluation of this abnormality?

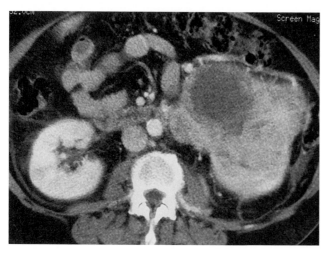 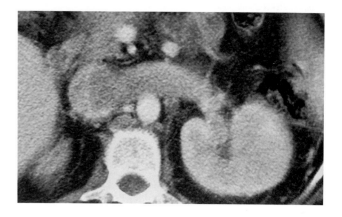

1. What is the most likely diagnosis?

2. What stage disease is shown?

3. What is the risk of a synchronous lesion in the right kidney?

4. What is the significance of the brightly enhancing tubular structures anterior to the renal mass?

CASE 7

Kidney: Calcified Renal Mass

1. Complicated renal cyst.

2. 20%.

3. Renal cell carcinoma.

4. CT or MRI.

Reference

Daniel WW Jr, Hartman GW, Witten DM, et al: Calcified renal masses: a review of ten years experience at the Mayo Clinic, *Radiology* 103:503–508, 1972.

Cross-Reference

Zagoria RJ, *Genitourinary Radiology: THE REQUISITES*, 2nd ed, pp 83–84.

Comment

The patient shown has a spherical, ball-shaped mass arising from the middle portion of the right kidney. This mass displaces the calyces with compression and splaying. There is a calcified rim around the upper half of this mass.

Of calcified renal masses, 60% are renal cell carcinoma. Overall, renal cell carcinomas calcify in approximately 20% to 30% of cases. Renal cysts calcify in 1% to 2% of cases. The diagnosis for this patient is renal cell carcinoma; however, the rim of calcification that is visible is more commonly seen with complicated cysts than with renal cell carcinoma. Of those masses in which the calcification is purely rimlike, as in this case, 80% are cysts that have been complicated with hemorrhage or infection. Significantly, 20% of those lesions are renal cell carcinomas, as shown here. The bottom line is that a calcified renal mass requires further evaluation because the risk of malignancy is high. Further imaging evaluation should be recommended for diagnosis and staging, if necessary. Although renal sonography is the standard test for evaluating noncalcified renal masses, CT before and after contrast material infusion is the standard technique for further characterization and possible staging of calcified renal masses. With CT or MRI, which are of comparable efficacy, the internal architecture of the mass can be better evaluated. If delicate, peripheral calcification is the only complex feature in an otherwise simple cyst, further evaluation is probably unnecessary. Alternatively, numerous septations, enhancement, or solid internal components would qualify this mass as a surgical renal mass, most likely a malignancy.

Notes

CASE 8

Kidney: Renal Cell Carcinoma with Extension into the Renal Vein and Inferior Vena Cava

1. Renal cell carcinoma.

2. Stage III.

3. 2%.

4. They represent collateral vessels draining or feeding the mass in the left kidney.

References

Catalano C, Fraioli F, Laghi A, et al: High-resolution multidetector CT in the preoperative evaluation of patients with renal cell carcinoma, *Am J Roentgenol* 180:1271–1277, 2003.

Zagoria RJ, Bechtold RE, Dyer RB: Staging of renal adenocarcinoma: role of various imaging procedures, *Am J Roentgenol* 164:363–370, 1995.

Cross-Reference

Zagoria RJ, *Genitourinary Radiology: THE REQUISITES*, 2nd ed, pp 96, 97, 99.

Comment

This patient has a large heterogeneous exophytic renal mass typical of renal cell carcinoma (RCC). RCC is hypervascular in 80% of cases. This hypervascularity often leads to enlargement of collateral arteries and veins around the kidney. RCC also has a predilection to grow contiguously into the venous system. The accurate diagnosis of venous extension of tumor is crucial for treatment planning. This diagnosis is most accurately made based on thin-section CT during bolus contrast material infusion or MRI. In this case the tumor thrombus is easily visible as a low-attenuation filling defect within and enlarging the left renal vein. The tumor extends into the inferior vena cava, filling approximately one half of the vena cava lumen. This finding is diagnostic of Robson stage III disease. Tumor thrombus within the renal vein also encourages the development of venous collaterals to drain the kidney and the renal tumor. When a renal mass such as this is detected, the extent of disease must be determined, particularly with regard to regional lymph nodes, the renal vein, the inferior vena cava, and areas where metastases commonly occur (e.g., the lungs, bones, and liver). Because surgery is the conventional mode of treatment for RCC, the other kidney should be scrutinized for synchronous lesions. RCC is bilateral in approximately 1% to 2% of nonfamilial cases.

Notes

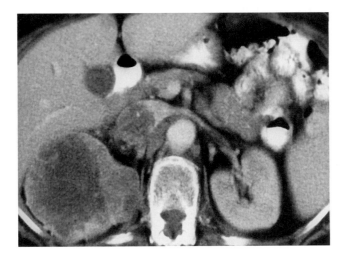 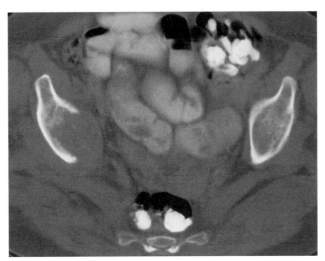

1. What is the most likely diagnosis?
2. What is the stage of this disease?
3. How does the radiologist differentiate caval invasion by tumor from inflow phenomenon?
4. How would you obtain a histologic diagnosis on this patient?

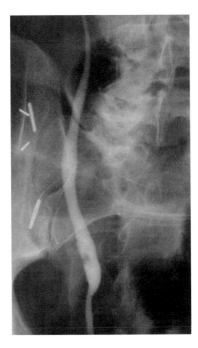 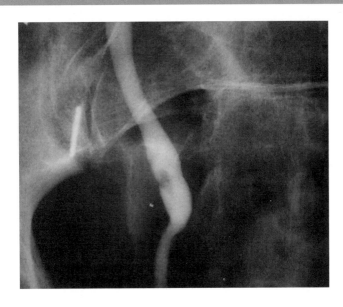

1. What are the major differential diagnoses for this filling defect?
2. When a ureteral transitional cell carcinoma is detected, what is the risk of a synchronous or metachronous transitional cell carcinoma elsewhere in the urinary tract?
3. Most radiolucent stones are composed of what substance?
4. What imaging characteristics of this mass suggest that it is a mucosal lesion?

C A S E 9

Kidney: Metastatic Renal Cell Carcinoma

1. Renal cell carcinoma associated with inferior vena cava invasion and osteolytic metastasis to the right ilium.

2. Stage IV.

3. Continuity of filling defect with ipsilateral renal vein, expansion of inferior vena cava, and persistent filling defect on delayed imaging.

4. CT-guided biopsy of iliac lesion.

Reference

Zagoria RJ, Bechtold RE, Dyer RB: Staging of renal adenocarcinoma: role of various imaging procedures, *Am J Roentgenol* 164:363–370, 1995.

Cross-Reference

Zagoria RJ, *Genitourinary Radiology: THE REQUISITES*, 2nd ed, pp 89–100.

Comment

Every year in the United States 35,000 new cases of renal adenocarcinoma are diagnosed. Men are afflicted twice as often as women, and the incidence peaks between the ages of 50 and 70 years. The terms *clear cell carcinoma* and *hypernephroma* were used in the past because of the similarity of the lesion's histologic characteristics to those of clear cells of the adrenal cortex and because of the original misconception that these tumors arose from the adrenal gland itself, hence the term *hypernephroma*. Renal adenocarcinoma arises from epithelial cells of the proximal tubules and often develops in the upper or lower poles of the kidney.

The appearance of renal cell carcinomas (RCCs) on CT varies, depending on the size of the lesion and the phase of contrast enhancement. Approximately 90% are exophytic masses, and all are hypodense compared with kidney during the tubular phase of enhancement. Of RCCs, 31% display calcification on CT. The calcification is typically central, diffuse, or coarse. Although 20% of RCCs are described as cystic, this number is deceiving. The majority of cystic RCCs have peripheral nodular enhancement or thickened, calcified septa.

Helical CT enables evaluation of the liver and kidney in different stages of enhancement. With dynamic imaging performed early in the cortical phase of enhancement, subtle renal masses can be overlooked. Imaging during the nephrographic phase of enhancement (approximately 120 seconds after the injection of contrast has begun) is optimal for detecting small renal masses.

Notes

C A S E 10

Pelvicalices and Ureter: Transitional Cell Carcinoma

1. Transitional cell carcinoma, radiolucent stone, blood clot, infectious debris, and air bubble.

2. 40%.

3. Uric acid.

4. It has acute margins with the wall of the ureter, and there is slight indentation of the ureter wall adjacent to the lesion.

Reference

Wong-You-Cheong JJ, Wagner BJ, Davis CJ Jr: Transitional cell carcinoma of the urinary tract: radiologic-pathologic correlation, *Radiographics* 18:123–142, 1998.

Cross-Reference

Zagoria RJ, *Genitourinary Radiology: THE REQUISITES*, 2nd ed, pp 191–197.

Comment

The most common causes of radiolucent filling defects seen in the urinary tract are radiolucent stones, followed by transitional cell carcinoma (TCC). Other causes include blood clots, infectious debris, air bubbles, sloughed papillae, indentation by an extrinsic mass, other urothelial neoplasms, and submucosal inflammation. The majority of these lesions are the result of radiolucent stones and ureteral tumors, mainly TCC. Closely scrutinizing the details of these lesions can often help in the diagnosis. Acute angles where the filling defect abuts the urothelium suggest an intraluminal or a mucosal process. Retraction of the ureteral wall, as seen in this case, indicates that this is a mucosal lesion and probably a TCC. Of TCCs, 90% develop in the bladder, with approximately 9% arising in the pyelocalyceal system. When a TCC develops in one of the more unusual sites, there is a markedly increased risk for synchronous or metachronous TCC developing elsewhere along the urothelial lining. The presence of a ureter TCC, the least common site for these tumors to develop, is associated with synchronous TCCs 40% of the time. The most common site for synchronous tumors is the bladder. Smokers, patients exposed to benzene compounds or some oncologic chemotherapy agents, patients with Balkan nephropathy, and analgesic abusers are at increased risk of developing TCC.

Notes

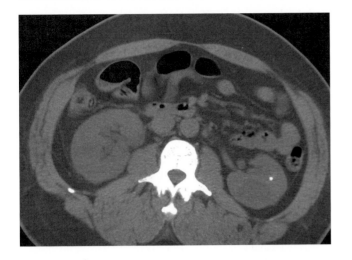

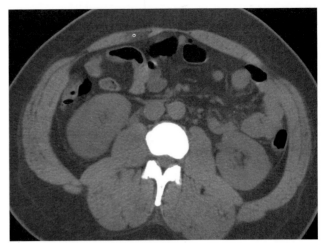

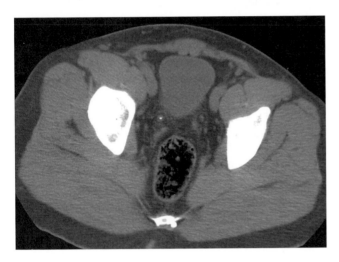

1. What is the cause for this patient's acute right flank pain?

2. What two secondary CT findings are most strongly indicative of ureterolithiasis?

3. What is the name commonly used to describe the collar of tissue around a ureteral stone seen on CT?

4. True or false: Uric acid stones are radiolucent on CT.

Pelvicalices and Ureter: Ureteral Stone

1. A ureteral stone in the lower right ureter.

2. Unilateral stranding around the ureter or kidney, and ipsilateral hydronephrosis.

3. Soft tissue rim sign.

4. False. Virtually all urinary tract calculi are radio-dense on CT.

References

Dalrymple NC, Casford B, Raiken DP, et al: Pearls and pitfalls in the diagnosis of ureterolithiasis with unenhanced helical CT, *Radiographics* 20:439–447, 2000.

Smith RC, Varanelli M: Diagnosis and management of acute ureterolithiasis: CT is truth. *Am J Roentgenol* 175:3–6, 2000.

Cross-Reference

Zagoria RJ, *Genitourinary Radiology: THE REQUISITES*, 2nd ed, pp 187–191.

Comment

This case shows mild right hydronephrosis with stranding around the right ureter. A small obstructing stone is shown in the lower right ureter, just above the ureterovesical junction.

Since it was first described in the mid 1990s, helical CT has become the standard way to diagnose ureteral stones. Virtually all stones in the urinary tract, except those composed of excreted chemicals like indinavir, are radiodense and clearly visible on unenhanced CT. This compares with detection of about 50% of urinary tract stones with standard radiography. CT is a rapid test that avoids the need for intravenous contrast material. A CT stone study is typically performed without any intravenous or oral contrast material.

When examining the urinary tract on a CT stone study, detection of secondary signs, signs caused by acute ureteral obstruction, are very helpful in making a diagnosis of ureterolithiasis. There is a greater than 90% positive predictive value for the presence of a ureteral stone when both unilateral soft tissue stranding around the kidney or the ureter and ipsilateral hydronephrosis are present. There is also a greater than 90% negative predictive value for a ureteral stone if both of these secondary signs are absent. The stranding and hydronephrosis may be subtle, as shown here, where the most obvious stranding is around the upper ureter. Other findings that can support the presence of a ureteral stone include ipsilateral renal enlargement, decreased attenuation of the kidney, and absence of the whiteness in the renal pyramids on the affected side. The latter two findings are thought to be caused by renal edema resulting from ureteral obstruction. The presence of nephrolithiasis also increases the likelihood of a ureteral stone.

In all cases where a ureteral stone is being considered, the course of each ureter should be carefully scrutinized. This is best done on an electronic monitor where "scrolling" through images can be performed. If a calcification is detected, its position in the ureter can be confirmed by following the ureteral course directly to the calcification. The presence of a "soft tissue rim" sign helps to confirm that the calcification is a ureteral stone, not a vascular calcification. The rim sign is due to edema of the ureteral wall surrounding the stone.

Notes

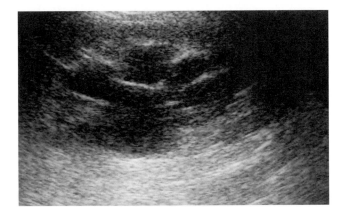

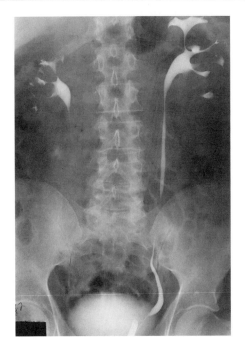

1. A sagittal sonogram of the left kidney is shown. What is the major finding and its differential diagnosis?

2. What examination is shown in the second image?

3. What is the correct diagnosis?

4. What other test (or tests) could be performed to confirm this diagnosis?

Pelvicalices and Ureters: Peripelvic Cysts

1. Multiple anechoic and echo-poor areas in the renal sinus. The differential diagnosis is pelvocaliectasis from obstruction or reflux and multiple peripelvic cysts.

2. Retrograde pyelogram.

3. Multiple, peripelvic renal cysts.

4. Contrast-enhanced CT, MRI, or intravenous urography

References

Carrim ZI, Murchison JT: The prevalence of simple renal and hepatic cysts detected by spiral computed tomography, *Clin Radiol* 58:626–629, 2003.

Israel GM, Hindman N, Bosniak MA: Evaluation of cystic renal masses: comparison of CT and MR imaging by using the Bosniak classification system, *Radiology* 231:365–371, 2004.

Minor TX, Yeh BM, Horvai AE, et al: Symptomatic perirenal serous cysts of mullerian origin mimicking renal cysts on CT, *Am J Roentgenol* 183:1393–1396, 2004.

Cross-Reference

Zagoria RJ, *Genitourinary Radiology: THE REQUISITES*, 2nd ed, pp 159–161.

Comment

Not all hypoechoic structures in the renal sinus represent hydronephrosis. The ultrasound image shows multiple echo-poor areas in the renal sinus. These areas could represent caliectasis resulting from ureteral obstruction or possibly from a ureteropelvic junction obstruction. The collecting system also may appear dilated when there is severe vesicoureteral reflux. However, with this degree of pelvocaliectasis resulting from reflux, a smaller kidney and cortical thinning over the upper and lower renal poles might be expected. The third consideration in this patient is multiple peripelvic cysts.

Renal sinus cysts can be classified as peripelvic or parapelvic, but the distinction between these is not critical because both are benign. Peripelvic cysts are common and are often multiple. Typically, peripelvic cysts insinuate themselves in the sinus fat. They are believed to be secondary to lymphatic obstruction. In contrast, parapelvic cysts originate from the renal parenchyma and extend into the renal sinus. They are usually larger than peripelvic cysts and are not as often multiple. Peripelvic cysts often distort the renal calyces and may stretch or attenuate the infundibuli, which is illustrated well on the retrograde pyelogram.

In this case a retrograde pyelogram was performed. A cystoscope was used to place a catheter in the distal ureter. Contrast material was then instilled by syringe or by drip infusion. This procedure requires cystoscopy and is routinely performed in the operating room with the patient under sedation. In contrast to the intravenous urogram, on a retrograde pyelogram the renal parenchyma is not opacified. Retrograde pyelography is commonly performed (1) to evaluate the ureters and intrarenal collecting system when they have not been completely imaged on CT urogram, (2) to evaluate a filling defect that is visible on either excretory urography or CT, and (3) to evaluate the patient for whom no explanation for hematuria has been found on other imaging studies. In addition, brushings of the ureter can be obtained for cytologic analysis during the cystoscopy.

Notes

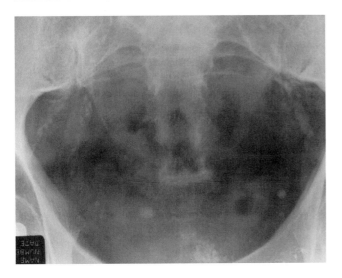 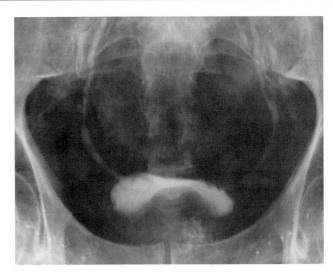

1. Name two causes of an immobile, off-midline stone in the bladder.

2. What is a pseudoureterocele?

3. What triad of findings on intravenous urography suggests the diagnosis of ureterocele on a duplex ureter?

4. Name three possible complications of intravesical ureteroceles.

Pelvicalices and Ureter: Calculus in an Orthotopic Ureterocele

1. Displacement of a bladder stone by a mass or an enlarged prostate, bladder diverticulum, or ureterocele.

2. A dilation of the intramural ureter secondary to contiguous bladder disease.

3. An upper pole renal mass, a radiolucent filling defect in the bladder, and ipsilateral or bilateral hydronephrosis.

4. Recurrent urinary tract infection, stone or milk of calcium formation, bladder outlet obstruction, and hydronephrosis.

Reference

Thornbury JR, Silver TM, Vinson RK: Ureteroceles vs. pseudoureteroceles in adults: urographic diagnosis, *Radiology* 122:81–84, 1977.

Cross-Reference

Zagoria RJ, *Genitourinary Radiology: THE REQUISITES*, 2nd ed, pp 163–165.

Comment

A ureterocele is a focal dilation of the distal end of the ureter and may be intravesical (simple) or ectopic. When the ureterocele and its orifice are both within the bladder, it is termed *intravesical*. The orifice of an intravesical ureterocele opens in the normal location but is stenotic. However, there is usually only slight dilation of the distal ureter above the ureterocele. Intravesical ureteroceles can be associated with single or duplex ureters. In contrast to those discovered in children, ureteroceles in adults usually form in single ureters that insert orthotopically, thus the term *adult ureterocele*. In most cases adult ureteroceles are incidentally discovered, but they may occur with (1) obstructive signs and symptoms, especially when large; (2) recurrent urinary tract infections; or (3) stones or milk of calcium formation.

Because renal function is typically normal, the intravesical ureterocele is distended with urine on intravenous urography, is shaped like a spring onion or cobra head, and protrudes into the lumen of the bladder. The wall of the ureterocele is visible as a lucent line or halo between the contrast-opacified urine in the ureterocele and the bladder lumen. In this case an impacted stone is isodense compared with the contrast-opacified urine in the ureterocele. On voiding cystourethrography the ureterocele often appears as a filling defect, but it can also intussuscept into the distal ureter and mimic a bladder diverticulum.

In contrast to the thin (1–2 mm) radiolucent halo associated with a ureterocele, a pseudoureterocele has an irregularly thick and nodular wall. The reported causes of pseudoureterocele include obstruction of the ureteral orifice caused by carcinoma of the bladder or cervix, a benign bladder tumor, radiation cystitis, a stone impacted in the intravesical portion of the ureter causing ureterovesical edema, or transurethral prostatic resection with ureteral orifice injury.

Notes

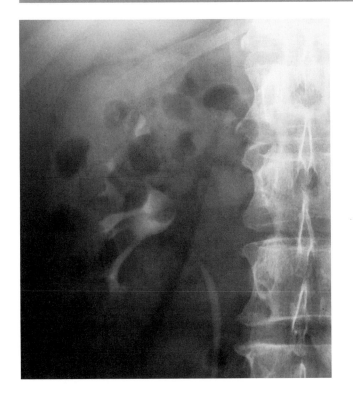 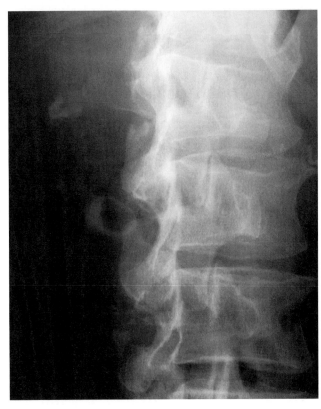

1. What is the most likely diagnosis for the filling defect shown?

2. What are the main differential diagnoses for radiolucent filling defects seen on intravenous urography?

3. What other imaging modalities could be used to better demonstrate the composition of this filling defect?

4. What chemical comprises most radiolucent urinary tract stones?

Pelvicalices and Ureter: Radiolucent Filling Defect

1. Radiolucent stone.

2. Radiolucent stones, transitional cell carcinoma, blood clot, infectious debris, sloughed papillae, and air bubbles.

3. Noncontrast CT or sonography.

4. Uric acid.

Reference

Fein AB, McClennan BL: Solitary filling defects of the ureter, *Semin Roentgenol* 21:201–213, 1986.

Cross-Reference

Zagoria RJ, *Genitourinary Radiology: THE REQUISITES*, 2nd ed, p 180.

Comment

Two films from an intravenous urogram demonstrate a relatively smooth radiolucent filling defect in the right renal pelvis. On the frontal view it is difficult to determine that this defect is not an overlying gas bubble in the colon, but its position in the renal pelvis is confirmed by the left posterior oblique view of the right kidney. Radiologists should be familiar with the common causes of radiolucent filling defects seen on intravenous urography. The most common cause is a radiolucent stone. This cause is followed closely by urothelial tumors, the majority of which are transitional cell carcinomas. Less common causes include blood clots, infectious debris, sloughed papillae, and air bubbles. The significance of these filling defects must not be underestimated. Every radiolucent filling defect should be further evaluated. This evaluation can be as simple as obtaining additional imaging studies (CT, sonography, or endoscopy). In this patient, who had a history of gross hematuria, the sharply defined radiolucent filling defect in the renal pelvis has a somewhat innocuous appearance. However, this defect was found to be a transitional cell carcinoma, and the patient underwent right nephroureterectomy.

When further imaging evaluation of a radiolucent filling defect is necessary, CT and sonography may be helpful. On noncontrast CT performed several days after any contrast-infused study, all urinary tract stones are radiodense. CT is particularly useful when the filling defect is in the ureter, an area that is difficult to examine with sonography. Nearly all radiolucent stones are composed of uric acid, with a small percentage formed from xanthine or nonmineralized matrix.

Notes

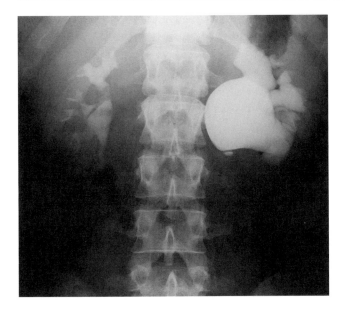
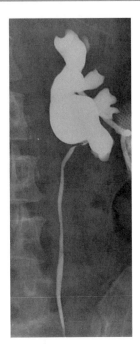

1. This condition is one of the most common causes of abdominal masses in neonates. What is the diagnosis?

2. How often are both kidneys involved?

3. What congenital urinary tract anomalies are associated with this condition?

4. How is this condition treated?

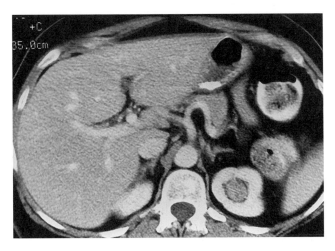
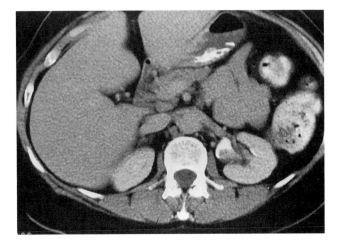

1. Two images from a CT scan of the abdomen are shown. What is the difference in the technique between these two images?

2. What is the diagnostic usefulness of the image on the right?

3. What are the three most common primary malignant neoplasms of the kidney in adults,?

4. What is the recommended treatment for this patient?

CASE 15

Pelvicalices and Ureter: Ureteropelvic Junction Obstruction

1. Congenital ureteropelvic junction obstruction.

2. In 20% of cases.

3. Horseshoe kidney, contralateral multicystic dysplastic kidney, contralateral renal agenesis, ureteral duplication, and vesicoureteral reflux.

4. Retrograde or antegrade endopyelotomy, or open pyeloplasty.

Reference

Park JM, Bloom DA: The pathophysiology of UPJ obstruction: current concepts, *Urol Clin North Am* 25:161–169, 1998.

Cross-Reference

Zagoria RJ, *Genitourinary Radiology: THE REQUISITES*, 2nd ed, pp 74, 75, 372–374.

Comment

Ureteropelvic junction (UPJ) obstruction can be defined as a functional or anatomic obstruction. This condition usually is caused by a deficiency and derangement of ureteral smooth muscle that results in a failure of normal peristalsis in the affected segment. UPJ obstruction is the most common genitourinary anomaly detected by antenatal ultrasonography and is the most common cause of urinary tract obstruction in childhood.

When UPJ obstruction is equivocal or when there is a discrepancy between the symptoms and the radiologic findings, a ureteral perfusion test (urodynamic antegrade pyelography or pressure-flow study of Whitaker) or diuretic renography can be performed to assess the functional significance of the obstruction. The ureteral perfusion test is used to measure the pressure differential between the renal pelvis and the bladder. For this test, a 21-gauge needle is placed into the intrarenal collecting system and a Foley catheter is placed into the bladder. Mild, moderate, and severe obstruction are suggested by differential pressures of 14 to 20 cm water, 21 to 34 cm water, and more than 34 cm water, respectively.

Open pyeloplasty has been the standard treatment for obstruction. However, advances in percutaneous and endourologic techniques have resulted in less invasive treatments, such as endoscopic pyelotomy. The most significant risk factor for endourologic procedures is the presence of crossing vessels at the UPJ, for which preoperative imaging with CT angiography, MR angiography, or endoluminal sonography can be performed.

Notes

CASE 16

Pelvicalices and Ureter: Transitional Cell Carcinoma of the Renal Pelvis

1. The image on the left was obtained in the portal venous phase of contrast enhancement, approximately 70 to 90 seconds after the start of intravenous contrast administration. The image on the right was obtained in the pyelographic phase of enhancement, 120 to 180 seconds after the start of contrast injection.

2. Allows evaluation of the contrast-opacified renal collecting system.

3. Renal cell carcinoma, transitional cell carcinoma, and squamous cell carcinoma.

4. Nephroureterectomy.

Reference

Wong-You-Cheong JJ, Wagner BJ, Davis CJ Jr: Transitional cell carcinoma of the urinary tract: radiologic-pathologic correlation, *Radiographics* 18:123–142, 1998.

Cross-Reference

Zagoria RJ, *Genitourinary Radiology: THE REQUISITES*, 2nd ed, pp 115–118, 180–188.

Comment

This is a classic case of transitional cell carcinoma (TCC) of the left renal collecting system. More than 90% of urothelial neoplasms are TCCs; the remaining 10% are squamous cell carcinomas. TCC occurs in the urothelial tissue in proportion to the surface area, so the most common location is the urinary bladder, followed by the renal pelvis, and the ureters. In the kidney a TCC presents as a unilateral soft tissue mass in the renal sinus, as in this case. If the infiltrating mass involves the renal parenchyma, it causes obliteration of the renal sinus fat and results in the so-called "faceless kidney," a presentation of more advanced disease.

With the advent of helical and multidetector CT, rapid imaging through the upper abdomen has become possible, and lesions in the kidneys can be overlooked because of the lack of sufficient renal and ureteral enhancement. For this reason delayed imaging through the kidneys during the pyelographic phase is recommended. As the figure on the right shows, the soft tissue mass is outlined by radiodense contrast in the left collecting system.

Of patients with TCC in the renal pelvis, 30% have multicentric disease. The treatment of choice for TCC is nephroureterectomy, as opposed to simple nephrectomy for renal cell carcinoma.

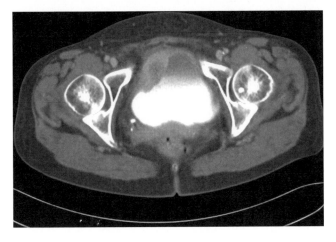 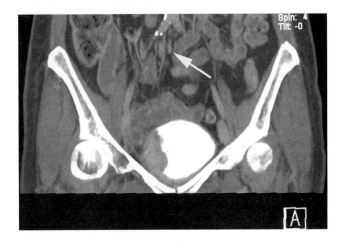

1. In the image on the left, what is the differential diagnosis of the abnormality?

2. True or false: Bladder carcinoma most often presents with dysuria.

3. True or false: The finding (*arrow*) in the image on the right constitutes presence of distant metastases.

4. Name three causes of hematuria.

Bladder: Transitional Cell Carcinoma

1. Bladder carcinoma, benign neoplasm, cystitis, fibrosis, adherent blood products.

2. False. It most often presents with hematuria.

3. False. Common iliac adenopathy constitutes N4, M0 disease.

4. Causes include cancer of the urinary tract, urinary tract infections, stone disease, renal diseases (e.g., glomerulonephritis, vasculitis, tubulointerstitial disease, etc.), and prostatic hypertrophy.

References

Webb, JA: Imaging in hematuria, *Clin Radiol* 52:167–171, 1997.

Yazgan C, Fitoz S, Atasoy C, et al: Virtual cystoscopy in the evaluation of bladder tumors, *Clin Imaging* 28:138–142, 2004.

Cross-Reference

Zagoria RJ, *Genitourinary Radiology: THE REQUISITES*, 2nd ed, pp 206–211.

Comment

Evaluation of the patient with hematuria involves clinical assessment and imaging to include the entire urinary tract. The imaging options include intravenous urography, CT urography, MRI, and ultrasonography. CT urography is advantageous because of its ability to demonstrate disease beyond the urinary tract, including distant metastases. The standard for evaluation of the bladder remains cystoscopy, which is both invasive and not without risk for complications (including iatrogenic bladder injury and urinary sepsis). CT virtual cystoscopy continues to increase in sensitivity as imaging technology improves and may play a larger diagnostic role in the future.

The bladder is the most common site of neoplastic disease in the urinary tract, and transitional cell carcinoma accounts for greater than 85% of bladder malignancies in Western countries. Bladder malignancy is increasing in incidence, probably because of increasing exposure to carcinogens. The incidence increases with age, and patients usually present with gross hematuria, which is more often painless in contrast to stone disease. Upon discovery, 70% of tumors are localized to the bladder. Transitional cell tumors are categorized as low or high grade, and the staging system mirrors its route of spread. The two noninvasive entities, papillary and flat (carcinoma in situ), are designated Ta and Tis. Invasion then proceeds sequentially through the wall of the bladder: lamina propria (T1), muscularis (T2), extravesical fat (T3), and into adjacent structures (T4).

Regional lymph node metastases are designated as unilateral regional (internal/external iliac N1), contralateral/bilateral regional (N2–3) and juxtaregional (common iliac or aortic, N4). Of note, nodes above the aortic bifurcation constitute distant metastases (M1).

Less common urothelial tumors include squamous cell carcinoma and adenocarcinoma. Squamous cell carcinoma is common outside of the United States due to its strong association with schistosomiasis infection, the sequela of which is the precursor lesion squamous metaplasia. Adenocarcinoma is rare and is known to arise in an urachal remnant, although it may originate from any location. Nonurothelial primary tumors of the bladder are rare and include sarcomas and lymphoma. These neoplastic processes may be simulated on imaging by inflammatory conditions including cystitis and fibrosis such that histologic confirmation is required.

Notes

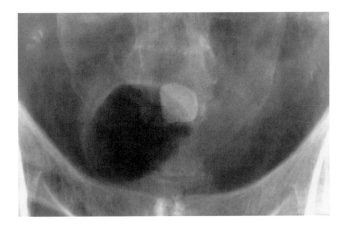
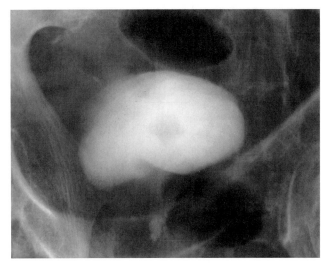

1. Name three risk factors for the development of bladder stones. Which one of these factors is probably the most prevalent?

2. Urinary infection with which bacterium is most often associated with bladder stones?

3. What are "hanging" bladder stones?

4. On a conventional radiograph of a supine patient, what is the significance of a bladder stone that is not in the midline?

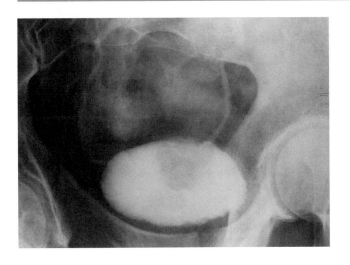
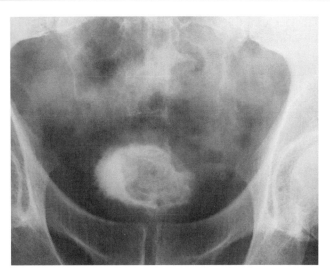

1. What is the purpose of the second radiograph?

2. Does a large amount of residual contrast material demonstrated on the postvoid radiograph indicate bladder dysfunction?

3. What is the differential diagnosis of this finding?

4. What other tests might be performed for further evaluation?

Bladder: Bladder Calculus

1. Urinary stasis, urinary tract infection, foreign body, intestinal mucosa in the urinary tract. Bladder outlet obstruction is probably the most common risk factor.

2. *Proteus* species.

3. Stones that form on nonabsorbable suture material can be suspended from the bladder wall.

4. The stone may be in a diverticulum or ureterocele or may be displaced by a bladder mass or an enlarged prostate.

Reference

Trevino R, Goldstein AMB, Vartanian NL, et al: Vesical bladder stones formed around nonabsorbable sutures and possible explanation for their delayed appearance, *J Urol* 122:849–853, 1979.

Cross-Reference

Zagoria RJ, *Genitourinary Radiology: THE REQUISITES*, 2nd ed, pp 226–227.

Comment

There are three main causes of vesical stone disease: (1) urinary stasis or presence of a foreign body, (2) primary endemic stone disease, and (3) migrant calculi from the kidney. In children and adults the most important risk factor is urinary stasis caused by bladder outlet obstruction, either mechanical or neurogenic causes. Most migrant calculi from the kidney are passed through the urethra unless the bladder outlet is relatively small, as in children, or is obstructed. Notice that the prostate gland is moderately enlarged in this case.

Foreign bodies, such as a long-term indwelling catheter, nonabsorbable suture material, pubic hairs, or fracture fragments, may form the nidus for stone formation and growth. Nonabsorbable suture material over time may migrate through the bladder wall, penetrate the mucosa, and act as a nidus. Stones formed in this manner may not change in position. In contrast, other bladder calculi are mobile. Mobility is an important distinguishing feature of bladder stones because neoplastic, inflammatory, and metabolic calcifications of the bladder wall are immobile.

On the excretory urogram, most calcified bladder stones produce filling defects in the contrast-filled bladder. As with ureteral stones, all bladder stones are radiopaque on CT. Bladder stones can be treated by cystoscopic removal, litholapaxy, chemolysis, or (when large) suprapubic cystolithotomy.

Notes

Bladder: Transitional Cell Carcinoma of the Bladder

1. The postvoid film is used to evaluate the bladder mucosa and also provides a crude measurement of bladder function.

2. Not necessarily. A large amount of contrast material in the bladder on a postvoid radiograph also may be due to a long delay between the initial radiograph and the postvoid film.

3. The finding is a focal filling defect in the bladder. The differential diagnosis is neoplasm, large calculus, blood clot, or, less likely, focal cystitis, ureterocele, or fungus ball.

4. Cystoscopy, CT, ultrasonography, or MRI.

Reference

Hillman BJ, Silvert M, Cook G, et al: Recognition of bladder tumors by excretory urography, *Radiology* 138:319–323, 1981.

Cross-Reference

Zagoria RJ, *Genitourinary Radiology: THE REQUISITES*, 2nd ed, pp 6, 228–230.

Comment

Bladder carcinoma accounts for 4% of all malignancies and has a peak incidence in the sixth to seventh decades of life. There is a 3:1 male predominance. Of malignant bladder neoplasms, 95% are carcinomas (88% are transitional cell carcinoma, 5% are squamous cell carcinoma, and 2% are adenocarcinoma). Seventy-five percent are superficial papillary lesions and 25% are invasive. Synchronous lesions occur in the upper urinary tract in approximately 2% of patients, and metachronous lesions occur in 7% of patients.

Intravenous urography has limited sensitivity for the detection of bladder neoplasms; small lesions are overlooked in up to 40% of patients with known bladder tumors. Early filling views and postvoid images of the bladder may be useful because the radiodense distended bladder may obscure subtle masses. CT and MRI are the imaging modalities of choice for staging known bladder neoplasms because they are most sensitive for detecting extramural extension and nodal metastases.

Notes

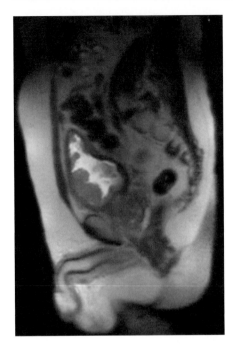

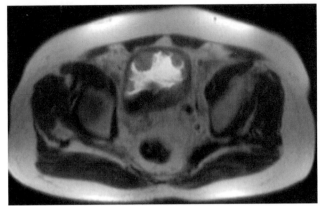

Both images reprinted with permission from Lee JKT, Sagel SS, Stanley RJ, Heiken P, *Computed Body Tomography with MRI Correlation*, ed 4, Philadelphia: Lippincott Williams and Wilkins, 2006.

1. Given the history of hematuria, what is the differential diagnosis?

2. What is the most common histologic subtype of bladder cancer?

3. What histologic subtype of bladder cancer is associated with urachal remnants?

4. What is the most important imaging feature of a bladder tumor in determining therapy and prognosis?

Bladder: MR Bladder Carcinoma

1. Differential diagnosis includes multifocal or bladder carcinoma, fungal infection, or focal proliferative cystitis.

2. Transitional cell carcinoma, accounting for 85% of primary bladder malignancy.

3. Adenocarcinoma.

4. Extension through the bladder wall.

Reference

Tekes A, Kamel I, Imam K, et al: Dynamic MRI of bladder cancer: evaluation of staging accuracy, *Am J Roentgenol* 184:121–127, 2005.

Cross-Reference

Zagoria RJ, *Genitourinary Radiology: THE REQUISITES*, 2nd ed, pp 213–214.

Comment

MRIs show multiple polypoid bladder masses without evidence of invasion through the muscular layer of the bladder wall.

Bladder cancer is the most common genitourinary malignancy. Risk factors include tobacco, artificial sweeteners, coffee, cyclophosphamides, and aromatic amines. The most commonly affected patient is in the sixth to seventh decade of life, and men are affected three times as often as women. Histologic subtypes of bladder cancer include transitional cell carcinoma (TCC), squamous cell carcinoma, adenocarcinoma, and spindle cell carcinoma.

TCC is by far the most common subtype, accounting for 88% of all bladder malignancies. TCC of the bladder is more than 50 times more common than TCC of the renal pelvis or ureter, and although bladder tumors often develop in patients with TCC of the ureter or renal pelvis, only 2% to 4% of patients with bladder carcinoma have ureteral TCC.

Both T1- and T2-weighted images are useful in the assessment of bladder carcinoma. T1-weighted images are recommended for determination of invasion into perivesical fat and adjacent organs (except the prostate) and for evaluation of nodal or bone marrow disease. T2-weighted images are useful in the evaluation of muscular extension and direct spread to the prostate gland. Primary bladder malignancy demonstrates enhancement on post-gadolinium imaging and tends to enhance earlier than normal surrounding bladder wall (i.e., within 5–15 seconds following injection).

A key distinction to make in the assessment of bladder cancer is discrimination between superficial (stage 1) disease and deep invasion of the muscular layer of the bladder wall (stage T3a) given their differing treatment options and associated differences in prognosis. T2-weighted images will demonstrate the muscular bladder wall as a clearly defined hypointense band. Stage Tis, T1, or T2 disease will demonstrate an intact muscular layer, whereas disease breaching the muscular layer is at least stage T3a.

Notes

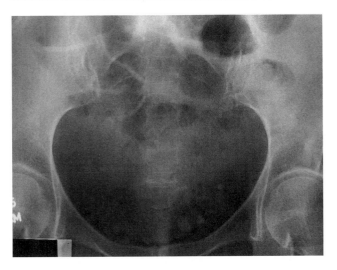
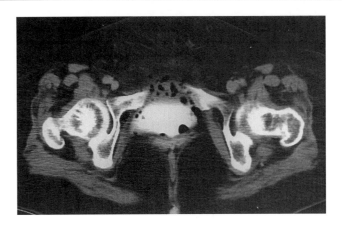

1. True or false: Bladder wall emphysema is equivalent to gangrenous cystitis and therefore should be treated as a life-threatening illness in all cases.

2. Name the two main risk factors for this disease.

3. What is the recommended treatment for this disease?

4. True or false: The most common causative organism is *Clostridium perfringens*.

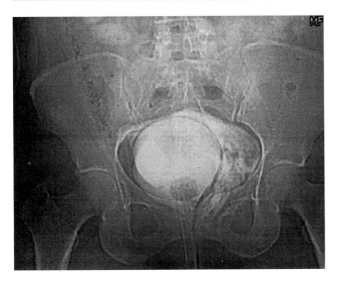
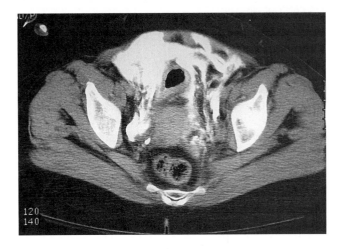

1. What radiologic examinations are commonly used to evaluate traumatic bladder injury?

2. What type of bladder rupture is associated with the collection of extravasated contrast media in the space of Retzius?

3. A "cloud-like" appearance of contrast on conventional cystography is associated with which type of bladder rupture?

4. If the distinction between intraperitoneal and extraperitoneal bladder rupture is still in question after CT cystography, what can be done?

CASE 21

Bladder: Emphysematous Cystitis

1. False.

2. Diabetes mellitus and bladder outlet obstruction.

3. First-line treatment includes antibiotic therapy, adequate bladder drainage, and treatment of hyperglycemia (if present).

4. False.

Reference

Quint EJ, Drach GW, Rappaport WD, Hoffman CJ: Emphysematous cystitis: a review of the spectrum of disease, *J Urol* 147:134–137, 1992.

Cross-Reference

Zagoria RJ, *Genitourinary Radiology: THE REQUISITES*, 2nd ed, pp 224–225.

Comment

Emphysematous cystitis (EC), or cystitis emphysematosa, is a rare infection in which pockets of gas form in the bladder wall. Risk factors include poorly controlled diabetes and urinary stasis (caused by neurogenic bladder or bladder outlet obstruction). Less commonly there is an association with subcutaneous emphysema, hemorrhagic cystitis, and alcoholic liver disease. *Escherichia coli* and *Enterobacter* species are the organisms most commonly isolated, but other bacteria, including *Clostridium perfringens* and *Nocardia* and *Candida* species, also have been linked to EC. Carbon dioxide gas bubbles form in the bladder wall or lumen when the infecting microbe ferments glucose. Because glucose is consumed in this process, the urine dipstick test may be negative for glucose. The clinical course of this rare cystitis is variable and unpredictable; the course can be benign and reversible, but rare fatalities have been reported. Emphysematous ureteritis, nephritis, and adrenalitis may coexist and cause a more life-threatening infection.

The radiologic appearance of EC may be confused with that of rectal air, pneumatosis cystoides intestinalis, emphysematous vaginitis, and gas gangrene of the uterus. The appearance of linear ring or ovoid clusters of gas in the bladder wall on CT is usually diagnostic. The bladder wall may be thickened or nodular. Treatment includes appropriate antibiotic therapy and adequate bladder drainage. Elimination of the infecting microorganisms results in gradual absorption of carbon dioxide. Bladder luminal gas without mural collections of gas, known as primary pneumaturia or pneumocystosis, is not synonymous with EC.

Notes

CASE 22

Bladder: Radiologic Diagnosis of Bladder Rupture

1. Conventional cystography and CT cystography.

2. Extraperitoneal.

3. Intraperitoneal.

4. Short of surgical exploration, delayed CT scanning or repeat scanning after direct instillation of contrast material into the bladder.

Reference

Sivit CJ, Cutting JP, Eichelberger MR: CT diagnosis and location of rupture of the bladder in children with blunt abdominal trauma: significance of contrast material extravasation in the pelvis, *Am J Roentgenol* 164:1243–1246, 1995.

Cross-Reference

Zagoria RJ, *Genitourinary Radiology: THE REQUISITES*, 2nd ed, pp 231–234.

Comment

This case demonstrates an extraperitoneal bladder rupture. The distinction between intraperitoneal and extraperitoneal bladder rupture has important surgical implications. Although conventional cystography is the time-honored method, CT cystography is as accurate and can be performed while the patient is being scanned for evaluation of other abdominopelvic injuries.

The distribution of extravasated contrast material or urine is critical for classifying full-thickness bladder ruptures. In cases of isolated extraperitoneal rupture, like that shown in this case, extravasated fluid or contrast is described as "flame-shaped" and may collect in the perivesical, anterior prevesical (space of Retzius), or retrorectal space. Remember that the prevesical space can extend superiorly to the level of the umbilicus. Extravasated intraperitoneal contrast medium is described as "cloud-like"; contrast or urine may collect in the rectouterine or rectovesical pouch or outline loops of small bowel. If the intraperitoneal leak is large, extravasated contrast may extend to the paracolic gutters or lateral pelvic recesses.

With CT cystography it can be difficult to evaluate extravasated urine or contrast material when there is lavage fluid or an extraperitoneal hematoma, or when abdominopelvic anatomy is distorted by traumatic injury. In difficult cases, delayed CT scanning (15–30 minutes) or repeat scanning after administration of additional intravenous or intravesical contrast material may help.

Notes

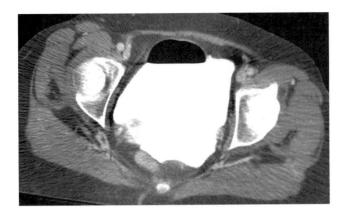
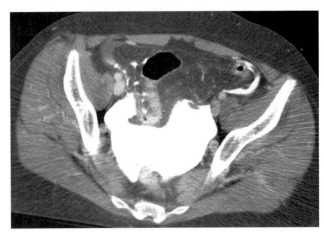
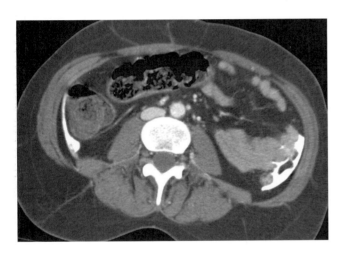
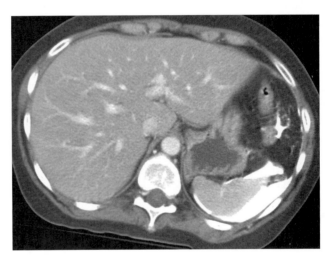

1. True or false: A CT cystogram can be performed by clamping a bladder catheter and allowing the bladder to fill with intravenous contrast excreted by the kidneys.

2. This CT cystogram shows a bladder rupture; which type?

3. Does a cystogram positive for rupture negate the need for a urethrogram since a urethral tear will be treated well with the catheter?

4. Which type of bladder rupture is usually treated with emergency surgical repair?

Bladder: Intraperitoneal Bladder Rupture

1. False. To exclude a bladder rupture, the bladder must be distended. This requires about 300 ml of contrast material infused by low-pressure gravity infusion.

2. Intraperitoneal.

3. No.

4. Intraperitoneal.

Reference

Peng MY, Parisky YR, Cornwell EE, et al: CT cystography versus conventional cystography in evaluation of bladder injury, *Am J Roentgenol* 173:1269–1272, 1999.

Cross-Reference

Zagoria RJ, *Genitourinary Radiology: THE REQUISITES*, 2nd ed, pp 231–234.

Comment

The CT cystogram shown was performed in this patient following a motor vehicle collision. There is contrast material leaking from the bladder into the peritoneal space. Images show contrast material in the space of Douglas, the paracolic gutters, and around the spleen. No contrast is seen in the extraperitoneal spaces. These findings are diagnostic of an intraperitoneal rupture of the bladder. These are usually treated as surgical emergencies and repaired through a laparotomy. Intraperitoneal bladder tears comprise about one third of bladder tears, with extraperitoneal rupture occurring about two thirds of the time. To maximize sensitivity for detection, either a standard cystogram or a CT cystogram should be performed in patients suspected of having this type of injury. Extravasated contrast material is the sine qua non of a bladder rupture. Once detected, a rupture must be classified accurately as either intraperitoneal, extraperitoneal, or both combined. This will guide treatment decisions, with extraperitoneal tears generally treated without emergent surgery, usually healing spontaneously if the bladder is kept decompressed with a catheter.

Male patients who have blunt pelvic trauma are also at risk for a urethral injury. Prior to placing a catheter for a cystogram, a urethrogram should be performed to evaluate the urethra for lacerations and transections, which could be exacerbated by attempted catheterization. If a catheter is in place at the time of cystography, it should not be removed until the urethra has been evaluated. This can be achieved by doing a pericatheter contrast urethrogram. About 5% of patients with bladder ruptures also have coexisting urethral tears. Urethral tears usually require surgery for definitive repair.

Notes

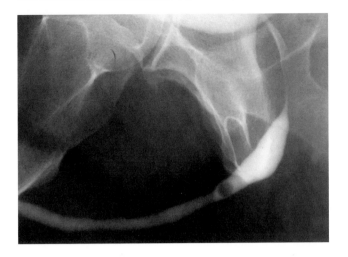
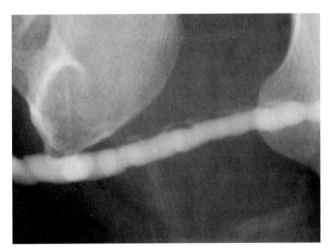
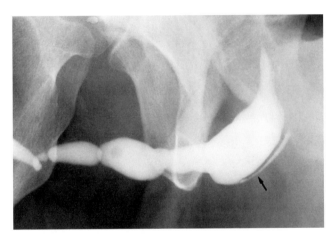

1. In the top two images, what causes the slightly irregular contour along the dorsal aspect of the anterior male urethra?

2. In the bottom image, what structure does the *arrow* point to?

3. Where is the gland for the structure marked by the *arrow* located?

4. True or false: The structure indicated by the *arrow* can be opacified normally on a voiding cystourethrogram or retrograde urethrogram.

Urethra: Glands and Ducts of the Anterior Male Urethra

1. Contrast fills the glands of Littre.

2. Cowper's duct.

3. It is embedded in the urogenital diaphragm lateral to the membranous urethra.

4. True.

Reference

Yaffe D, Zissin R: Cowper's glands duct: radiographic findings, *Urol Radiol* 13:123–125, 1991.

Cross-Reference

Zagoria RJ, *Genitourinary Radiology: THE REQUISITES*, 2nd ed, pp 203–204.

Comment

The mucosa of the penile urethra shows many recesses, which continue into deeper-branching tubular mucous glands (glandulae urethrales urethrae masculinae) that are particularly numerous on the dorsal aspect. These small mucous glands were named by the French surgeon Alexis Littre (1654–1725) and bear his name. Although Littre's glands may sometimes opacify normally, they are more often demonstrated when the glands become inflamed in the setting of acute or chronic urethritis (littritis).

The glandula bulbourethralis bear the name of the English surgeon William Cowper (1666–1709). Cowper's glands are each about 1 cm in diameter (but like everything else, atrophy with age), are embedded in the substance of the sphincter of the urethra, and are located just posterolateral to the membranous part of the urethra. The excretory duct of each gland (Cowper's duct) is almost 3 cm in length and passes obliquely forward to open on the floor of the bulbar urethra. The third figure of this case shows opacification of Cowper's duct resulting from serial urethral strictures. Opacification of a minimally dilated duct on a retrograde or voiding urethrogram is of no clinical significance, but occasionally ductal stenosis may result in dilation of the more proximal duct or Cowper's gland (imperforate syringocele or retention cyst).

Notes

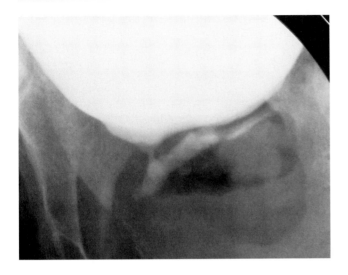
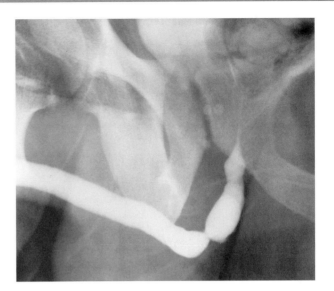

1. A cystourethrogram (the image on the left) was performed in this patient who had contracture of the bladder neck and had just undergone attempted, but failed, bladder catheterization. What is the abnormal finding, and what might have caused it?

2. What are some of the causes for the lesion shown on the retrograde urethrogram (the image on the right), which was performed on another patient?

3. What causes "watering can" perineum?

4. Should squamous cell carcinoma of the bulbar urethra be included in the differential diagnosis for the lesion shown on the retrograde urethrogram?

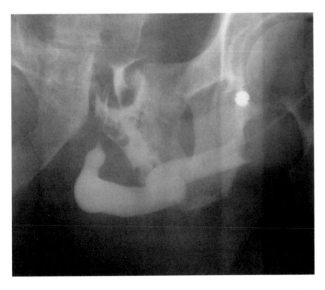

1. Name the two segments of the posterior male urethra.

2. The membranous urethra is contained within what critical anatomic structure?

3. What is the most common mechanism of traumatic injury to the posterior male urethra?

4. True or false: The posterior urethral injury demonstrated on this urethrogram is the most common type encountered after traumatic injury.

CASE 25	CASE 26

Urethra: Iatrogenic Urethral Injuries

1. "False passage" caused by repeated attempts to pass a transurethral catheter.

2. Focal urethral stricture can be caused by infection, noninfectious urethritis, iatrogenic injury, or traumatic injury.

3. Chronic infection of the perineum may result in urethral obstruction, periurethral abscess, and fistula formation.

4. No.

Reference

Shaver WA, Richter PH, Orandi A: Changes in the male urethra produced by instrumentation or transurethral resection of the prostate, *Radiology* 116:623–628, 1975.

Cross-Reference

Zagoria RJ, *Genitourinary Radiology: THE REQUISITES*, 2nd ed, pp 246–247.

Comment

Iatrogenic injury to the urethra may result from open surgery, instrumentation, or catheter placement. Extravasation of contrast material indicates a urethral laceration. Urethral strictures have been reported in 3% to 17% of patients who have had transurethral prostatectomy. The majority of strictures in children are iatrogenic; the patient with the stricture on retrograde urethrogram had repetitive cystoscopy as a child. Any indwelling transurethral catheter predisposes a patient to urethritis and increases the risk for stricture. Iatrogenic stricture is most common at the penoscrotal junction and membranous urethra; the meatus and bladder neck also are common sites. Iatrogenic strictures are usually focal and short. Other causes of urethral stricture include nongonococcal and gonococcal infection (in the bulbous urethra or just proximal to the meatus), noninfectious inflammation (chemical irritation or Reiter's syndrome), traumatic injury (solitary strictures that develop more quickly than inflammatory strictures), or neoplasm (usually causes a long, irregular stricture).

False passages may be created after failed attempts to pass a catheter or other instrument. Failed catheter placement can produce a tract posterior to the prostatomembranous or bulbar urethra that may enter the prostate or penetrate the bladder. An even more ominous injury results when the Foley catheter balloon is placed in the membranous urethra and inflated; this mishap is more likely to occur in the patient with spinal cord injury who lacks functioning perineal sensory fibers.

Urethra: Blunt Traumatic Injury of the Posterior Urethra

1. Membranous and prostatic urethra.

2. Urogenital diaphragm.

3. Blunt traumatic injury resulting in pelvic fracture, especially those involving the anterior arch.

4. False.

Reference

Goldman SM, Sandler CM, Corriere JN Jr, McGuire EJ: Blunt urethral trauma: a unified, anatomical mechanical classification, *J Urol* 157:85–89, 1997.

Cross-Reference

Zagoria RJ, *Genitourinary Radiology: THE REQUISITES*, 2nd ed, pp 246–247, 328.

Comment

Traumatic urethral injury (TUI) has been classified in a number of ways. Before 1977 TUI was divided into anterior and posterior urethral injuries. Posterior urethral tears are virtually always secondary to pelvic fractures and most often occur after motor vehicle accidents. Blunt injury of the anterior male urethra usually involves the bulbous urethra and often results from a straddle-type injury; the pelvis usually is not fractured.

In 1977 Colapinto and McCallum presented a classification system that divided urethral injuries into three types. In type I injuries the urethra is elongated but intact. The membranous urethra is ruptured above the urogenital diaphragm in type II injuries, and more extensive urethral injuries involving the membranous and bulbar urethrae and the urogenital diaphragm are classified as type III.

The most recent classification is presented in the referenced article. Goldman and colleagues divide TUI into five types. Types I, II, and III are the same as in the Colapinto and McCallum classification. Type IV injuries involve the bladder neck and extend into the prostatomembranous urethra, and type IVA injuries involve the bladder base but spare the urethra. Type IVA was added to the classification system because on urethrography extravasated contrast material may pool in the periurethral space in type IVA injuries, thereby mimicking type IV tears. Partial or complete tears of the anterior urethra are designated as type V injuries.

This case shows a type II TUI. Several studies have shown that only 15% of urethral injuries are type I or II, and the majority of urethral injuries are not isolated to the posterior urethra but extend into the adjacent bulbous urethra (type III).

Notes

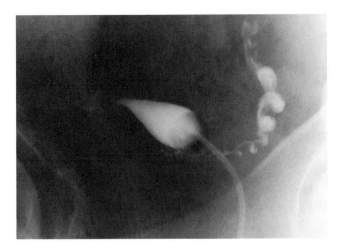
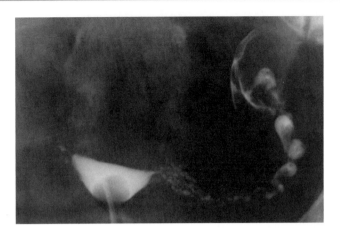

1. What is the differential diagnosis for the hysterosalpingogram shown? How often is tubal patency demonstrated?

2. What are the major clinical complications associated with this disease?

3. Given a referral for primary infertility, state at least two reasons for not doing a hysterosalpingogram.

4. What are the major differences between the water-soluble and oil-soluble types of contrast media used for hysterosalpingograms?

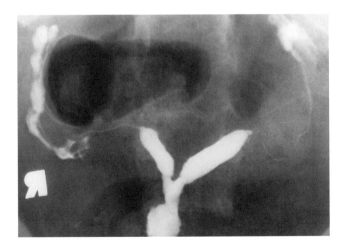
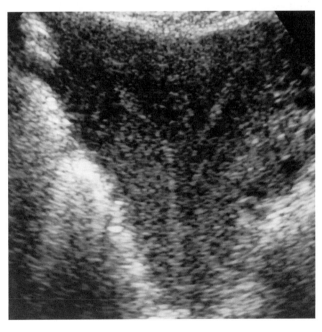

1. What is the most likely diagnosis in this case?

2. This represents a malformation of what embryonic genital duct system?

3. In men, what causes regression of this duct system?

4. What are the diagnostic criteria for this malformation on hysterosalpingography?

Ob/Gyn: Salpingitis Isthmica Nodosa

1. Salpingitis isthmica nodosa, tuberculosis of the fallopian tube, and tubal adenomyosis. "Free spill" of contrast is seen in about one fourth of all cases.

2. Infertility and ectopic uterine gestation.

3. Active menstrual bleeding, acute pelvic inflammatory disease, within 4 days of dilation and curettage, and pregnancy.

4. Image detail and peritoneal absorption.

Reference

Creasy JL, Clark RL, Cuttino JT, Groff TR: Salpingitis isthmica nodosa: radiologic and clinical correlates, *Radiology* 154:597–600, 1985.

Cross-Reference

Zagoria RJ, *Genitourinary Radiology: THE REQUISITES,* 2nd ed, pp 13–15, 285–286.

Comment

The term *salpingitis isthmica nodosa* (SIN) was coined by German pathologist Hans Chiari in 1887 to describe the predominant location, pathologic appearance, and presumed cause of a disease typified by epithelial inclusions within the walls of the fallopian tube. The classic findings of SIN on hysterosalpingogram (HSG) include numerous, small diverticular outpouchings in the isthmic part of one or both fallopian tubes. Tubal patency is observed in about 25% of cases. The cause of SIN has been debated, but a medical history of genital infection is frequently obtained, and the development of SIN after exposure to gonococci has been reported.

The clinical importance of this condition is its association with both infertility and extrauterine gestation. In the report referenced earlier, the prevalence of SIN was 4% in a group of women referred for HSG because of infertility. These authors also report a high rate of ectopic pregnancy (9.4%)

Tuberculous salpingitis and tubal adenomyosis are in the differential diagnosis of findings attributed to SIN.

The authors recommend water-soluble contrast mediums for HSG because they provide better mucosal detail than the oil-based contrast agents and are more readily taken up by the peritoneal epithelium. Oil-soluble contrast material gained popularity after initial reports of an association between use of this material and successful impregnation after HSG. However, these oily contrast agents are not absorbed as well and have been linked to the development of fibrosis or granulomatosis.

Notes

Ob/Gyn: Septate Uterus on Ultrasonography and Hysterosalpingography

1. Septate uterus.

2. Müllerian or paramesonephric.

3. Müllerian inhibiting factor (produced by the testes).

4. Intercornuate distance less than 4 cm and intercornual angle less than or equal to 75 degrees.

Reference

Troiano RN, McCarthy SM: Müllerian duct anomalies: imaging and clinical issues, *Radiology* 233:19–34, 2004.

Cross-Reference

Zagoria RJ, *Genitourinary Radiology: THE REQUISITES,* 2nd ed, pp 263–264.

Comment

Through fusion, the müllerian or paramesonephric ducts form the upper vagina, uterus, and fallopian tubes in the female embryo. A müllerian inhibiting or suppression factor is secreted by the embryonic testes and suppresses the development of the paramesonephric ducts. Thus, phenotypic women with testicular feminization syndrome (androgen insensitivity caused by abnormal testosterone receptors) do not have an internal female genital tract because the normal but often undescended testes produce müllerian regression factor and androgens. In contrast, phenotypic women with gonadal dysgenesis (failure of testicular differentiation) usually have female internal genital ducts because the abnormal gonads do not retain the ability to secrete this factor.

This case illustrates a septate uterus on transvaginal sonography and hysterosalpingography (HSG). Septate uterus represents the most common anomaly of müllerian duct fusion and is classified as a class V anomaly in the American Fertility Society system. Various degrees of failure of absorption of the midline septum can be observed in this anomaly. Complete failure gives rise to a complete septate uterus; the septum can extend from the fundus to the endocervical canal. Partial absorption failure results in a septum that is confined to the endometrial cavity (subseptate uterus). Spontaneous abortion may occur in as many as 90% of patients with septate uteri because a fertilized ovum quickly outgrows the blood supply of the poorly vascularized septum. Some of the diagnostic features of a septate uterus on transvaginal ultrasonography and HSG include a convex, flat, or minimally concave uterine fundal contour; intercornual distance less than or equal to 4 cm; and intercornual angle less than or equal to 75 degrees.

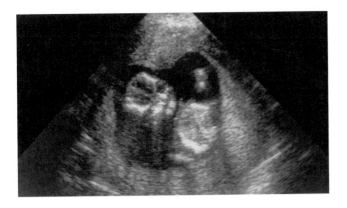 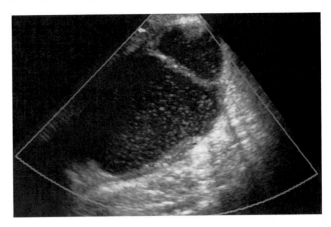

1. After what time in pregnancy (weeks' gestational age) are corpus luteum cysts expected to resolve?

2. As a general rule, what is the size threshold (diameter) below which simple ovarian cysts can be managed conservatively when discovered during pregnancy?

3. If removal is indicated, during which trimester is elective excision of an ovarian mass recommended?

4. True or false: The majority of complex ovarian cysts discovered during pregnancy are malignant.

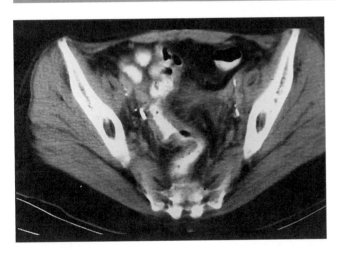 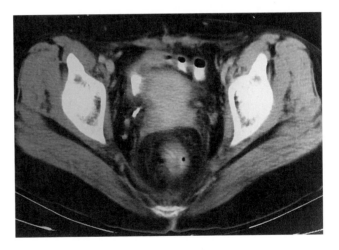

1. This patient received radiation therapy for stage IIB cervical carcinoma. What is the most likely diagnosis?

2. What thickness of the distended rectal wall is considered abnormal?

3. True or false: The frequency of radiotherapy-associated complications is much higher in patients with cervical cancer than in those with endometrial cancer.

4. True or false: Injury to the ascending colon as a result of radiation therapy for cervical cancer is common.

Ob/Gyn: Ovarian Cystadenoma in Pregnancy

1. Approximately 16 weeks' gestational age.

2. 5 cm.

3. Second trimester.

4. False. Only about 2% to 5% of adnexal masses removed during pregnancy are malignant.

Reference

Hill LM, Connors-Beatty MA, Norwak A, Tush B: The role of ultrasonography in the detection and management of adnexal masses during the second and third trimesters of pregnancy, *Am J Obstet Gynecol* 179: 703–707, 1998.

Cross-Reference

Zagoria RJ, *Genitourinary Radiology: THE REQUISITES,* 2nd ed, pp 287–297.

Comment

Cystadenoma is one of the most commonly encountered benign ovarian neoplasms. Serous tumors are often unilocular and commonly contain "simple" fluid. In contrast, mucinous cystadenomas are multilocular and have uniformly thin (less than 3 mm) septations. Fluid within individual loculi may be "complex" because of proteinaceous debris, hemorrhage, or both. Papillary projections are unusual and, if present, should suggest a borderline malignancy or cystadenocarcinoma.

When discovered during pregnancy, ovarian cysts less than 5 cm in diameter tend to resolve between 13 and 30 weeks. It has been recommended that all cysts greater than 10 cm in diameter be removed; controversy exists regarding the appropriate management of cysts between 5 and 10 cm in diameter. Elective excision (before symptoms develop) of an ovarian mass that persists beyond 16 weeks' gestation and avoidance of surgery in the first and third trimesters help to decrease the risk for pregnancy termination and preterm labor.

Serous cystadenoma must be differentiated from a functional ovarian cyst, hydrosalpinx, paratubal cyst, peritoneal pseudocyst, and tuboovarian abscess. Functional ovarian cysts are common in women of child-bearing age and may represent follicular cysts, corpus luteum cysts, or corpora albicans cysts. Hydrosalpinx appears as a tortuous, fluid-filled mass containing mucosal infoldings. Paratubal cysts are usually small and are among the most common conditions of the fallopian tubes that can mimic an ovarian cyst. Peritoneal pseudocysts are collections of ascitic fluid trapped within mesothelium-lined cavities. These fluid collections are often associated with endometriosis or prior surgery.

Ob/Gyn: Colitis after Radiation Treatment of Cervical Carcinoma

1. Proctocolitis secondary to radiation treatment.

2. 4 mm or more.

3. True.

4. False.

Reference

Blomlie V, Rofstad EK, Trope C, Lien HH: Critical soft tissues of the female pelvis: serial MR imaging before, during, and after radiation therapy, *Radiology* 203: 391–397, 1997.

Cross-Reference

Zagoria RJ, *Genitourinary Radiology: THE REQUISITES,* 2nd ed, pp 307–309.

Comment

For patients with cervical cancer that involves the parametrial tissues, lower third of the vagina, or pelvic sidewall, radiation therapy is the treatment of choice. Radiation injury to the rectosigmoid colon or to the lower urinary tract may be confused with recurrent disease. Adverse effects occur significantly more often in patients who have cervical cancer compared with those who have endometrial cancer because of higher rectal doses from intracavitary radiation sources. Injury to the rectal wall usually occurs before injury to the bladder; the mean time is 20 to 24 months after the completion of radiation therapy.

Although rectovaginal fistula is the most significant complication, radiation enterocolitis occurs more often, yet still affects fewer than 5% of patients. Patients may complain of abdominal or rectal cramping, diarrhea, or rectal bleeding. Radiation enteritis is less common than proctosigmoiditis, but the patient whose small intestine is fixed in the pelvis by surgical adhesions or who has other pelvic pathologic conditions is at increased risk. Several findings on CT may suggest the diagnosis of radiation proctosigmoiditis. Colon wall thickness of 4 mm or more is considered abnormal and is the most common sign of radiation colitis. Like ischemic colitis, which shares the common pathophysiologic finding of an occlusive arteriopathy, radiation colitis has been associated with pneumatosis. Rarely, there is perirectal fibrofatty proliferation.

Pelvic hydroureter may occur because of parametrial cellulitis, trigonal ulceration, or periureteral fibrosis but is transient in about half of cases. Gas in the urinary bladder is a harbinger of vesical fistula, but after cystoscopy it may remain in the irradiated bladder for more than 1 week because of poor bladder emptying.

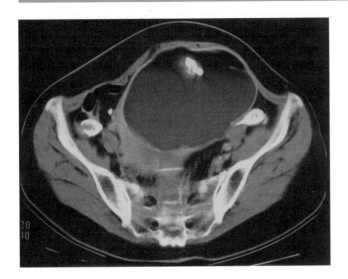 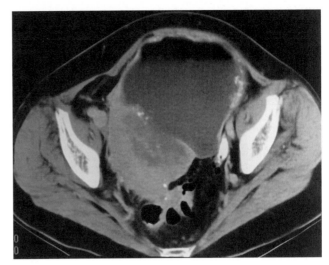

1. What is the most common complication associated with a dermoid cyst?

2. Name three other complications.

3. What is the most common malignancy associated with a dermoid cyst?

4. What findings on CT or MRI suggest malignant transformation?

Ob/Gyn: Mature Cystic Teratoma with Malignant Transformation

1. Torsion.

2. Trauma, infection, rupture or slow leak, autoimmune hemolytic anemia, perforation into a hollow viscus, and malignancy.

3. Squamous cell carcinoma.

4. Rapid growth, infiltration of adjacent tissues, extensive adhesions, and peritoneal implants.

References

Case records of the Massachusetts General Hospital, *N Engl J Med* 332:1631–1636, 1995.

Rha SE, Byun JY, Jung SE, et al: Atypical CT and MRI manifestations of mature ovarian cystic teratomas, *Am J Roentgenol* 183:743–750, 2004.

Cross-Reference

Zagoria RJ, *Genitourinary Radiology: THE REQUISITES,* 2nd ed, p 289.

Comment

In its pure form, the dermoid cyst is always benign. However, rarely (in 2% of cases) malignant transformation occurs. This transformation occurs only in lesions larger than 5 cm in diameter. This case illustrates an ovarian squamous cell carcinoma, the most common malignancy (accounting for 80% of cases) arising from epidermal dysplasia or from squamous metaplasia of the respiratory tract epithelium in a dermoid cyst. However, any of the mature tissues in a dermoid cyst may undergo malignant transformation, which is reflected in the variety of tumors reported (i.e., adenocarcinoma of the intestinal epithelium, carcinoid tumor, thyroid carcinoma, basal cell carcinoma, malignant melanoma, leiomyosarcoma, and chondrosarcoma).

Although dermoid cysts are most often discovered in women of childbearing age, malignant transformation usually occurs in postmenopausal women. Clinical evidence of transformation includes pain, weight loss, and rapid tumor growth. When infiltration into adjacent tissues, extensive adhesions, or peritoneal metastases are evident on imaging or at laparoscopy, malignancy should be suspected. Note the eccentric, necrotic mass along the dextrolateral wall of the cystic teratoma in this patient. Occasionally, paraaortic and pelvic lymphadenopathy are reported, but hematogenous metastasis is rare. Poor prognostic factors include ascites, rupture, and malignant invasion of the dermoid wall. Overall, the 5-year survival rate is 15% to 31%.

Notes

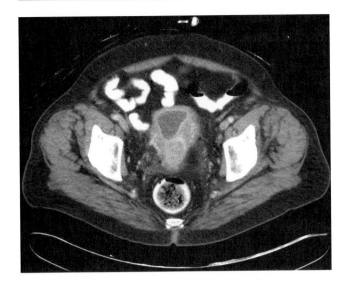
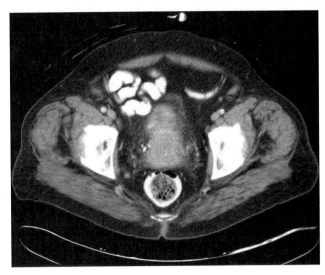

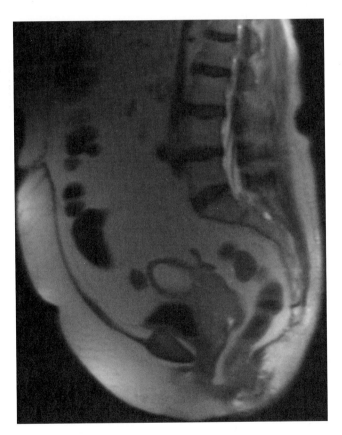

1. On CT images, the presence of hydronephrosis indicates what clinical T stage?

2. On MRIs, extension of disease beyond the black cervical stroma indicates extension of disease into what structures?

3. Among cervical, ovarian, and endometrial cancer, which has the lowest incidence in the United States?

4. Why is MRI the best test for local extension of disease?

Ob/Gyn: Cervical Cancer

1. T3A—usually due to involvement of the ureter or ureterovesical junction.

2. The parametria—the veins, arteries and nerves supplying and draining the cervix.

3. Cervical carcinoma.

4. The high spatial contrast allows identification of disease beyond the confines of the cervical stroma. This determines both therapy and prognosis.

Reference

Scheidler J, Heuck AF: Imaging of cancer of the cervix, *Radiol Clin North Am* 40:577–590, 2002.

Cross-Reference

Zagoria RJ, *Genitourinary Radiology: THE REQUISITES,* 2nd ed, pp 307–309.

Comment

Cervical cancer is a usually a disease of women of menstrual age that plateaus at age 40 in American women. Approximately 13,000 new cases are diagnosed each year. Causality by human papillomavirus has been generally accepted, and the vast majority of tumors are of squamous cell origin. Patients are usually asymptomatic, and detection is usually via the Papanicolaou smear. The majorities of cancers are confined to the cervical canal when discovered and are stage 1 disease. Any cervical mass that is greater than 1.5 cm should be examined using MRI to determine whether the patient is a candidate for surgical therapy. CT scanning lacks the contrast resolution necessary for primary staging of relatively low volume disease, with overall staging accuracy reportedly ranging from 60% to 80%. In cases of advanced disease, CT is preferred. It is quick to perform and read and has a higher spatial resolution than MRI.

On MRIs, cervical cancer is usually hyperintense to the dark cervical stroma on T2-weighted images. The preservation of the black ring of the cervical stroma, no matter how thin, virtually excludes parametrial extension. These patients are candidates for surgical cure (T2A). Those in whom the black line is broken and a mass extends beyond the expected confines of the cervix have an 85% likelihood of parametrial invasion and are usually treated primarily with brachytherapy (T2B). It is generally agreed that the administration of intravenous gadolinium-diethylenetriamine-pentaacetic acid (Gd-DTPA) improves staging accuracy to between 85% and 90%. In cases of advanced disease, sagittal T2-weighted and/or Gd-DTPA-enhanced T1-weighted images will show invasion of the rectum, bladder, and vaginal fornices (T4). In this case, clinical staging was IIA and confined to the cervix; treatment was surgical.

Notes

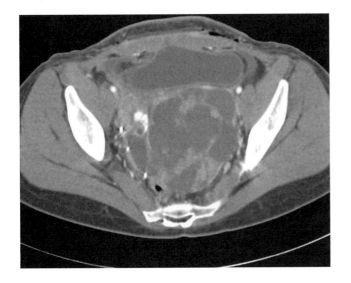 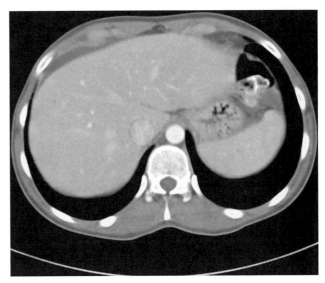

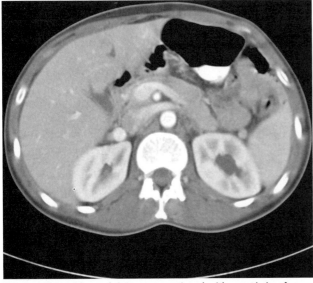

Upper right and lower left images reprinted with permission from Lee JKT, Sagel SS, Stanley RJ, Heiken P, *Computed Body Tomography with MRI Correlation*, ed 4, Philadelphia: Lippincott Williams and Wilkins, 2006.

1. What is the most common CT appearance of an ovarian cystadenocarcinoma?

2. How is it differentiated from a tumor of low malignant potential such as a cystadenoma?

3. Why is it important to identify peritoneal implants?

4. What does hydronephrosis indicate regarding therapy?

Ob/Gyn: Ovarian Carcinoma

1. Mixed fluid and soft tissue density ovarian mass with enhancing nodules, usually accompanied by ascites.

2. Low malignant potential tumors have gracile septa and no enhancing wall nodules.

3. The larger the solid tumor burden outside of the pelvis, the more likely the patient will require chemotherapy prior to or instead of surgery.

4. Most oncologists prefer two functioning kidneys prior to beginning chemotherapy; a stent may be required.

Reference

Kurtz AB Tsimikas JV, Tempany CMC, et al: Diagnosis and staging of ovarian cancer: comparative values of Doppler and conventional US, CT, and MR imaging correlated with surgery and histopathologic analysis—report of the Radiology Diagnostic Oncology Group, *Radiology* 212:19–27, 1999.

Cross-Reference

Zagoria RJ, *Genitourinary Radiology: THE REQUISITES,* 2nd ed, pp 287–288.

Comment

Ovarian cancer is a disease of perimenopausal women, with its peak between ages 45 and 55 years. Approximately 23,000 new cases are identified each year. Risk factors include a family history of ovarian carcinoma and, in some cases, breast cancer. The majority of tumors are of epithelial origin and are serous or mucinous cystadenocarcinomas. Unfortunately, no effective screening examination exists, and the majority of women (60%) present with advanced disease extending beyond the pelvis. Cystadenocarcinoma, as in this patient, usually appears on contrast-enhanced CT images as a large, predominantly cystic mass with a nodular, enhancing wall and thick, enhancing septa. Ascites, hydronephrosis, omental and peritoneal implants are common accompaniments. Enlarged lymph nodes are less common but do occur. Cystadenocarcinoma with ascites and minimal implant formation is treated with an extensive surgery. The procedure is comprised of hysterectomy, bilateral salpingo-oophorectomy, lymphadenectomy, ascites and peritoneal sampling, omentectomy, and manual examination of the surface of the liver. On imaging examinations it is important to identify solid implants prior to therapy because a large solid tumor burden is best treated with chemotherapy rather than primary debulking surgery.

Notes

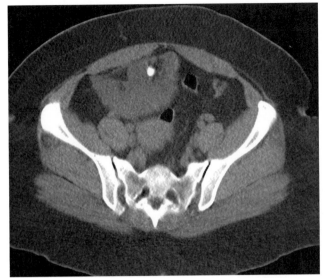

Both images reprinted with permission from Lee JKT, Sagel SS, Stanley RJ, Heiken P, *Computed Body Tomography with MRI Correlation*, ed 4, Philadelphia: Lippincott Williams and Wilkins, 2006.

1. What is the Rokitansky nodule?

2. What is the most sensitive and specific CT feature of mature cystic teratoma?

3. What percentage of mature cystic teratomas contain calcium?

4. Why is surgical resection recommended for this benign lesion?

Ob/Gyn: Ovarian Dermoid Cyst

1. The mural nodule that contains most of the solid teratomatous elements.

2. Fat attenuation within the cyst.

3. 55% to 60%.

4. Increased risk for ovarian torsion and rarely malignant transformation.

References

Jabra AA, Fishman EK, Taylor GA: Primary ovarian tumors in the pediatric patient: CT evaluation, *Clin Imaging* 17:199–203, 1993.

Outwater EK, Siegelman ES, Hunt JL: Ovarian teratomas: tumor types and imaging characteristics, *Radiographics* 21:475–490, 2001.

Cross-Reference

Zagoria RJ, *Genitourinary Radiology: THE REQUISITES,* 2nd ed, p 290.

Comment

Mature cystic teratomas are the most common ovarian neoplasm. The term *teratoma* implies that these masses contain internal components of all three primitive germ cell layers, while *dermoid cyst* describes the presence of skin and dermal appendages in the lining of the cystic mass. These neoplasms are usually asymptomatic and are incidentally discovered in young or middle-aged women. They are bilateral in 15% to 25% of patients.

Dermoid cysts have a characteristic pathologic appearance. They are unilocular in 85% of cases and lined with squamous epithelium. Hair follicles, skin glands, muscle, and other tissues lie within the wall. The cystic component represents sebaceous material, which is liquid at body temperature. There is usually a raised protuberance projecting into the cyst cavity known as the Rokitansky nodule. Most of the hair, bone, or teeth tend to be located within this nodule.

The ultrasound appearance of these lesions is variable, but the most common manifestation is a cystic lesion with a densely echogenic tubercle (Rokitansky nodule) projecting into the cyst lumen. At CT, fat attenuation within a cyst, with or without calcification in the wall, is diagnostic. This fat/fluid level effectively excludes other rare lipomatous pelvic tumors such as lipoma and liposarcoma. Fat is reported in 93% of cases and teeth or other calcifications in 56%.

Dermoids grow slowly, at an average rate of 1.8 mm per year. They are typically resected because they predispose to ovarian torsion and rarely undergo malignant transformation into squamous cell or other carcinomas.

Notes

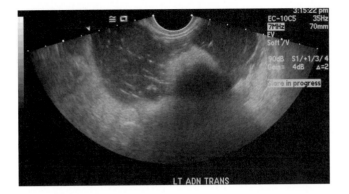

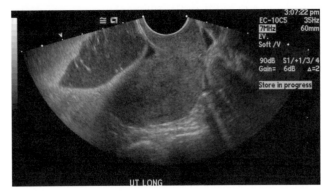

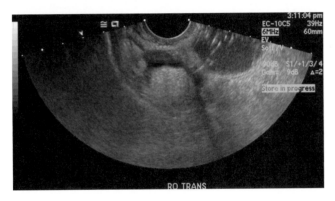

1. What is the "tip of the iceberg sign" as seen in these images?

2. How often is this entity seen bilaterally?

3. True or false: Most patients have symptoms associated with this entity?

4. The mural nodule associated with this cystic mass is called what?

Ob/Gyn: Bilateral Ovarian Dermoids

1. An echogenic mass that fades into acoustic shadowing due to sound absorption.

2. 10%.

3. False.

4. Rokitansky nodule, also dermoid plug.

References

Kim KA, Park CM, Lee JH, et al: Benign ovarian tumors with solid and cystic components that mimic malignancy, *Am J Roentgenol* 182:1259–1265, 2004.

Outwater EK, Siegelman ES, Hunt JL: Ovarian teratomas: tumor types and imaging characteristics, *Radiographics* 21:475–490, 2001.

Cross-Reference

Zagoria RJ, *Genitourinary Radiology: THE REQUISITES,* 2nd ed, pp 289, 290.

Comment

Mature cystic teratomas, often called dermoid cysts, are tumors composed of well-differentiated derivations of at least two of the three germ cell layers (ectoderm, mesoderm, and endoderm). They generally affect younger people, with a mean patient age of 30 years. Mature cystic teratoma is the most common germ cell neoplasm. Mature cystic teratomas are usually asymptomatic, although abdominal pain and other nonspecific symptoms can occur. In 10% of cases, mature cystic teratomas are bilateral. Simple resection is used for those requiring removal.

Squamous epithelium lines the wall of the cyst. Hair, muscle, and other tissues can lie within the wall. Bone and teeth can also be found within the cyst. A raised protuberance is sometimes found that projects into the cyst cavity and is known as the Rokitansky nodule. This is also referred to in some texts as a dermoid plug.

The characteristic appearance on ultrasonography is a cystic mass with complex fluid and a mural nodule. Fluid-fluid levels are common. Another classic appearance is the "tip of the iceberg sign," an echogenic mass that fades into dense acoustic shadowing due to sound absorption. CT imaging is more sensitive for fat and findings are more straightforward. Fat attenuation within an ovarian cyst is diagnostic of mature cystic teratoma.

Notes

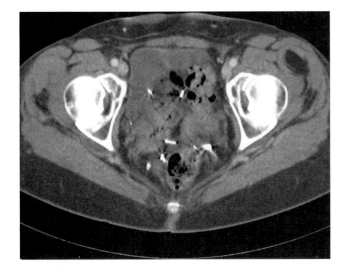

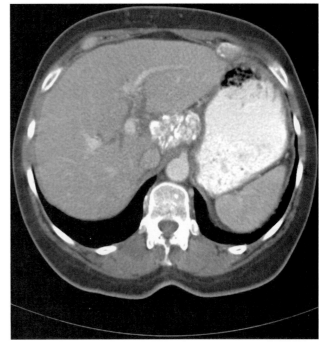

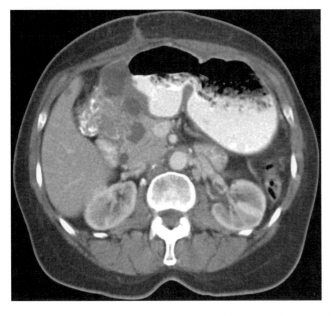

1. According to FIGO recommendations, what method should be used to primarily stage this disease?

2. What is the most common route of spread of this tumor?

3. Can metastatic implants calcify?

4. What is the sensitivity of CT scan for the detection of peritoneal implants?

Ob/Gyn: Recurrent Ovarian Carcinoma

1. Laparotomy with total abdominal hysterectomy and bilateral salphingo-oophorectomy, omentectomy, peritoneal washings and wall sampling, and lymph node sampling.

2. Intraperitoneal dissemination via ascites.

3. Yes.

4. In most recent studies sensitivity ranges from 85% to 93%.

Reference

Coakley FV, Choi PH, Gougoutas CA, et al: Peritoneal metastases: detection with spiral CT in patients with ovarian cancer, *Radiology* 223:495–499, 2002.

Cross-Reference

Zagoira RJ, *Genitourinary Radiology: THE REQUISITES,* 2nd ed, pp 47–48, 297.

Comment

Ovarian cancer is the second most common cancer among gynecologic malignancies and causes more deaths than any other cancer of the female reproductive tract. Staging is performed surgically and is based on recommendations from the International Federation of Gynecology and Obstetrics (FIGO). CT is useful in surgical planning and follow-up after treatment. In stage I, the cancer is confined to the ovaries. In stage II, spread is limited to the true pelvis. Extrapelvic peritoneal implants or abdominopelvic lymph node metastases are found in stage III. In stage IV there is hematogenous spread to distant organs. Ovarian cancer is treated with debulking surgery, which can be curative if the disease in confined to the ovaries. Disseminated disease is treated with cytoreduction surgery with the goal to leave deposits no more than 1 cm in diameter because chemotherapy is more successful with smaller masses.

Intraperitoneal dissemination via ascites is the most common route of spread of ovarian cancer. The omentum, subphrenic spaces, mesentery, and pericolic gutters are most commonly involved. Most ovarian metastases to the peritoneum are low in attenuation and some may be cystic. They enhance after contrast administration. Serous carcinoma implants may calcify as shown here in the perihepatic metastasis. The sensitivity of CT for the detection of peritoneal implants ranges from 85% to 93% in recent studies with multidetector scanners. However, sensitivity drops to less than 50% for lesions smaller than 1 cm.

Ovarian cancer can also spread through the lymphatic system via retroperitoneal lymph nodes, obturator and internal iliac lymph nodes, and external iliac and inguinal lymph nodes. The sensitivity of CT for the detection of involved lymph nodes is approximately 50%. Adenopathy is defined as lymph nodes measuring greater than 1 cm in the short axis.

Stage IV ovarian cancer consists of hematogenous metastases and most commonly affects the liver. It is important to differentiate peritoneal implants around the liver from intraparenchymal liver metastases due to prognostic implications and differences in treatment. Ovarian cancer may also metastasize to the pleura, lungs, adrenal glands, bone, and brain.

Notes

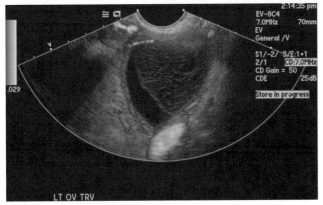
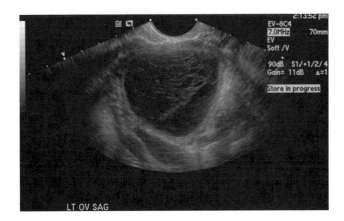

See also Color Plate

1. What is the classic presentation for the symptomatic patient with this finding?

2. The above may mimic what other pathologic processes?

3. What is the classic pattern seen on ultrasonography?

4. True or false: This entity is usually associated with fever and leukocytosis.

C A S E   3 7

Ob/Gyn: Ovarian Hemorrhagic Cyst

1. Pelvic or abdominal pain that may wake the person from sleep.

2. Tuboovarian abscess and ectopic pregnancy.

3. Lace-like pattern with no flow in septations.

4. False.

References

Jain KA: Sonographic spectrum of hemorrhagic ovarian cysts, *J Ultrasound Med* 21:879–886, 2002.

Swire MN, Castro-Aragon I, Levine D: Various sonographic appearances of the hemorrhagic corpus luteum cyst, *Ultrasound Q* 20:45–58, 2004.

Cross-Reference

Zagoria RJ, *Genitourinary Radiology: THE REQUISITES,* 2nd ed, pp 282–284.

Comment

Patients with hemorrhagic ovarian cysts (HOCs) can be symptomatic or asymptomatic. The classic history for the symptomatic patient is the abrupt onset of pelvic or lower abdominal pain which may wake the person from sleep. If the cause of the pelvic pain is HOCs, it should be tender to direct pressure with transvaginal ultrasonography (US). If not, other causes of pelvic pain should be considered. HOCs are not associated with fever or leukocytosis. If a patient presents with acute pelvic pain and has imaging findings compatible with a classic small hemorrhagic cyst, no further follow-up is needed. If the cyst is atypical or larger than 3 cm, follow-up US at 6 weeks is recommended.

Transvaginal US is the imaging modality of choice for diagnosis. HOC can mimic tuboovarian abscess and ectopic pregnancy. In these instances, clinical symptoms and presentation along with urine pregnancy test may help to distinguish one from the other. Hemorrhagic cysts evolve slowly into various stages of acute hemorrhage, clot formation, and clot retraction. This gives rise to changing sonographic appearances as they regress. Fresh blood is usually anechoic. In the subacute stages when clot forms, it becomes echogenic. The echogenicity of the HOC diminishes with time as the red cells undergo hemolysis. A classic appearance of an HOC on US is an adnexal mass with associated good through-transmission. Within this mass are fine interdigitating septations, which give a sponge like or lacelike appearance. As shown in this case, the septations do not show flow on Doppler and the findings are virtually diagnostic of a hemorrhagic cyst. Another common appearance is a retracting blood clot. As blood clot retracts, it forms acute angles, distinguishing if from tumor. On CT, hemorrhagic cysts appear thin-walled. Internal density may be near water or higher depending on the physical state of blood products.

Notes

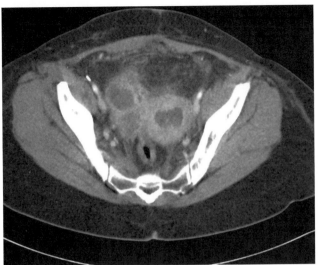
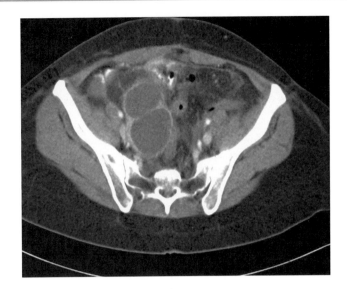

Both images reprinted with permission from Lee JKT, Sagel SS, Stanley RJ, Heiken P, *Computed Body Tomography with MRI Correlation*, ed 4, Philadelphia: Lippincott Williams and Wilkins, 2006.

1. What is the primary imaging modality for suspected tuboovarian abscess?

2. True or false: Internal gas bubbles are a common CT finding.

3. Name at least three differential diagnoses for the CT appearance of tuboovarian abscess.

4. Describe the pathogenesis of tuboovarian abscess.

Ob/Gyn: Tuboovarian Abscess

1. Ultrasonography.

2. False.

3. Endometriosis, ovarian tumors and cysts, and abscesses from other sources within the abdomen and pelvis.

4. Tuboovarian abscess is a complication of pelvic inflammatory disease, which commonly occurs as a result of *Chlamydia trachomatis* or *Neisseria gonorrhoeae* infection of the cervix or vagina that then spreads into the endometrium, fallopian tubes, ovaries, and adjacent structures.

References

Hiller N, Sella T, et al: Computed tomographic features of tuboovarian abscess, *J Repro Med* 50:203–208, 2005.

Wilbur AC, Aizenstein RI, Napp TE: CT findings in tuboovarian abscess, *Am J Roentgenol* 158:575–579, 1992.

Cross-Reference

Zagoria RJ, *Genitourinary Radiology: THE REQUISITES,* 2nd ed, pp 273–275.

Comment

Tuboovarian abscess (TOA) is a common complication of pelvic inflammatory disease (PID), which results from ascending vaginal or cervical infection that progresses to endometritis and salpingitis. TOA occurs in reportedly one third of patients hospitalized for salpingo-oophoritis. The infection is typically polymicrobial and usually affects women in the third and fourth decades of life. Less common etiologies include the sequelae of pelvic surgery and complications of an intraabdominal process, such as appendicitis or diverticulitis.

Ultrasonography is the primary imaging modality used to confirm a suspected diagnosis of TOA. Typical sonographic findings include a complex, cystic mass with debris, septations, and an irregular, thick wall. CT may be used if the diagnosis of TOA is not clinically suspected or ultrasound examination is equivocal. As seen here, the most common CT characteristics include a multilocular fluid-density mass in an adnexal location. The wall is typically thick and uniform, and demonstrates enhancement. Ancillary findings include haziness of the surrounding fat and thickening of the mesosalpinx. Anteriorly located abscesses often displace the mesosalpinx anteriorly. Thickening of the uterosacral ligaments and increased density of the presacral and perirectal fat are features of posteriorly located TOAs. Differential diagnoses include endometriosis, ovarian tumors and cysts, and abscesses from other sources within the pelvis and abdomen. Internal gas bubbles are the most specific radiologic sign of abscess, but this is reportedly a rare finding in TOA.

Although these abscesses generally remain localized to the ovary and fallopian tubes, rupture may result in a life-threatening generalized peritonitis. Treatment modalities for TOA include antibiotics, image-guided drainage, and surgery.

Notes

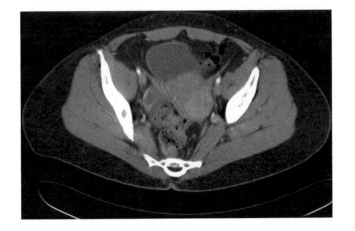
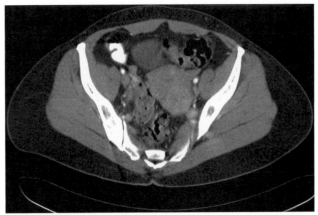

Upper right image reprinted with permission from Lee JKT, Sagel SS, Stanley RJ, Heiken P, *Computed Body Tomography with MRI Correlation*, ed 4, Philadelphia: Lippincott Williams and Wilkins, 2006.

1. Describe the abnormality in the uterus by its location and enhancement.

2. Name the various types of these primary uterine lesions based on their locations.

3. Which imaging modality is the most sensitive in their detection and characterization?

4. True of false: The malignant form of this lesion is easily differentiated by MRI.

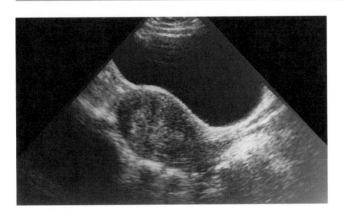
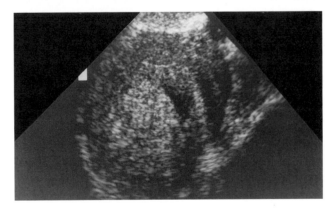

1. What are the risk factors for endometrial carcinoma?

2. True or false: An endometrial thickness of 4 mm or less, even in women with bleeding, is associated with endometrial atrophy.

3. True or false: For a postmenopausal woman with vaginal bleeding and an endometrial thickness of 7 mm, endometrial biopsy should be performed.

4. In postmenopausal women on cyclic hormone replacement therapy, at what point in the cycle should pelvic ultrasonography be performed?

CASE 39

Ob/Gyn: Uterine Fibroids

1. An intramural, mildly enhancing uterine mass.

2. Submucosal, intramural, subserosal, intraligamentous, intratubal, and pedunculated.

3. MRI.

4. False. Degenerating fibroids can mimic leiomyosarcomas.

Reference

Murase E, Siegelman ES, Outwater EK, et al: Uterine leiomyomas: histopathologic features, MR imaging findings, differential diagnosis and treatment, *Radiographics* 19:1179–1197, 1999.

Cross-Reference

Zagoria RJ, *Genitourinary Radiology: THE REQUISITES,* 2nd ed, pp 276–278.

Comment

Uterine leiomyomas (fibroids) are benign neoplasms of smooth muscle. They are the most common pelvic tumors in females and are more frequent in the reproductive years.

Leiomyomas enlarge the uterus and cause contour abnormalities. Submucosal, intramural, and subserosal are the most common types, although extrauterine forms such as pedunculated, intraligamentous (broad ligament), and intratubal (fallopian tubes) can occur.

Leiomyomas enlarge in response to hormonal increases and regress with menopause. They can calcify and undergo various types of degeneration (red, cystic, and hyaline/myxoid) if they outgrow their blood supply. Exophytic (subserosal) or pedunculated leiomyomas can undergo torsion and subsequently degenerate.

Diagnosis is usually made by pelvic examination and confirmed with imaging. By ultrasonography (US), leiomyomas are predominantly hypoechoic. US is limited in detecting small (smaller than 2 cm) or very large lesions. CT is limited as well in detection since leiomyomas appear isodense to the uterus and have variable enhancement.

MRI is the most sensitive modality in detecting and characterizing uterine leiomyomas. Simple fibroids appear as well-defined masses with homogeneous low T1 and T2 signal relative to the myometrium. Mildly delayed homogeneous enhancement occurs. Degenerating fibroids are variable in appearance with heterogeneous high T2 signal and irregular enhancement. Consequently, they are difficult to distinguish from the more worrisome leiomyosarcoma.

Notes

CASE 40

Ob/Gyn: Endometrial Measurements on Ultrasonography in Postmenopausal Women

1. Nulliparity, late menopause, greater than 20 pounds overweight, diabetes, hypertension, unopposed estrogen, tamoxifen therapy, oral contraceptives.

2. True.

3. True.

4. Ideally, ultrasonography is performed when the endometrium is thinnest, either at the end of cycle following bleeding or early in the cycle.

References

Davidson KG: Ultrasonographic evaluation of the endometrium in postmenopausal vaginal bleeding, *Radiol Clin North Am* 41:769–780, 2003.

Gull B: Can ultrasound replace dilation and curettage? *Am J Obstet Gynecol* 23:137–150, 2003.

Cross-Reference

Zagoria RJ, *Genitourinary Radiology: THE REQUISITES*, 2nd ed, pp 257–258, 298–302.

Comment

More than 70% of women with endometrial carcinoma are postmenopausal, and the majority (greater than 75%) present with bleeding. Most patients have been exposed to excess estrogen, which can lead to hyperplasia.

Postmenopausal patients with bleeding and endometrial thickness of 4 mm or less have endometrial atrophy, which is the most common cause of postmenopausal bleeding. In postmenopausal women with bleeding, either with or without hormone replacement therapy (HRT), endometrial thickness of 5 mm or greater may prompt biopsy. For postmenopausal women on HRT without bleeding, an endometrial thickness of less than 8 mm does not require biopsy, as hormonal influences cause endometrial proliferation. Ultrasonography early (before day 13) or late (after day 23) in the cycle is optimal for evaluation of women on HRT because the endometrium is thinnest at these times, and a measurement over 8 mm at these times is more likely to indicate endometrial pathology. Endometrial biopsy may result in false-negative results, requiring further evaluation.

Causes of postmenopausal bleeding for women with endometrial thickness greater than 4 mm include endometrial hyperplasia, polyps, fibroids, endometrial carcinoma, or estrogen withdrawal.

Sonohysterography allows more detailed evaluation of the endometrium, and can better depict polyps or submucosal fibroids that may cause bleeding.

Notes

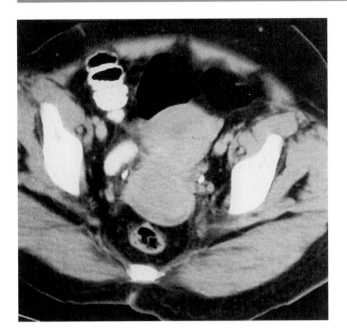 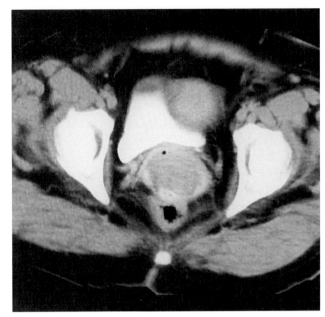

1. What is the most likely type and stage of this tumor?

2. What are the International Federation of Gynecology and Obstetrics (FIGO) guidelines for staging this tumor?

3. Has the incidence of this disease increased or decreased over the past 30 years?

4. What are the risk factors associated with this disease?

Ob/Gyn: Cervical Carcinoma

1. Stage IIa.

2. Clinical staging of cervical carcinoma requires bimanual pelvic examination, chest radiography, excretory urography, cystoscopy, and radiographic examination of the lungs and skeleton.

3. The incidence of invasive carcinoma is decreasing as a result of increased patient awareness and routine Papanicolaou smear screening. However, the overall incidence of cervical dysplasia is increasing, presumably as a result of the increased incidence of sexually transmitted diseases.

4. Low socioeconomic status, multiple sexual partners, immunosuppression, and human papillomavirus infection.

References

Kaur H, Silverman PM, Iyer RB, et al: Diagnosis, staging, and surveillance of cervical carcinoma, *Am J Roentgenol* 180:1621–1631, 2003.

Okamoto Y, Tanaka YO, Nishida M, et al: MR imaging of the uterine cervix: imaging-pathologic correlation, *Radiographics* 23:425–445, 2003.

Cross-Reference

Zagoria RJ, *Genitourinary Radiology: THE REQUISITES,* 2nd ed, pp 305–310.

Comment

Cervical carcinoma is the third most common gynecologic malignancy, after endometrial and ovarian carcinomas. Clinically, the patient with advanced cervical cancer may have abnormal vaginal discharge or vaginal bleeding, but preinvasive cervical cancer is usually asymptomatic. The diagnosis is confirmed most often by a cervical biopsy or by Papanicolaou testing. In situ disease (stage 0) requires no imaging. Biopsy-confirmed invasive disease requires staging. The goal of imaging is to accurately stage disease and direct therapy. Stage I cervical cancer is confined to the cervix. In stage II disease the cancer extends beyond the cervix, and in stage III disease the tumor spreads to the pelvic sidewall or causes ureteral obstruction. Stage IV cervical cancer invades the bladder or rectum directly or extends beyond the true pelvis.

Patients with a superficial cervical carcinoma can undergo a transvaginal cone excision (in which the tumor is excised and the uterus is left in place). Patients with stage Ib and IIa usually undergo radical hysterectomy with preoperative radiation therapy. Patients who have parametrial invasion (stage IIb and higher) are treated with radiation therapy in combination with radiation-sensitizing chemotherapy. The take-home point about cervical cancer staging recalls Shakespeare, "To be or not to be, that is the question...." With respect to treatment options, stage IIb is an important staging threshold. Critical imaging observations in the staging of cervical carcinoma include parametrial invasion, pelvic lymphadenopathy, hydroureter, and extrapelvic metastatic disease. The presence of any of these findings connotes advanced disease and precludes surgery. Hydronephrosis is an important diagnosis that upstages the classification to stage IIIb. Either CT or MRI can be used to stage cervical carcinoma.

Notes

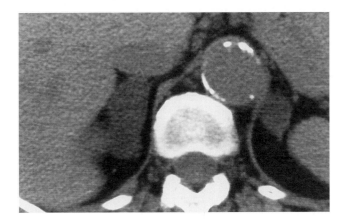

1. What is the most likely diagnosis?

2. What is the physiologic basis for the imaging findings?

3. What is the role of MRI in evaluating these findings?

4. What is the significance of mass size and density?

Adrenal: Evaluation of Adrenal Masses: Size versus Density

1. Bilateral adrenal adenomas.

2. Intracellular lipid is present in adrenal adenomas but almost never in metastases, carcinomas, or pheochromocytomas.

3. Chemical shift MRI is specific for differentiating an adenoma from a metastasis when non-contrast-enhanced CT is equivocal. The role of MRI has lessened with the advent of washout calculations of intravenous CT contrast. MRI is particularly useful when the Hounsfield unit measurement is borderline on a non-contrast-enhanced CT.

4. The low density is more important than the adrenal size.

References

Israel GM, Korobkin M, Wang C, et al: Comparison of unenhanced CT and chemical shift MRI in evaluating lipid-rich adrenal adenomas, *Am J Roentgenol* 183: 215–219, 2004.

Mayo-Smith WW, Boland GW, Noto RB, Lee MJ: State of the art adrenal imaging, *Radiographics* 21:995–1012, 2001.

Cross-Reference

Zagoria RJ, *Genitourinary Radiology: THE REQUISITES,* 2nd ed, pp 355–356.

Comment

Adrenal adenoma is one of the more common incidentally discovered masses; these benign tumors are discovered in 1% to 8% of autopsy cases and in 1% of patients undergoing abdominal CT examination. Adenomas are typically less than 3 cm in diameter and can be bilateral. The differential diagnosis for bilateral adrenal masses includes bilateral adenomas, metastases, hemorrhage (bilateral in 10% of neonates and 20% of adults), granulomatous adrenalitis, and pheochromocytomas (10% are bilateral).

This case demonstrates the typical findings of bilateral adrenal adenomas (bilateral, well-circumscribed, low-density masses without other evidence of metastases). The low density (less than 10 Hounsfield units) is caused by cytoplasmic lipid, which also explains signal loss on opposed-phase chemical shift MRI. While the presence of intracytoplasmic lipid is considered diagnostic of adrenal adenoma, some metastases, such as clear cell renal adenocarcinoma can also contain cytoplasmic lipid. Adenomas enhance vigorously with the administration of intravenous contrast material, and the contrast material washes out of the gland on delayed imaging. This washout is greater in adenomas than in metastases. An absolute washout value of more than 60% contrast washout on 15-minute delayed CT or more than 50% on 10-minute delayed CT has been used to differentiate adenomas from metastases. Other washout parameters are discussed elsewhere in this book. For equivocal findings, either MRI or follow-up CT can be performed. If immediate pathologic diagnosis is required, adrenal biopsy using CT guidance is safe and accurate.

Notes

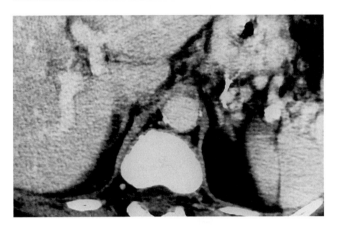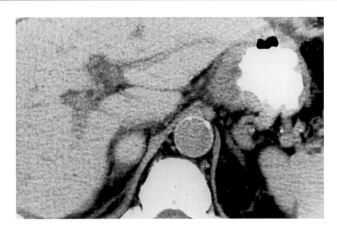

1. What is the finding on the image on the right (which was obtained from a CT scan performed 1 week after the image on the left was taken)?

2. How often is this lesion bilateral?

3. Which modality is most specific for this diagnosis: ultrasonography, CT, or MRI?

4. What degree of enhancement would be expected with administration of intravenous contrast?

Adrenal: Acute Adrenal Hemorrhage on CT

1. Acute adrenal hemorrhage.

2. In up to 20% of cases.

3. MRI.

4. No enhancement.

References

Mayo-Smith WW, Boland GW, Noto RB, Lee MJ: State-of-the-art adrenal imaging [Review], *Radiographics* 21:995–1012, 2001.

Kawashima A, Sandler CM, Ernst RD, et al: Imaging of nontraumatic hemorrhage of the adrenal gland [Review], *Radiographics* 19:949–963, 1999.

Cross-Reference

Zagoria RJ, *Genitourinary Radiology: THE REQUISITES,* 2nd ed, pp 366, 369.

Comment

Adrenal hemorrhage can be a complication of blunt abdominal trauma, sepsis, coagulopathy, anticoagulation therapy, surgery, or adrenal venography. Spontaneous adrenal hemorrhage is less common. Some of the clinical situations with which spontaneous hemorrhage is associated are septicemia (Waterhouse-Friderichsen syndrome), severe physiologic stress, hypotension, surgery, and adrenal tumors. Metastatic melanoma can be associated with adrenal hemorrhage. Adrenal hemorrhage is usually asymptomatic, but symptoms can include abdominal pain or hypotension. Up to 20% of the cases are bilateral.

The radiologist should be aware of the appearance of acute adrenal hemorrhage on cross-sectional imaging. On ultrasonography, adrenal hemorrhage may appear as a hyperechoic mass. The echogenicity gradually decreases as the hematoma resolves, and the eventual appearance may mimic that of an adrenal cyst. On unenhanced CT the adrenal gland is enlarged and has increased attenuation as a result of acute blood products (as in this case). MRI is the most accurate imaging modality for detecting and characterizing adrenal hemorrhage because of imaging features that are sensitive and specific for blood products. As a result of the presence of methemoglobin, signal intensity is increased in acute adrenal hemorrhage on T1W images. On T2W images, serpiginous, linear low signal within an area of heterogeneous signal may be visible, depending on the age of the bleed. In older hemorrhages a cystic area of T2-hyperintense fluid surrounded by a dark rim may be present as a result of hemosiderin within macrophages

(as shown in Figure 9-15 on page 369 of *Genitourinary Radiology: THE REQUISITES,* 2nd ed).

Notes

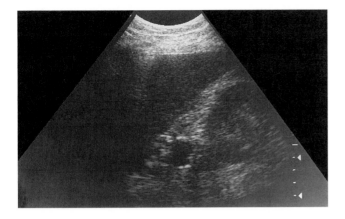

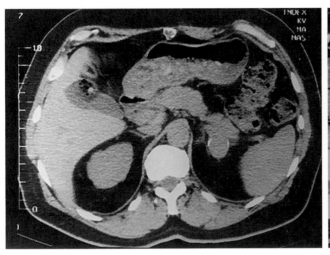

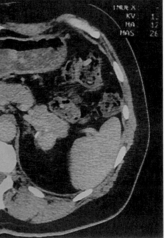

1. A sagittal sonogram of the left kidney and a composite figure of two noncontrast CT images are shown. What is included in the differential diagnosis?

2. What is the most common cause of an adrenal pseudotumor on CT?

3. True or false: Most adrenal pseudotumors occur on the right side.

4. True or false: Many adrenal pseudotumors are vascular lesions.

Adrenal: Adrenal Pseudotumor

1. Splenic artery aneurysm or pseudoaneurysm.

2. Exophytic renal cyst.

3. False.

4. True.

References

Brady TM, Gross BH, Glazer GM, Williams DM: Adrenal pseudomasses due to varices: angiographic-CT-MRI-pathologic correlations, *Am J Roentgenol* 145:301–304, 1985.

Lawler LP, Horton KM, Fishman EK: Peripancreatic masses that simulate pancreatic disease: spectrum of disease and role of CT, *Radiographics* 23:1117–1131, 2003.

Cross-Reference

Zagoria RJ, *Genitourinary Radiology: THE REQUISITES*, 2nd ed, pp 77–78, 369–374.

Comment

Normal periadrenal viscera or a vascular lesion may mimic an adrenal mass. Pseudolesions of the adrenal gland occur more frequently on the left side. Causes of a left adrenal pseudotumor include vessels, a splenule, left renal mass (most commonly an exophytic upper pole renal cyst), pancreatic body or tail mass, adjacent small bowel, gastric diverticulum, and redundant gastric fundus. Pseudotumor that is caused by bowel may be diagnosed by repeating the radiologic or ultrasound study after oral contrast is administered. Vascular adrenal pseudomasses include a tortuous splenic artery, splenic artery aneurysm or pseudoaneurysm, and periadrenal venous collaterals in portal hypertension. Right adrenal pseudotumors are less common and may be caused by tortuous renal vessels or exophytic renal and hepatic masses.

In this case a splenic artery aneurysm mimicked a left adrenal mass on abdominal sonography. Aneurysms of the splenic artery are the most common cause of visceral artery aneurysms. They occur in women twice as frequently as in men, and 90% of women with splenic pseudoaneurysms have been pregnant at least twice. The most common complication of splenic artery aneurysms is rupture, which carries a high mortality rate. Treatment is stenting, embolization, or resection, which should be performed when the aneurysm reaches 2 cm or greater in diameter. Calcification in the aneurysm wall is present in two thirds of cases. Notice the linear focus of mural calcification on both the ultrasound and noncontrast CT examinations.

Notes

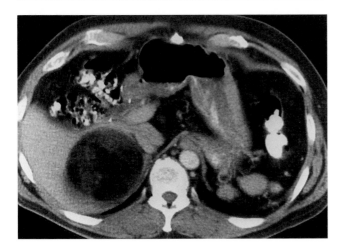 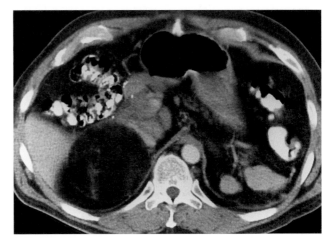

1. What suprarenal lesions may contain areas of mature adipose tissue?

2. What is the most common clinical presentation of myelolipoma?

3. Is there a correlation between tumor size and symptoms?

4. True or false: Most myelolipomas increase in size over time.

Adrenal: Natural History of Myelolipoma

1. Adrenal myelolipoma, exophytic renal angiomyolipoma, retroperitoneal lipoma, and retroperitoneal liposarcoma.

2. Incidentally discovered asymptomatic suprarenal mass.

3. Usually not. However, very large myelolipomas may hemorrhage causing pain.

4. False.

References

Elsayes KM, Mukundan G, Narra VR, et al: Adrenal masses: MR imaging features with pathologic correlation, *Radiographics* 24(Suppl 1):73–86, 2004.

Han M, Burnett AL, Fishman EK, Marshall FF: The natural history and treatment of adrenal myelolipoma, *J Urol* 157:1213–1216, 1997.

Cross-Reference

Zagoria RJ, *Genitourinary Radiology: THE REQUISITES*, 2nd ed, pp 360–361.

Comment

Adrenal myelolipoma is a rare benign neoplasm, and as illustrated here is composed of mature adipose and hematopoietic tissues. Although there is no consensus as to the etiology of this tumor, the most widely held theory is that it is caused by adrenocortical metaplasia of reticuloendothelial cells in response to nonspecific stimuli.

Although these tumors may cause abdominal or flank pain, most adrenal myelolipomas are asymptomatic, and the great majority are hormonally inactive. At the time of discovery, these tumors may range from several centimeters to more than 30 cm in diameter. There is no clear correlation between tumor size and symptoms relating to mechanical compression, retroperitoneal hemorrhage, or tumor necrosis. When followed over a period of up to 10 years, these tumors may increase in size, but growth is slow and is not necessarily related to the development of symptoms or hemorrhage. Growth alone therefore should not be an indication for resection.

The recommended management of adrenal myelolipoma is conservative; surgical removal is indicated only if the patient is symptomatic.

Notes

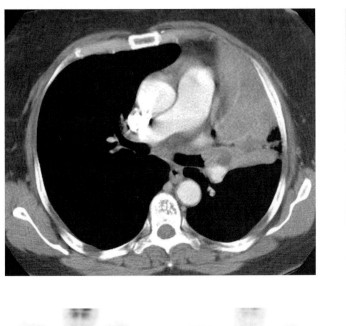
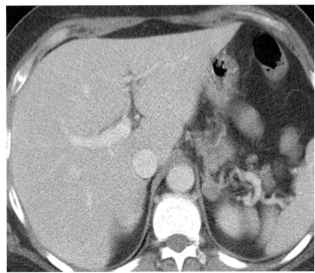

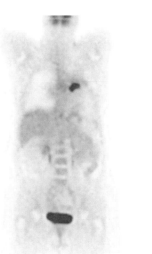
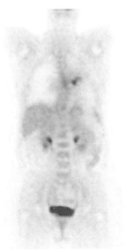
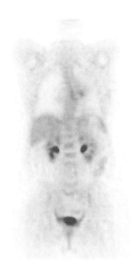
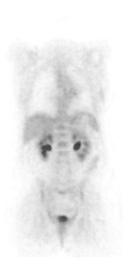

1. What are the findings on the CT and PET images?

2. Based on the PET, is the left adrenal mass benign or malignant?

3. Are additional imaging studies necessary to evaluate the left adrenal mass?

4. What is the main advantage of using PET instead of CT or MRI for evaluation of an adrenal mass in a patient with lung cancer?

C A S E   4 6

Adrenal: Lung Cancer and Benign Left Adrenal Mass on PET

1. CT: Mass in left distal mainstem bronchus resulting in left upper lobe collapse. Indeterminate left adrenal mass. PET: Intense uptake corresponding to mass in left distal mainstem bronchus and mild uptake in collapsed lung. No uptake in left adrenal mass.

2. Benign.

3. No.

4. Detecting additional sites of metastatic disease.

References

Gupta N, Graeber GM, Tamim WJ, et al: Clinical utility of PET-FDG imaging in differentiation of benign from malignant adrenal masses in lung cancer, *Clin Lung Cancer* 3:59–64, 2001.

Kumar R, Xiu Y, Yu JQ, et al: 18F-FDG PET in evaluation of adrenal lesions in patients with lung cancer, *J Nucl Med* 45: 2058–2062, 2004.

Cross-Reference

Zagoria RJ, *Genitourinary Radiology: THE REQUISITES*, 2nd ed, pp 354–358.

Comment

In this case, the lung cancer seen on CT is intensely fluorodeoxyglucose (FDG)–avid on PET. There is also mild uptake in the left upper lobe on PET due to left upper lobe collapse. No uptake is seen in the left adrenal mass, indicating it is a benign lesion.

PET has changed the way adrenal masses are worked up in patients with lung cancer. The advantages of PET over CT or MRI are detection of additional sites of metastases and evaluation of the biologic activity of the primary malignancy. PET findings are considered positive when the uptake in the adrenal mass is greater than background liver activity.

Published PET studies on patients with lung cancer and adrenal masses have shown sensitivity of 93% to 100% and specificity of 80% to 100% for adrenal metastases. False-positive PET results have been reported in pheochromocytomas and adrenal adenomas. False-negative PET results have been reported in necrotic adrenal masses and metastases from neuroendocrine and bronchioloalveolar cancer. CT and MRI still have an important role in evaluating incidentally detected indeterminate adrenal masses in patients without history of malignancy, but PET examinations have proven useful to characterize adrenal masses in patients with lung carcinoma. In this patient, despite the enlarged adrenal on CT, the decreased activity on PET and the absence of other metastases rendered this patient an operative candidate.

Notes

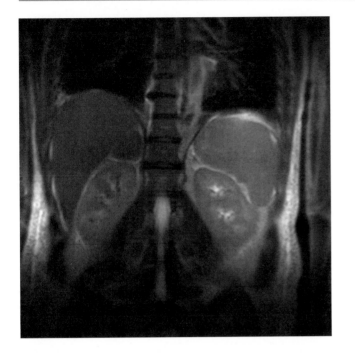

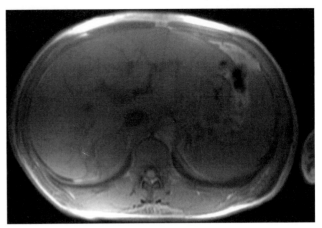

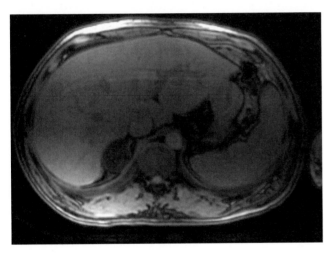

1. What is the diagnosis?

2. What MR technique has been used to make this diagnosis?

3. What percentage drop in density is considered diagnostic for a benign adenoma when using the CT washout technique?

4. What material within the lesion causes the signal drop to occur on chemical shift MRI?

Adrenal: Adrenal Adenoma

1. Adrenal adenoma.

2. Chemical shift imaging.

3. Greater than or equal to 50% at 10 minutes.

4. Intracellular lipid.

Reference

Elsayes KM, Mukundan G, Narra VR, et al: Adrenal masses: MR imaging features with pathologic correlation, *Radiographics* 24(Suppl):73–86, 2004.

Cross-Reference

Zagoria RJ, *Genitourinary Radiology: THE REQUISITES*, 2nd ed, pp 355–357.

Comment

This case demonstrates a mass involving the right adrenal gland that is homogeneous and relatively isointense to liver on T1- and T2-weighted images. The most characteristic finding is a drop in signal intensity on the out-of-phase images. These findings are typical of an adrenal adenoma.

The evaluation of a suspected hyperfunctioning adrenal mass such as a pheochromocytoma or aldosteronoma should begin with an appropriate biochemical evaluation. CT or MRI can be utilized for further evaluation of these and other adrenal masses. The CT criteria utilized for diagnosis of an adrenal adenoma include both histologic and physiologic parameters. Attenuation less than 10 Hounsfield units (HU) on nonenhanced CT is diagnostic. If this criterion is not met, contrast-enhanced CT can be obtained and a washout value calculated. One technique that has been utilized is to obtain imaging at approximately 1 minute and 10 minutes following contrast administration. Relative washout is calculated with the following formula: [(initial HU − delayed HU)/initial HU] times 100%. Fifty percent or greater relative washout is specific for adenoma. MRI is another powerful tool in the characterization of a problematic adrenal mass. Its reliability is in part due to the same principle used for nonenhanced CT evaluation. This principle is that most adrenal adenomas contain intracytoplasmic lipid, but metastases do not. On comparison of T1-weighted in- and out-of-phase images, the adrenal adenoma can be seen to drop in signal intensity on the out-of-phase image. This drop in signal intensity is often judged in comparison with the spleen, because the liver may be infiltrated with fat and thus also demonstrates loss of signal intensity. This loss of signal intensity occurs because of the chemical environment of protons in fat and water, which results in different resonance frequency rates. This difference is exploited by choosing TE intervals that produce a net loss of signal from voxels containing both lipid and water. In equivocal cases, PET scan or biopsy may be required.

Notes

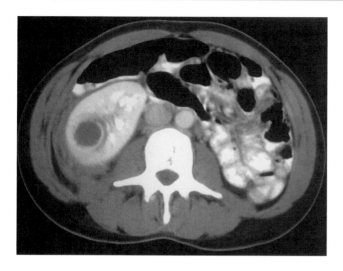 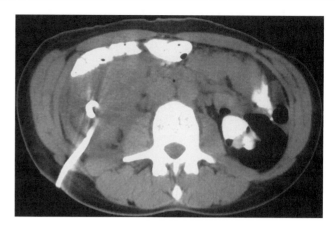

1. What is the most likely diagnosis in this patient with right flank pain and fever lasting 1 week?

2. Is this renal lesion usually symptomatic?

3. What treatment is best for patients with this disease?

4. What is the likely cause of this lesion?

Vascular and Interventional: Percutaneous Drainage of a Renal Abscess

1. Renal abscess.

2. Yes.

3. A combination of systemic antibiotics and percutaneous drainage.

4. Acute pyelonephritis.

Reference

Siegel JF, Smith A, Moldwin R: Minimally invasive treatment of renal abscess, *J Urol* 155:52–55, 1996.

Cross-Reference

Zagoria RJ, *Genitourinary Radiology: THE REQUISITES,* 2nd ed, p 399.

Comment

In a patient with signs and symptoms of acute pyelonephritis and a complex fluid collection within the kidney, the diagnosis of renal abscess should be made. The patient shown has a complex, thick-walled cystic mass in the right kidney, thickening of Gerota's fascia, perinephric fluid, and stranding. Heterogeneous enhancement of the right kidney indicates associated pyelonephritis. Renal abscesses generally develop in patients who have pyelonephritis. In turn, the pyelonephritis usually results from an ascending infection from the bladder. In a minority of cases, renal abscesses develop as a result of hematogenous spread of infection. Renal abscesses, like abscesses elsewhere in the body, usually do not resolve with simple antibiotic management. Percutaneous drainage of renal abscesses combined with systemic antibiotics has become the standard treatment.

The second image demonstrates placement of a pigtail catheter in this renal abscess. Typically, using CT or ultrasound guidance, the radiologist places a needle percutaneously in the fluid collection. Fluid is aspirated and usually confirms the diagnosis of abscess. Then, using either the trocar or Seldinger technique, the radiologist places a drainage catheter. The abscess should be evacuated at the time of drainage. Renal abscesses usually resolve in less than 1 week after initiation of treatment with percutaneous drainage and systemic antibiotics. After resolution of symptoms and cessation of drain output, the percutaneous drain can be removed.

Notes

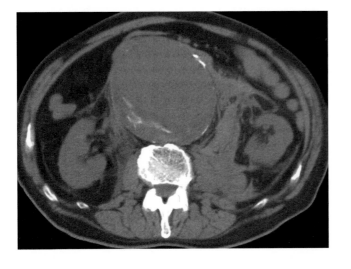
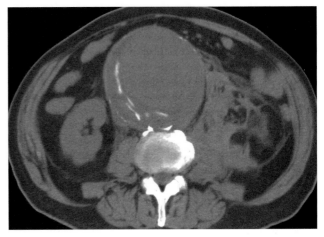

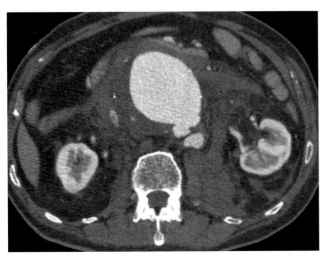
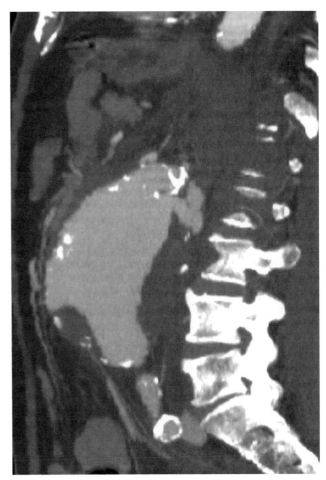

1. What is the significance of the high-density material in the pararenal and perinephric spaces bilaterally?

2. What is the significance of the high-attenuation crescent in the lumen of the aorta?

3. What is the diagnosis in this elderly patient with back pain?

4. Can the site of bleeding be identified?

Retroperitoneum: Ruptured Abdominal Aortic Aneurysm

1. It represents acute hemorrhage.

2. This is a sign of acute or impending rupture of an abdominal aortic aneurysm.

3. Ruptured abdominal aortic aneurysm.

4. Yes, it is seen extending posterolaterally from the aneurysm on the sagittal image of the contrast enhanced scan.

Reference

Mehard WB, Heiken JP, Sicard GA: High-attenuating crescent in abdominal aortic aneurysm wall at CT: a sign of acute or impending rupture, *Radiology* 192:359–362, 1994.

Cross-Reference

Zagoria RJ, *Genitourinary Radiology: THE REQUISITES,* 2nd ed, pp 74–79.

Comment

The images show a large abdominal aortic aneurysm (AAA) with high-attenuation fluid surrounding it. High-attenuation fluid on a noncontrast CT represents blood, proteinaceous fluid, or contrast material. In this case no oral contrast material was given, and the only reasonable explanation for the fluid is bleeding from the AAA. When searching for acute retroperitoneal hemorrhage, a non-contrast-enhanced CT is usually adequate. A CT with contrast may also be obtained to look for other pathology. The reformatted contrast study shows a site of rupture in the wall of the AAA. This may be helpful in planning repair of this aneurysm.

Most patients with a ruptured AAA die before they present to the hospital, and the operative mortality rate is high for those who do undergo reparative surgery. When AAAs exceed 5 cm in diameter, they are more likely to rupture and prophylactic repair may be undertaken. Approximately 40% of AAAs larger than 5 cm in diameter rupture within 5 years. In addition to the size of the aneurysm, the presence of an intraluminal high-density crescent has been associated with acute or impending rupture of an AAA. This sign is illustrated in this case. This crescent is thought to represent acute hemorrhage in the wall or in thrombus around the aneurysm. This is sometimes associated with acute onset of back pain. The crescent has also been observed in cases where acute rupture has occurred.

Notes

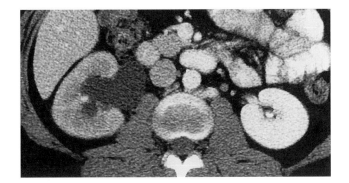 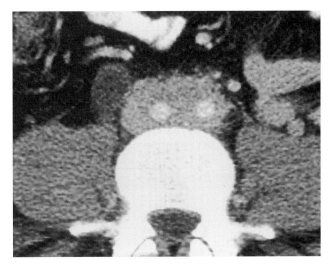

1. What is causing the delayed nephrogram and nephromegaly of the right kidney?

2. What is the likely cause of the soft tissue around the aorta and iliac arteries?

3. What is the fluid-containing structure to the right of the abnormal soft tissue?

4. What is the treatment for this type of hydronephrosis?

Retroperitoneum: Retroperitoneal Fibrosis

1. Ureteral obstruction.

2. Retroperitoneal fibrosis.

3. Hydroureter.

4. This condition may be managed temporarily with ureteral stents. Definitive therapy usually requires surgical dissection of the ureter.

Reference

Amis ES: Retroperitoneal fibrosis, *Am J Roentgenol* 157:321–329, 1991.

Cross-Reference

Zagoria RJ, *Genitourinary Radiology: THE REQUISITES,* 2nd ed, pp 170, 183, 186.

Comment

Retroperitoneal fibrosis (RPF) includes both idiopathic (Ormond's disease) and secondary proliferation of non-neoplastic fibrotic tissues. RPF tends to be centered around the aorta initially, but with progression it encases the inferior vena cava and ureters. RPF is usually centered near the L4–5 level of the spine, but it may arise or extend the entire length of the retroperitoneum, including the renal sinus. Approximately 50% of RPF cases involve both ureters. RPF is one of the most common causes of bilateral ureteral obstruction. Obstruction of the ureter is caused by encasement of the ureter by the surrounding RPF. This encasement causes a narrowed, aperistaltic segment of ureter and resulting hydronephrosis. Only limited success in reversing RPF has been achieved using systemic steroids and chemotherapeutic agents, definitive treatment of the hydronephrosis usually requires surgical intervention, moving the ureter away from the fibrosis and insulating it with protective peritoneum or omentum, thus preventing further progression of the RPF.

Secondary RPF is associated with numerous other entities, including aortic aneurysms, aortic and iliac graft procedures, retroperitoneal hematomas, urinomas, infections, inflammatory bowel disease, sclerosing cholangitis, and fibrosing mediastinitis, and with use of certain drugs, most notably ergot alkaloids.

Lymphoma can present with a similar or identical appearance. Surgical biopsy is often required to obtain adequate tissue to exclude lymphoma. There are no "absolute" imaging characteristics to differentiate RPF from retroperitoneal lymphoma, although extensive soft tissue proliferation behind the aorta strongly suggests lymphoma rather than RPF.

Notes

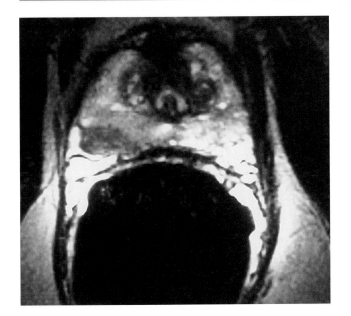
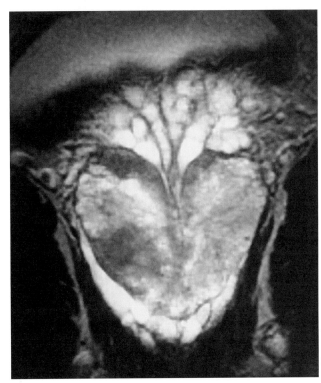

1. True or false: The majority of prostate adenocarcinomas arise from the peripheral zone.

2. Nodules of benign prostate hyperplasia arise from which zone of the prostate?

3. What is the clinicopathologic significance of the neurovascular bundle?

4. The ejaculatory ducts are located in which zone of the prostate?

Prostate and Seminal Vesicles: Zonal Anatomy of the Prostate on MRI

1. True.

2. The transitional zone.

3. It is a common site where adenocarcinoma transgresses the prostatic capsule.

4. The central zone.

References

Claus FG, Hricak H, Hattery RR: Pretreatment evaluation of prostate cancer: role of MR imaging and 1H MR spectroscopy, *Radiographics* 24(Suppl):167–180, 2004.

McNeal JE: Normal anatomy of the prostate and changes in benign prostatic hypertrophy and carcinoma, *Semin Ultrasound CT MR* 9:329–334, 1988.

Cross-Reference

Zagoria RJ, *Genitourinary Radiology: THE REQUISITES*, 2nd ed, pp 337–339.

Comment

On these turbo spin-echo T2W images the cancer is a hypointense area in the right side of the peripheral zone at the mid-gland level. At surgery, there was microscopic spread of adenocarcinoma through the capsule and into the right neurovascular bundle.

Prostate anatomy was redefined more than a decade ago through the meticulous analysis of the microscopic structure of the acinar and ductal patterns of the glandular prostate. Discrete glandular "zones" of the prostate were defined and have impacted our understanding of prostate adenocarcinoma and benign prostatic hyperplasia (BPH). The central zone consists of an acinar-ductal system that empties into the verumontanum, close to the orifices of the ejaculatory duct. Its branches ramify proximally to the base of the prostate gland (i.e., closer to the bladder neck) and surround the ejaculatory ducts. The other major glandular zone, the peripheral zone, has no contact with the verumontanum but is more extensive; it extends from the prostatic apex inferiorly to the base of the gland superiorly. Together, the ducts of the peripheral and central zones compose roughly 95% of the glandular tissue of the prostate. Acinar mucin traps water and is what gives the peripheral and central zones their high signal intensity on long TR/TE MRI. The preprostatic segment of the urethra is proximal to the verumontanum and is surrounded by a smaller glandular system called the transitional zone. This zone contributes negligibly to prostate function.

Benign prostatic hyperplasia has been found to be a disease exclusively of the preprostatic region; nodules arise from either the transition zone or the submucosal tissues of the periurethral gland. The central zone is relatively immune from disease, but the peripheral zone is the site of chronic inflammatory processes, atypical hyperplasias, and most prostatic carcinomas. Rarer transition zone cancers arise in BPH nodules.

Notes

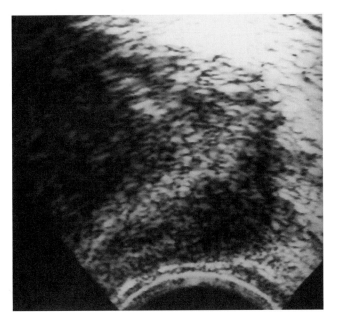
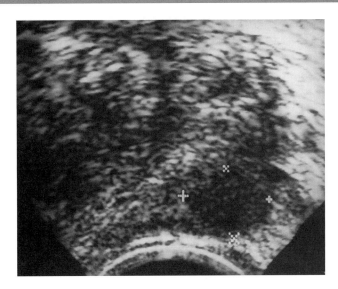

1. What is the differential diagnosis for this abnormality?

2. On transrectal prostate sonography, what percentage of prostate carcinomas are hypoechoic?

3. Where do carcinomas arise in the prostate gland?

4. What are important predictors of aggressive behavior for prostate cancer?

Prostate and Seminal Vesicles: Hypoechoic Lesion on Prostate Ultrasonography

1. Differential diagnosis for a hypoechoic nodule in the prostatic peripheral zone includes prostate carcinoma, atypical hyperplasia, focal prostatitis, nodule of benign prostatic hyperplasia, focal atrophy, and prostatic cyst.

2. About 70% (30% are isoechoic and 1% hyperechoic).

3. Of prostate carcinomas, 85% are located in the peripheral zone, 10% in the transitional zone (usually found in the chips of tissue after transurethral resection of the prostate), and 5% in the central zone surrounding the ejaculatory ducts.

4. Gleason grade (higher grade has worst prognosis). Tumor size and elevated prostate-specific antigen levels.

References

Hittelman AB, Purohit RS, Kane CJ: Update of staging and risk assessment for prostate cancer patients [Review], *Curr Opin Urol* 14:163–170, 2004.

Kuligowska E, Barish MA, Fenlon HM, Blake M: Predictors of prostate carcinoma: accuracy of gray-scale and color Doppler US and serum markers, *Radiology* 220:757–764, 2001.

Cross-Reference

Zagoria RJ, *Genitourinary Radiology: THE REQUISITES*, 2nd ed, pp 329–332.

Comment

In the United States, prostate cancer is the most common malignancy in men and the second most common cause of cancer-related death after lung carcinoma. Serum prostate-specific antigen (PSA), digital rectal examination (DRE), and transrectal ultrasonography of the prostate play an important role in the diagnosis of prostate carcinoma. Modern high-frequency transducers have improved anatomic definition, and refinements in equipment have allowed for ultrasound-guided biopsy. Ultrasound guidance improves the yield of prostate needle biopsy over that of digital-guided procedures.

One limitation of transrectal ultrasonography is the low specificity of a hypoechoic, peripheral zone lesion. Although prostatic adenocarcinoma can appear hypoechoic, there are benign causes, including atypical hyperplasia, focal prostatitis, and prostatic cyst. In addition, approximately 30% of prostate carcinomas are isoechoic to normal prostate gland on transrectal ultrasonography and cannot be detected reliably unless there is distortion of the contour of the gland. Although 40% of hypoechoic lesions are malignant, the positive predictive value increases to 60% when there is a corresponding nodule on DRE. The positive predictive value increases to 70% when the DRE is abnormal and serum PSA level is elevated. The main role for prostatic ultrasonography is to provide imaging guidance for prostatic biopsy when there is a palpable nodule or an elevated PSA level.

PSA density is calculated by dividing the serum PSA level by clinical prostatic volume (calculated from ultrasound results). PSA density is an attempt to increase the specificity of PSA levels by adjusting for prostate gland size. Biopsy is recommended when PSA density exceeds 0.1 to 0.14.

Notes

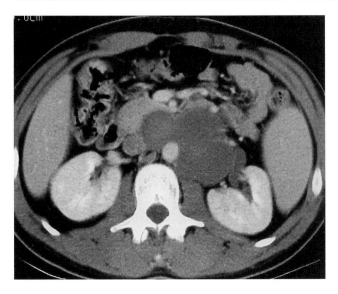

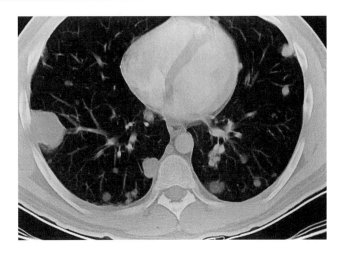

1. What is the most common route through which testicular carcinoma is spread?

2. Where is the "sentinel" node for a primary malignancy of the left testicle? Where is it for a malignancy of the right testicle?

3. What are the staging implications of testicular cancer that invades the epididymis or the scrotal wall?

4. Which testicular cancers are associated with alpha-fetoprotein levels? Which are associated with elevated human chorionic gonadotropin levels?

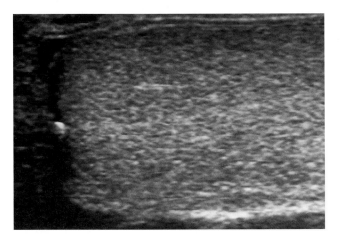

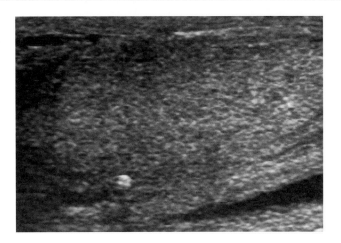

1. What is the most likely diagnosis?

2. Is this lesion intratesticular or extratesticular? What is the significance of this distinction?

3. Is this a benign or a premalignant condition?

4. What is one common associated condition?

Scrotum: Staging of Testicular Cancer

1. Via the lymphatics to the retroperitoneal nodes first, and then hematogenously to the lungs, liver, bone, and brain.

2. Left: Renal perihilar, just inferior to the renal vein. Right: Paracaval, inferior to the right renal artery.

3. Change in the lymph nodal drainage pattern.

4. Alpha-fetoprotein: Yolk sac carcinoma, embryonal cell carcinoma, and mixed tumors (teratocarcinoma). Human chorionic gonadotropin: pure seminoma, embryonal cell carcinoma, and choriocarcinoma.

Reference

Sheinfeld J: Nonseminomatous germ cell tumors of the testis: current concepts and controversies, *Urology* 44:2–10, 1994.

Cross-Reference

Zagoria RJ, *Genitourinary Radiology: THE REQUISITES*, 2nd ed, pp 322–325.

Comment

The staging of germ cell testicular neoplasms is based on the tendency for these tumors to spread to the retroperitoneal nodes first, and then the mediastinal nodes and lung parenchyma. Later, hematogenous spread to the lungs, liver, bones, and brain may occur. In addition to serum assays of elevated alpha-fetoprotein (AFP), human chorionic gonadotropin (hCG), and lactate dehydrogenase, staging usually includes chest radiography; CT of the chest, abdomen, and pelvis; and a radionuclide bone scan. The paracaval, interaortocaval, and right common iliac node groups are considered the primary sites of spread (sentinel node groups) for right-sided tumors. For left-sided testicular tumors, interaortocaval, left paraaortic, and left common iliac nodes are sentinel nodes. Local spread of the testicular neoplasm to the epididymis may result in metastatic external iliac lymphadenopathy, and spread to the scrotal wall may result in inguinal node involvement.

It is important to distinguish between pure seminomatous and mixed or nonseminomatous germ cell tumors (i.e., embryonal cell carcinoma, teratoma, yolk sac tumor, and choriocarcinoma) because this can dramatically alter the optimal treatment regimen. Serum markers are important for the management of testicular cancers after radical orchiectomy. AFP is produced by endodermal sinus cells of the yolk sac and has a half-life of 5 days; hCG is a glycoprotein secreted by placental cells and has a half-life of 30 hours. Failure of the markers to normalize appropriately, based on their serum half-life, implies the patient probably has metastatic disease.

Scrotum: Scrotal Pearl

1. Scrotal calculus, or scrotal pearl.

2. Extratesticular. It is unlikely to be malignant.

3. Benign.

4. Hydrocele.

Reference

Linkowski GD, Avvelone A, Gooding GAW: Scrotal calculi: sonographic detection, *Radiology* 156:484, 1985.

Cross-Reference

Zagoria RJ, *Genitourinary Radiology: THE REQUISITES*, 2nd ed, p 325.

Comment

Scrotal calculi, also called scrotal pearls or fibrinoid loose bodies, are benign and mobile concretions found between the membranes of the tunica vaginalis. Pathologically there is a central nidus of hydroxyapatite surrounded by fibrinoid material. The calculi can be single or multiple and may be larger than 4 mm in diameter (as large as 10 mm). Scrotal calculi may be the result of a nonspecific inflammatory process of the tunica vaginalis or torsion of a testicular appendage. Nonspecific scrotal inflammation may cause granulation tissue to form from exfoliated vaginal endothelial cells. With time, a fibrinoid nidus develops and gradually calcifies. Alternatively the scrotal pearl may form as a result of calcification of a torsed and infarcted appendix testis or epididymis. In either case, secondary hydroceles are commonly associated with scrotal pearls.

A large calcification in the tunica vaginalis must be distinguished from a peripheral intratesticular calcification. Testicular microliths are usually multiple and smaller than 3 mm in diameter. Larger parenchymal calcifications may be associated with old testicular trauma or a testicular neoplasm. For instance, large focal calcifications have been reported in cases of "burned out" primary testicular neoplasms and large cell calcifying Sertoli cell tumors of the testis. The latter is a rare tumor that has been associated with gynecomastia, sexual precocity, and Carney's complex (cardiac myxoma, pigmented skin lesions, cutaneous myomas, myxoid mammary fibroadenomas, primary pigmented nodule adrenocortical disease, and pituitary adenoma).

Notes

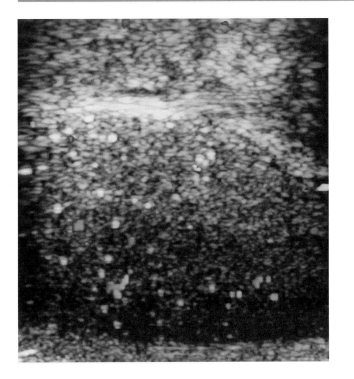

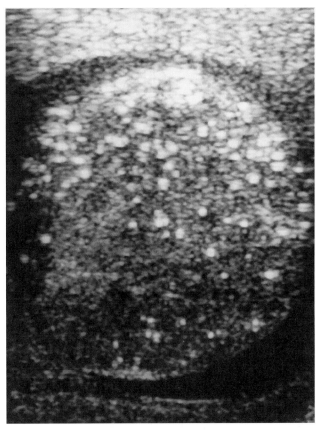

1. Two images from a testicular sonogram are shown. What is the most likely diagnosis?

2. What is the clinical significance of this lesion?

3. Name three causes of calcification in the testes.

4. True or false: The calcifications of testicular microlithiasis always shadow.

Scrotum: Testicular Microlithiasis

1. Testicular microlithiasis.

2. An association with primary testicular neoplasm.

3. Testicular neoplasms, resolved infections, hematomas, and infarcts.

4. False.

References

Backus ML, Mack LA, Middleton WD, et al: Testicular microlithiasis: imaging appearances and pathologic correlation, *Radiology* 192:781–785, 1994.

Rashid HH, Cos LR, Weinberg E, Messing EM: Testicular microlithiasis: a review and its association with testicular cancer [Review], *Urol Oncol* 22:285–289, 2004.

Cross-Reference

Zagoria RJ, *Genitourinary Radiology: THE REQUISITES*, 2nd ed, p 325.

Comment

Testicular microlithiasis is a benign condition typified by the presence of multiple (from 5 to more than 60), small punctate intratesticular calcifications. These calcifications measure 1 to 3 mm in diameter and are located in the seminiferous tubules. The condition usually affects both testicles but may be asymmetric. The calcifications do not all shadow on testicular ultrasonography.

Testicular microlithiasis has been associated with a number of other diseases, including cryptorchid testes, testicular atrophy, and infertility. An association between ultrasound-detectable testicular microlithiasis and germ cell tumors was noted in 20% to 45% of patients in one study, which has led to extensive follow-up of patients with incidentally discovered microlithiasis. In that study, the associated testicular masses were separate from the microlithiasis. Follow-up of patients with isolated microlithiasis has resulted in a lower incidence of neoplasia than originally suspected, suggesting that the entities may have been coexistent and that microlithiasis was not necessarily a precursor to neoplasia. The recommendations for follow-up of incidentally discovered microlithiasis in asymptomatic patients without a mass are controversial. Some urologists will follow patients with yearly ultrasound examinations up to age 40 (when the overall incidence of testicular cancer decreases). Tumor markers for testicular cancer are not generally recommended as a screening tool in asymptomatic patients with incidentally discovered testicular microlithiasis. Tumor markers are used when the patient has a known testicular mass, prior to orchiectomy for a baseline value. If the tumor markers are elevated at the time of diagnosis of the mass, they can be used to evaluate for recurrent disease after surgical resection of the tumor.

Notes

Fair Game

Case scenario: You are staffing an outpatient imaging center and a technologist comes to you with a patient concern. She asks for your help.

1. What should be done prior to a contrast-enhanced CT scan if the patient has a history of having had an adverse reaction during a prior contrast material injection?

2. What should be done prior to a contrast-enhanced CT scan if the patient is taking metformin?

3. What should be done if contrast material that was injected for a CT has extravasated into the patient's arm?

4. What should be done if the patient is suddenly feeling sick after a contrast-enhanced CT scan?

Contrast Material Problems

1. The patient should be questioned to determine the type and severity of his or her previous reaction. If it was severe, he or she should not receive intravenous contrast material without pretreatment, unless it is an emergency. An inpatient setting is preferable for contrast material injection, even after pretreatment, in these patients.

2. The patient should be instructed to discontinue metformin for at least the next 48 hours and until contrast-induced renal failure has been excluded with a blood test.

3. The patient should be assessed for tissue damage and neuromuscular function. The limb should be elevated and cold compresses applied. Further management will depend on the volume and type of contrast material that extravasated.

4. The patient should be assessed immediately. Treatment (see below) of an adverse reaction should commence if more than a minor reaction is occurring.

Reference

Committee on Drugs and Contrast Media of the American College of Radiology: *Manual on Contrast Media*, 5th ed, Reston, VA, 2004, American College of Radiology.

Cross-Reference

Zagoria RJ, *Genitourinary Radiology: THE REQUISITES*, 2nd ed, pp 4–6.

Comment

Prevention and treatment of adverse reactions related to the injection of contrast materials is critical for radiologists. While of no therapeutic value, iodinated radiographic contrast materials (RCMs), like other drugs, can cause unwanted side effects. Radiologists must be knowledgeable about how to avoid and treat these adverse reactions.

Prior to administering RCM, it should be determined if the patient is at a substantially increased risk for an adverse reaction. Patients who have had a previous reaction to contrast material have a greatly increased risk for having another reaction. If the previous reaction was minor, such as a sense of heat, or a headache, no pretreatment is indicated. However, if the previous reaction was serious, then a full pretreatment regimen should be administered prior to injecting RCM. One approach, proven to be beneficial in preventing repeated reactions, is to postpone the scan, and have the patient take 50-mg prednisone tablets every 6 hours, starting at least 13 hours before the RCM injection.

In addition, 50 mg of diphenhydramine should be given orally 30 minutes to 1 hour or intravenously 10 minutes before the RCM injection. Only low osmolar contrast agents should be used in these patients for intravascular injections, and an inpatient setting is preferable for the contrast material injection.

Other preventive measures should be taken in patients with renal insufficiency, due to their increased risk for developing contrast-induced nephrotoxicity. If a patient's renal function is decreased, contrast material should be avoided, when possible. If required, then intravenous hydration before and after RCM administration is the best prophylaxis for nephrotoxicity avoidance.

If a patient is taking a medication containing metformin, other precautions are needed. Metformin excretion requires functioning kidneys, and life-threatening lactic acidosis can occur if metformin concentrations exceed therapeutic levels due to continued intake with decreased renal excretion. Since RCM can cause renal failure, the coadministration of metformin and RCM poses a small risk for a serious reaction. While metformin can be taken safely up until the time of RCM injection, its use should be discontinued until RCM-induced renal insufficiency has been excluded. This is accomplished by having your patient discontinue metformin intake for at least 48 hours after RCM injection. This allows time for manifestations of RCM-induced nephrotoxicity to develop. Prior to reinstituting metformin, the patient should have normal renal function confirmed with a standard serum analysis of creatinine.

Once RCM has been injected, adverse reactions are not rare. One of the more common adverse events is extravasation of contrast material into the soft tissues near the injection site. While the vast majority of these extravasation events do not result in significant injury, some injuries can result in substantial morbidity. Keys to treating extravasation injuries include accurate assessment and follow-up. Larger volumes of low-osmolar contrast material can be extravasated without injury than when using high-osmolar agents. Our policy is to monitor every patient with any significant extravasation of RCM in the radiology department for at least 1 hour. During the period of observation, cold compresses are applied and the limb is elevated, if possible. If symptoms are stable or diminishing during the period of observation, no evidence of tissue necrosis has developed, and neuromuscular function is intact in the affected limb, the patient is discharged with instructions on how to contact a healthcare provider should symptoms worsen. The severity of soft tissue injury peaks about 48 hours after RCM extravasation, making it impossible to accurately assess the degree of damage in the period immediately after extravasation. If a major extravasation (more than 100 mL of low-osmolar RCM) has occurred, or the patient develops neuromuscular deficits, increasing symptoms, or obvious evidence of tissue necrosis, then the patient is immediately referred to a surgeon with expertise in soft tissue injuries.

When a patient feels "sick" after RCM injection, he or she should be assessed immediately. The patient should be asked to specify his or her symptoms, and vital signs should be measured. If there is extensive urticaria, hypotension, or dyspnea, treatment should be initiated immediately. A working intravenous access should be maintained. Widespread hives are usually responsive to intravenous diphenhydramine, but cimetidine and epinephrine can be used in refractory cases. Intravenous normal saline should be administered rapidly, if hypotension is present. For hypotension and dyspnea, oxygen should be administered in addition to intravenous fluids. Dyspnea that requires further treatment can be remedied with beta-agonist inhalants. Epinephrine should be administered if symptoms are worsening or are refractory to inhalant therapy. Medications may be needed to reverse hypotension and the radiologist should be prepared to treat this life-threatening problem. In addition to giving intravenous fluids and oxygen, placing the patient in the Trendelenburg position can be helpful. Further management will be guided by vital signs and patient symptoms. Hypotension with bradycardia indicates a vasovagal reaction. The first-line drug for treatment of this condition is intravenous atropine. If the hypotension is accompanied by tachycardia, then the intravenous administration of epinephrine is indicated. Radiologists should be very familiar with the doses and routes of administration of these drugs. These are described in more detail in the textbook and the reference listed above.

Notes

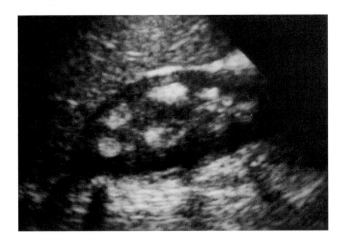

1. What are the most common causes for this finding? If the other kidney is normal, what is the most likely diagnosis?

2. What is the most common complication associated with this condition?

3. True or false: In patients with this condition, renal function is usually impaired.

4. How is this condition treated?

Kidney: Medullary Nephrocalcinosis

1. Hyperparathyroidism, distal renal tubular acidosis, and medullary sponge kidney. Medullary sponge kidney is the most likely diagnosis if the other kidney is normal.

2. Urolithiasis.

3. False. However, renal insufficiency may be seen in patients with severe, long-standing hypercalcemia and renal tubular acidosis.

4. Treatment is directed to the underlying cause of the nephrocalcinosis.

Reference

Shultz PK, Strife JL, Strife CF, McDaniel JD: Hyperechoic renal medullary pyramids in infants and children, *Radiology* 181:163–167, 1991.

Cross-Reference

Zagoria RJ, *Genitourinary Radiology: THE REQUISITES*, 2nd ed, pp 70, 147–151.

Comment

Medullary nephrocalcinosis is calcification in the tubules of the medullary pyramids and accounts for 95% of all cases of nephrocalcinosis. It is typically bilateral and symmetric because it is often the result of a metabolic disorder, although it may be unilateral or segmental in cases of medullary sponge kidney. On ultrasonography the pyramids are echogenic, and there may or may not be shadowing, depending on the size of the calcifications.

The most common causes of medullary nephrocalcinosis are hyperparathyroidism, benign tubular ectasia (medullary sponge kidney), and distal renal tubular acidosis (RTA). Other etiologies include the various other causes of hypercalcemia and hypercalciuria, papillary necrosis, use of certain medications (e.g., furosemide and amphotericin), and diseases that cause hyperoxaluria or hyperuricosuria. Unlike cortical nephrocalcinosis, medullary nephrocalcinosis is potentially reversible. Urolithiasis is the most common complication. Progressive renal insufficiency may be found in some cases of severe, long-standing hypercalcemia or RTA.

Medullary sponge kidney is common (signs were found on 0.5% of intravenous urograms in one study), and in some cases there is an autosomal-dominant inheritance pattern. It is believed to result from idiopathic dilation of the collecting ducts in the inner medulla and papillae. Bilateral renal involvement is seen in 70% of cases, but not all papillae are equally affected.

Notes

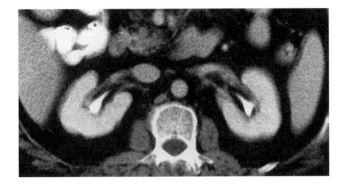
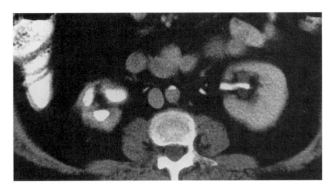
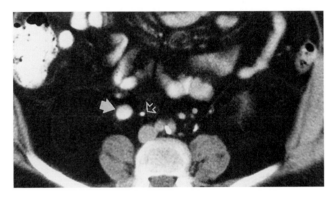

1. Three consecutive images from an abdominal CT examination are shown. In the third image, what structures are indicated by the *solid* and *open arrows?*

2. What is the significance of the size discrepancy indicated by the *arrows?*

3. How can the appearance of the right kidney be explained?

4. What other imaging study could be performed to confirm the diagnosis?

Kidney: Reflux Nephropathy in a Duplicated Collecting System

1. Duplicated right ureters.

2. One ureter is dilated as a result of ureterovesical reflux or obstruction.

3. Reflux nephropathy in the lower pole of a duplex system (the "nubbin" sign).

4. Voiding cystourethrogram.

References

Claudon M, Ben-Sira L, Lebowitz RL: Lower pole reflux in children: uroradiologic appearances and pitfalls, *Am J Roentgenol* 172:795–801, 1999.

Curtis JA, Pollack HM: Renal duplication with a diminutive lower pole: the Nubbin sign, *Radiology* 131: 327–331, 1979.

Cross-Reference

Zagoria RJ, *Genitourinary Radiology: THE REQUISITES*, 2nd ed, pp 126–128.

Comment

Ureteral duplications are common congenital anomalies, occurring in 1% to 10% of the population, and affect women twice as frequently as men. Duplications are described as "partial" when the two ureters join along their course and are described as "complete" when there is separate entry of each ureter into the bladder. Ureteral duplications are associated with other genitourinary tract anomalies in 30% of cases. These anomalies include ureteropelvic junction obstruction, ureterocele, hydronephrosis, and ureterovesical reflux. Atrophy of the lower pole moiety can simulate a solid renal mass; thus, to avoid this diagnostic error, recognition of ureteral duplication is important.

The Weigert-Meyer rule states that the lower end of the upper pole ureter inserts inferior and medial to the lower pole ureter. The upper pole ureter is subject to obstruction and at urography may result in the "drooping lily sign" (i.e., inferior displacement of the lower pole collecting system by an unopacified dilated upper moiety). Ectopic insertion of the upper pole ureter below the external sphincter may manifest as urinary incontinence, and insertion in the vagina can result in persistent drainage, recurrent infection, and eventual obstruction. Insertion of the upper pole ureter below the external sphincter is extremely rare in men, but ectopic insertion can occur in the vas deferens or seminal vesicles. There is an increased incidence of ureteroceles at the insertion of the upper pole ectopic ureter.

Vesicoureteral reflux may occur in the lower pole moiety and is most likely the result of an aberrant insertion of the ureter into the bladder. Reflux may result in dilation of the lower pole ureter and atrophy of the lower pole cortex, leaving a "nubbin" of renal tissue constituting the scarred lower pole. If the ureteral duplication is partial, the "yo-yo" phenomenon, in which urine produced in the upper pole refluxes into the lower pole ureter and causes reflux nephropathy in the lower pole moiety, can occur. The diagnostic feature of reflux nephropathy is broad parenchymal renal scars centered over dilated calyces.

Notes

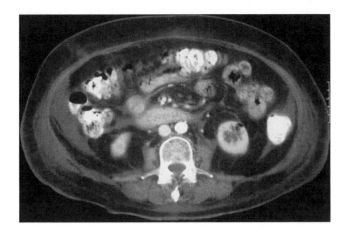 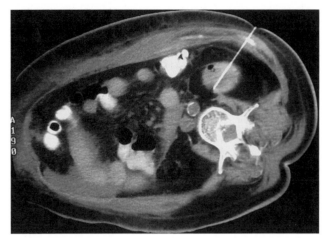

1. A contrast-infused CT in an elderly patient with urosepsis is shown. What is the most likely diagnosis?

2. Is the involvement localized or diffuse?

3. What systemic disease usually predisposes patients to this type of urinary tract infection?

4. What type of bacteria usually causes this disease?

Kidney: Localized Emphysematous Pyelonephritis

1. Emphysematous pyelonephritis.

2. Localized.

3. Diabetes mellitus.

4. A strain of *Escherichia coli*.

References

Cardinael AS, De Blay V, Gilbeau JP: Emphysematous pyelonephritis: successful treatment with percutaneous drainage, *Am J Roentgenol* 164:1554–1555, 1995.

Wan YL, Lee TY, Bullard MJ, Tsai CC: Acute gas-producing bacterial renal infection: correlation between imaging findings and clinical outcome, *Radiology* 198:433–438, 1996.

Cross-Reference

Zagoria RJ, *Genitourinary Radiology: THE REQUISITES*, 2nd ed, pp 136–139, 399.

Comment

This elderly patient with diabetes mellitus had septicemia and evidence of a urinary tract infection. The contrast-infused CT scan demonstrates ascites resulting from chronic congestive heart failure. More importantly, there is an inhomogeneous appearance of the lower pole of the left kidney. Centrally there is a small fluid collection with a locule of air clearly visible within the renal parenchyma. In a patient with urinary tract infection, gas within the renal parenchyma is diagnostic of emphysematous pyelonephritis. This infection is an aggressive variant of acute pyelonephritis and is seen almost exclusively in patients with diabetes mellitus. It is most commonly caused by a strain of *E. coli*. However, strains of *Proteus* and *Klebsiella* species and some fungi can also lead to gas production within the renal parenchyma. Until recently, conventional treatment for emphysematous pyelonephritis in the United States consisted of radical nephrectomy. Radical nephrectomy was performed to remove the source of infection and because the kidney was often irreversibly damaged by the aggressive infectious process. Since the widespread application of cross-sectional imaging techniques, some refinements in diagnosis and treatment of this disease have occurred. When this infectious process involves only one area within the kidney, it can be classified as localized emphysematous pyelonephritis. On numerous occasions this condition has been treated successfully with a combination of percutaneous drainage and systemic antibiotic therapy. Since these patients usually have other diseases that put the contralateral kidney at risk, such as diabetes, there is incentive to avoid nephrectomy. When applying percutaneous treatment for renal infections, the clinician must ensure that ureteral obstruction, if coexisting, is resolved to facilitate antibiotic treatment combined with infection drainage.

Untreated localized emphysematous pyelonephritis can progress very rapidly to a diffuse renal infection. Cases of diffuse emphysematous pyelonephritis almost always require radical nephrectomy, and this procedure carries a significant associated risk for morbidity in these severely ill patients.

Notes

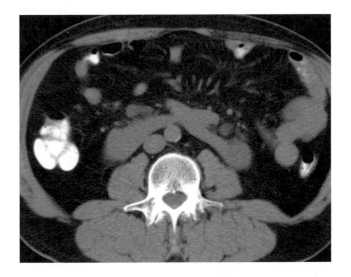 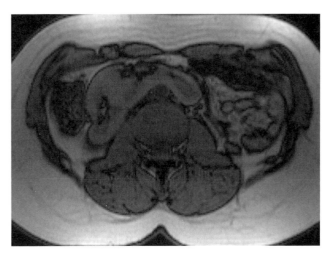

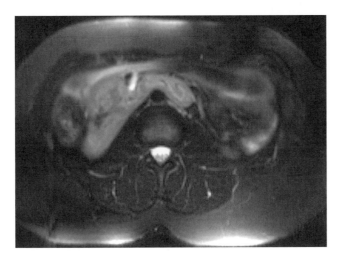

1. These are two different patients with the same diagnosis. What is the diagnosis?

2. What is the embryologic abnormality?

3. What is the significance of this finding?

4. What is the typical level of the midline fusion?

C A S E 6 0

Kidney: Horseshoe Kidney

1. Renal parenchyma extending across the midline: horseshoe kidney.

2. Abnormal contact of the developing metanephric blastema.

3. To reliably establish the benign diagnosis (e.g., not confuse it with a tumor or mass). Patients with horseshoe kidneys have an increased incidence of renal calculi and infection and are more susceptible to renal injury from blunt trauma due to the fusion adjacent to the vertebral bodies.

4. The inferior mesenteric artery.

References

Bauer SB, Perlmutter AD, Retik AB: Anomalies of the upper urinary tract. In Walsh PC, Retik AB, Vaughan ED Jr, Wein AJ, eds: *Campbell's Urology*, Vol 2, 6th ed, Philadelphia, 1992, Saunders, pp 1376–1381.

Gay SB, Armistead JP, Weber ME, Williamson BR: Left infrarenal region: anatomic variants, pathologic conditions, and diagnostic pitfalls [Review], *Radiographics* 11:549–570, 1991.

Cross-Reference

Zagoria RJ, *Genitourinary Radiology: THE REQUISITES*, 2nd ed, pp 60–61.

Comment

Horseshoe kidney has a 2:1 male to female predominance and is the most common renal fusion anomaly, occurring in 1:400 live births. A horseshoe kidney develops early in fetal life as the result of abnormal contact of the developing metanephric tissues. In 90% of cases, the fused portion is the inferior pole and may be a functioning renal parenchyma or a nonfunctioning band of fibrous tissue. The isthmic portion of a horseshoe kidney is usually located in the midline just inferior to the inferior mesenteric artery, which is believed to arrest the cranial migration of the kidney. Most horseshoe kidneys have multiple, bilateral renal arteries. Vascular supply is variable and aberrant vessels may arise from the superior mesenteric artery or iliac arteries as well. This anomaly is associated with increased incidence of ureteropelvic junction obstruction, duplication anomalies, recurrent infection, stone formation, and injury secondary to blunt trauma. There is a slight increased risk for transitional cell carcinoma, likely secondary to urinary stasis. In most cases, horseshoe kidneys are an incidental finding, are asymptomatic, and no treatment is recommended.

Notes

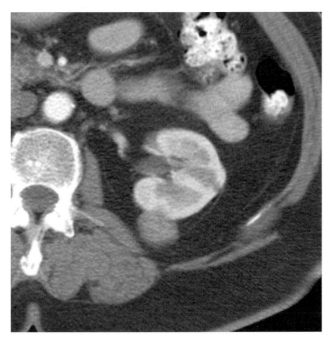

1. Describe the findings and give a differential diagnosis.

2. What stage renal cell carcinoma would this be?

3. Discuss the role of percutaneous biopsy of the solid renal mass.

4. What percentage of angiomyolipomas do not contain visible fat on CT?

Kidney: Lipid Poor Angiomyolipoma

1. Solid enhancing mass in the left kidney. Renal cell carcinoma, oncocytoma, lipid-poor angiomy-olipoma, metastasis. (From this single image on a contrast-enhanced CT, this exophytic lesion could represent a hemorrhagic cyst, but it was shown to enhance.)

2. Stage I.

3. Historically, biopsy has played a limited role in the workup of a solid renal mass, and its role remains controversial. However, with improving histologic techniques, increased numbers of patients with multiple primary neoplasms, and advances in image-guided tumor ablation, the role of biopsy may expand.

4. 5%.

References

Israel GM, Bosniak MA: How I do it: evaluating renal masses, *Radiology* 236:441–450, 2005.

Jinzaki M, Tanimoto A, Narimatsu Y, et al: Angiomyolipoma: imaging findings in lesions with minimal fat, *Radiology* 205:497–502, 1997.

Cross-Reference

Zagoria RJ, *Genitourinary Radiology: THE REQUISITES*, 2nd ed, pp 105–108, 400–401.

Comment

The widespread use of cross-sectional imaging has led to a marked increase in the number of incidentally detected solid renal masses. In addition to increasing detection, contrast-enhanced multiphase CT and MRI have dramatically improved the ability to characterize solid renal masses. Not all solid enhancing renal masses are renal cell carcinoma. Simple macroscopic fat on CT or lipid-sensitive MRI sequences reliably establish a diagnosis of angiomyolipoma. Conversely, the presence of retroperitoneal lymphadenopathy or thrombus extending into the renal vein makes renal cell carcinoma a much more likely diagnosis.

Some small (less than 1.5 cm) incidentally discovered enhancing renal masses continue to be a diagnostic dilemma. It may be difficult to demonstrate the presence of fat in small angiomyolipomas despite the use of narrow collimation as in this case. In addition, approximately 5% of angiomyolipomas will have no identifiable fat on CT or MRI. Small oncocytomas will also have an imaging appearance that is indistinguishable from renal cell carcinoma.

Certain patient populations may benefit from percutaneous biopsy prior to treatment. They include poor surgical candidates, patients undergoing image-guided tumor ablation, and patients with an existing primary malignancy to exclude renal metastasis.

Notes

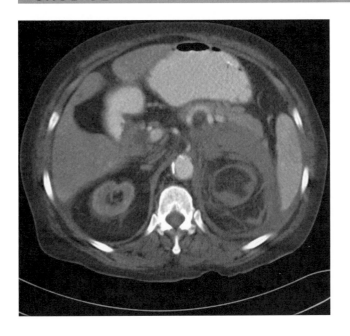 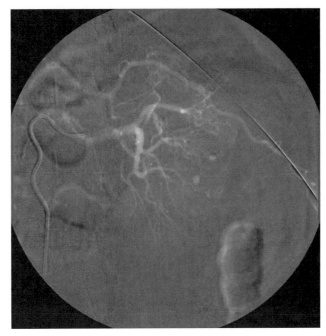

1. What percentage of angiomyolipomas are sporadic? What percentages are associated with tuberous sclerosis?

2. At what size are angiomyolipomas considered more likely to hemorrhage and therefore considered for excision or embolization?

3. What are some of the presenting symptoms?

4. What renal masses may present with internal renal fat?

Kidney: Angiomyolipoma with Spontaneous Perinephric Hemorrhage

1. 80%, 20%.

2. 4 cm.

3. Small ones are usually asymptomatic, larger masses may present with acute flank or abdominal pain, retroperitoneal hemorrhage with potential shock, hematuria, and a palpable mass.

4. Renal cell carcinoma, usually when it engulfs adjacent hilar fat, liposarcoma, Wilms' tumor, and lipoma.

References

Kim J, Park S, Shon J, Cho K: Angiomyolipoma with minimal fat: differentiation from renal cell carcinoma at biphasic helical CT, *Radiology* 230:677–684, 2004.

Zhang JQ, Fielding JR, Zou KH: Etiology of spontaneous perirenal hemorrhage: a meta-analysis, *J Urol* 167:1593–1596, 2002.

Cross-Reference

Zagoria RJ, *Genitourinary Radiology: THE REQUISITES*, 2nd ed, pp 106–108.

Comment

The images show a patient with a perinephric hemorrhage surrounding a fat-containing renal mass. Approximately 60% of these hemorrhages are due to an underlying renal cell carcinoma (RCC) or angiomyolipoma (AML), and 15% to vasculitides, particularly polyarteritis nodosa. Assuming that the perinephric hemorrhage is not life threatening, a follow-up contrast-enhanced CT scan is obtained in 6 to 8 weeks to search for a renal mass. If no mass is detected, then a renal angiogram should be obtained to exclude a vasculitis or vascular malformation. AMLs are benign hamartomas of the kidney composed of various proportions of vascular, smooth muscle and fatty components. Arteries supplying AMLs often develop small aneurysms, which is a characteristic finding on angiography. Demonstration of small aneurysms, however, is not pathognomonic for AML because it can occur with other tumors, including RCC. Intratumoral fat is the key to the imaging diagnosis of AML. Cases of RCC with intratumoral fat have been reported, but are rare. Typical AMLs are easily diagnosed with CT or MRI; however, approximately 5% of AMLs have no demonstrable fat on CT or MRI. AML with minimal fat may mimic RCC on imaging and require surgical excision for diagnosis.

Once intratumoral fat has been confirmed via CT or MRI, sonographic follow-up should be performed to assess growth. AMLs may enlarge over time. This is particularly true in patients with tuberous sclerosis.

Enlarging AMLs, particularly those that exceed 4 cm in diameter, may require prophylactic excision, ablation, or embolization.

Notes

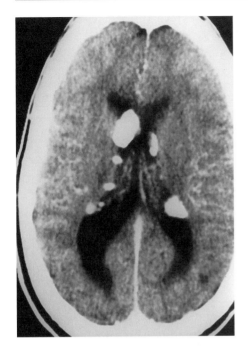
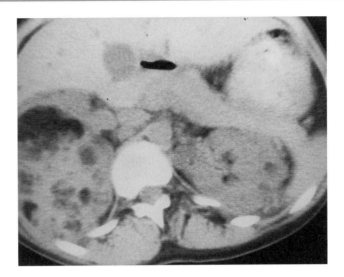

1. Of the three-tiered diagnostic criteria for this disease, there are six "primary" features. Name three of them.

2. What is the most common presenting symptom of this disease, and how does it impact the likelihood of another common feature of this disease?

3. Name two of the three skin lesions that are associated with this disease.

4. What combination of renal lesions is characteristic for this disease?

Kidney: Angiomyolipoma and Tuberous Sclerosis

1. Facial angiofibromas, multiple ungual fibromas, cortical tuber, subependymal nodule or giant cell astrocytoma, multiple calcified subependymal nodules protruding into the ventricle, and multiple retinal astrocytoma.

2. Myoclonic seizures that begin in infancy or early childhood. Patients who manifest seizures before the age of 5 years are more likely to have mental impairment than those who develop seizures at a later age.

3. Adenoma sebaceum (adenofibroma), nevus depigmentosus (ash leaf spots), café au lait spots.

4. Multiple angiomyolipomas together with renal cystic disease.

References

Choyke PL, Glenn GM, Walther MM, et al: Hereditary renal cancers, *Radiology* 226:33–46, 2003.

Seidenwurm DJ, Barkovich AJ: Understanding tuberous sclerosis, *Radiology* 183:23–24, 1992.

Takahashi K, Honda M, Okubo RS, et al: CT pixel mapping in the diagnosis of small angiomyolipomas of the kidneys, *J Comput Assist Tomogr* 17:98–101, 1993.

Cross-Reference

Zagoria RJ, *Genitourinary Radiology: THE REQUISITES*, 2nd ed, pp 105–108, 113–114.

Comment

The unenhanced renal CT image shows multiple very black masses in both kidneys. This low attenuation is diagnostic of fat, but it should be confirmed by measuring the Hounsfield units (HU) in one of the lesions. The brain CT shows periventricular calcifications. Within the genitourinary system, the most common and characteristic manifestation of tuberous sclerosis is the renal angiomyolipoma. Of patients with tuberous sclerosis, 80% develop angiomyolipomas, and they are frequently multifocal bilateral lesions. Angiomyolipomas have a tendency to hemorrhage spontaneously when larger than 4 cm in diameter. Even though the finding of a discrete echogenic renal mass on ultrasonography likely represents an angiomyolipoma, CT is still recommended because there have been reports of small echogenic renal cell carcinomas. Thin-section CT using narrow collimation through the renal mass should be performed. In equivocal cases a pixel histogram through the mass that demonstrates three contiguous pixels measuring less than -20 HU is diagnostic for fat within an angiomyolipoma. Patients with tuberous sclerosis also develop renal cysts, and the findings of renal cyst and renal angiomyolipoma strongly suggest the diagnosis of Bourneville's disease. There is now thought to be a small increased risk for renal cell carcinoma in patients with tuberous sclerosis.

The presence of an angiomyolipoma alone does not imply tuberous sclerosis because 80% of these hamartomas are discovered sporadically, usually in middle-aged adults who do not have tuberous sclerosis. The majority of patients in this cohort are women, the tumor is often asymptomatic, and the hamartoma is usually solitary. Symptoms resulting from local mass effect or hemorrhage may occur if the mass enlarges. Renal hemorrhage from an angiomyolipoma can be treated with arterial embolization.

Notes

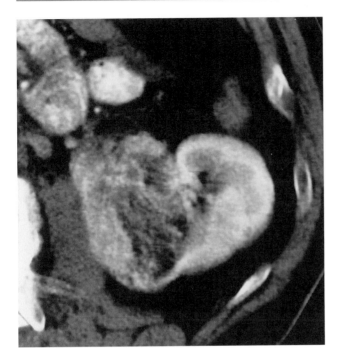 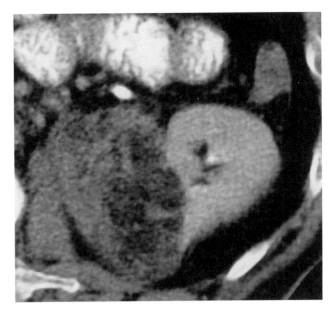

1. What is the most likely diagnosis for the renal mass shown?

2. What renal masses may contain internal fat?

3. What is the major complication associated with the type of mass shown?

4. What is the risk for distant metastases with the lesion shown?

Kidney: Renal Angiomyolipoma

1. Angiomyolipoma.

2. Angiomyolipoma or, rarely, lipoma, liposarcoma, Wilms' tumor, and renal cell carcinoma.

3. Spontaneous hemorrhage.

4. None.

Reference

Kim JK, Park S-Y, Shon J-H, Cho K-S: Angiomyolipoma with minimal fat: differentiation from renal cell carcinoma at biphasic helical CT, *Radiology* 230: 677–684, 2004.

Cross-Reference

Zagoria RJ, *Genitourinary Radiology: THE REQUISITES*, 2nd ed, pp 105–108.

Comment

The patient shown has a fat-containing, heterogeneous exophytic mass extending from the left kidney. The presence of fat in a renal mass should be considered diagnostic of angiomyolipoma. Rare lesions that may contain fat include renal lipoma, liposarcoma, dedifferentiated Wilms' tumor, and renal cell carcinoma that grows to engulf renal sinus or perinephric fat. Other than angiomyolipoma, fat-containing renal lesions are exceedingly rare and should not be considered unless there are features suggesting an alternative diagnosis. Angiomyolipomas are benign hamartomas of the kidney composed of vascular, smooth muscle, and fatty components. Approximately 95% of angiomyolipomas contain an adequate amount of fat to be visualized with CT. The major complication associated with angiomyolipoma is spontaneous hemorrhage. This complication is rare when lesions are smaller than 4 cm in diameter. Smaller, asymptomatic angiomyolipomas usually are not treated and may be followed with periodic sonographic monitoring. Larger lesions may be treated with surgery or prophylactically embolized.

Of patients with angiomyolipomas, 20% suffer from tuberous sclerosis. These patients usually develop multiple angiomyolipomas and also may develop renal cysts. Angiomyolipomas in tuberous sclerosis patients often grow rapidly and may become large. The remaining angiomyolipomas are considered idiopathic, and they tend to grow very slowly, if at all. Rapid increase in the size of a fat-containing tumor suggests an alternative diagnosis or evidence of complication related to the angiomyolipoma and may lead to surgical resection.

Notes

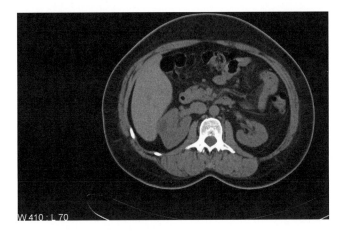

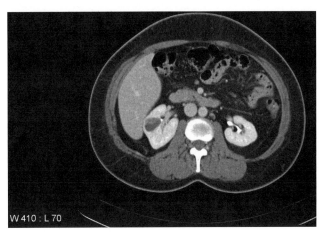

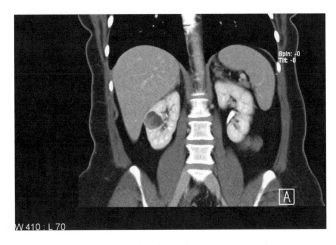

1. Using the Bosniak classification, in what category does this lesion fall?

2. What is the likelihood that this lesion is a malignant lesion?

3. What would be the appropriate therapy, if any?

4. What increase in Hounsfield units (HU) indicates the presence of a vascular neoplasm?

Kidney: Bosniak IV Cystic Renal Mass

1. Category IV.

2. Greater than 90%.

3. Surgical removal or, in the case of a poor surgical candidate, percutaneous ablation.

4. 15 HU.

Reference

Curry NS, Cochran ST, Bissada NK: Cystic renal masses: accurate Bosniak classification requires adequate renal CT, *Am J Roentgenol* 177:339–342, 2000.

Cross-Reference

Zagoria RJ, *Genitourinary Radiology: THE REQUISITES*, 2nd ed, pp 87–89.

Comment

The CT scans show a round cystic mass in the right kidney with an enhancing solid component along one wall: a Bosniak IV mass. The CT criteria for a simple cyst are as follows: fluid density, lack of internal architecture such as nodules or septations, an imperceptible free wall, and lack of significant enhancement upon administration of a contrast agent. With newer generation multirow CT scanners and associated increased beam-hardening effects, significant enhancement is now considered to be at least 15 HU. Simple cysts are considered Bosniak category I lesions and require no follow-up. Category II lesions contain a few (usually considered three or less) fine septations and may have thin rim calcification, or may be high density, but do not demonstrate enhancement. These lesions rarely contain cancerous elements and can usually be ignored. The more complicated the architecture and the greater the enhancement of a renal lesion, the more likely it is to be a cancer. Category III lesions may have thick walls, multiple septations, and coarse calcifications, while category IV lesions demonstrate enhancing elements. Category III lesions have a 25% to 45% likelihood of containing cancer, while category IV lesions are virtually always malignant tumors.

While these guidelines work very well, there are invariably difficult lesions with mixed features, such as minimal enhancement (15 HU) but many septations. In these cases it is best to get additional imaging studies such as ultrasonography and MRI, and to use the most worrisome feature to guide therapy.

Notes

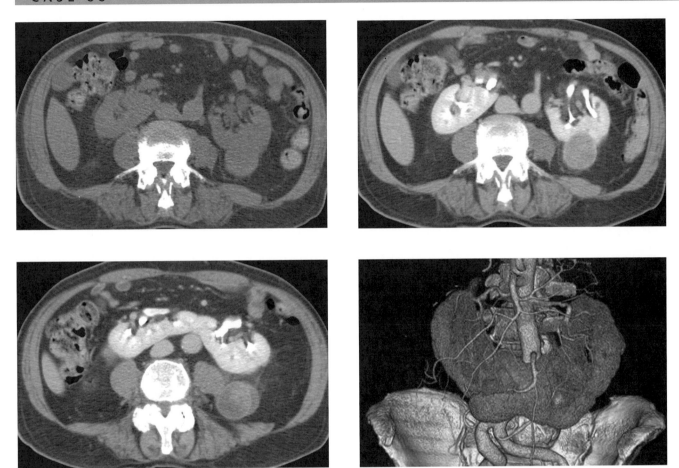

1. List two major kidney abnormalities shown in this case.

2. Are they causally related?

3. Does the congenital anomaly affect treatment of the acquired lesion?

4. What pathology occurs with increased incidence with this congenital anomaly?

Kidney: Renal Cell Carcinoma in Horseshoe Kidney

1. Horseshoe kidney and renal cell carcinoma.

2. No. Patients with horseshoe kidney have no increased incidence of renal cell carcinoma development.

3. Yes. Horseshoe kidneys almost always have aberrant vascular supply and drainage. This is often important when performing surgical resection of renal tumors.

4. Infections, stones, ureteropelvic junction strictures, and transitional cell carcinomas.

References

Bauer SB, Perlmutter AD, Retik AB: Anomalies of the upper urinary tract. In Walsh PC, Retik AB, Vaughan ED Jr, Wein AJ, eds: *Campbell's Urology*, Vol 2, 6th ed, Philadelphia, 1992, Saunders, pp 1376–1381.

Gay SB, Armistead JP, Weber ME, Williamson BR: Left infrarenal region: anatomic variants, pathologic conditions, and diagnostic pitfalls [Review], *Radiographics* 11:549–570, 1991.

Cross-Reference

Zagoria RJ, *Genitourinary Radiology: THE REQUISITES*, 2nd ed, pp 60–61.

Comment

The CT scans show a horseshoe kidney with fusion of the lower poles. The isthmus of tissue is functioning renal parenchyma, the usual form of a horseshoe kidney. The kidney is positioned low in the abdomen, also typical of horseshoe kidneys. This is thought to be due to arrested ascent of the kidney during fetal development since the isthmus of the kidney gets trapped below the inferior mesenteric artery. The CT also shows a spherical exophytic tumor arising from the upper pole of the left side of the fused kidney. This mass contains no visible fat, is solid, and enhances. These CT features imply a presumptive diagnosis of renal cell carcinoma (RCC).

Regardless of the underlying congenital anomaly shown here, detection of a renal mass requires characterization of the mass. A simple and highly reliable rule for imaging of renal tumors is that an exophytic mass arising from the kidney that is not a simple or minimally complex (Bosniak category I and II) cyst by imaging criteria, and does not contain fat, is an RCC. Use of this rule will result in a correct diagnosis for about 90% of RCCs. Of course, thorough imaging should be aimed at excluding fat in a tumor and in determining if the lesion is a simple cyst or a more ominous tumor. Once an RCC is diagnosed, findings to aid treatment planning should be gathered. This includes staging information, tumor size, metastatic disease presence, venous extension, and lymph node involvement. The status of the other kidney should be carefully evaluated since a nephrectomy of the involved kidney is standard treatment for RCC. Finally, the presence of vascular anomalies may help in surgical planning. Horseshoe kidneys rarely have standard single renal arteries. More often they are fed by multiple accessory renal arteries, often originating from the lower aorta and iliac arteries, and less commonly they originate from mesenteric and lumbar vessels.

Notes

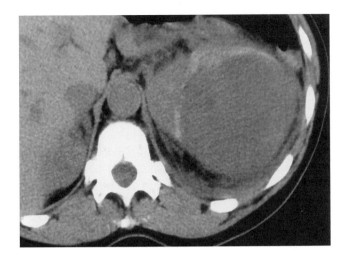
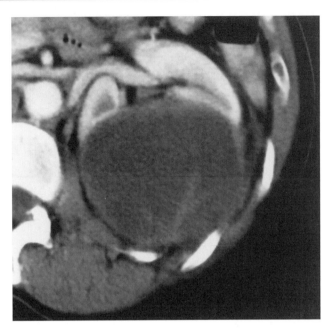

1. What is the material layering posteriorly in the left perinephric space?

2. Is spontaneous perinephric hemorrhage usually idiopathic?

3. What is the most likely diagnosis of the left renal mass?

4. What causes the internal enhancement in this mass?

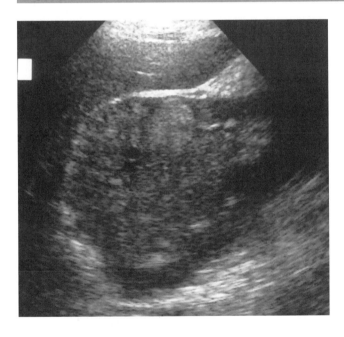
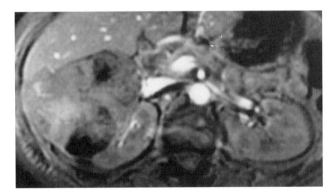

1. What is the most likely diagnosis for this renal mass?

2. Is the mass more or less echogenic than the normal kidney?

3. What are the main differential diagnostic considerations?

4. Using the Robson classification system, is this more likely a stage II or stage III tumor?

CASE 67

Kidney: Renal Cell Carcinoma with Spontaneous Perinephric Hemorrhage

1. Hemorrhage.

2. No. In nearly all cases there is an underlying abnormality, most commonly neoplasm.

3. Renal cell carcinoma.

4. Enhancing tumor tissue.

Reference

Zagoria RJ, Dyer RB, Wolfman NT: Radiology in the diagnosis and staging of renal cell carcinoma, *Crit Rev Diagn Imaging* 31:81–115, 1990.

Cross-Reference

Zagoria RJ, *Genitourinary Radiology: THE REQUISITES*, 2nd ed, pp 83, 90–100.

Comment

Spontaneous perinephric hemorrhage indicates hemorrhage into the perirenal and pararenal spaces unrelated to trauma. Although this hemorrhage is spontaneous, it is not idiopathic. In nearly all cases an identifiable underlying cause can be found. In approximately 60% of cases the underlying cause is neoplasm. The neoplasm may be either a renal cell carcinoma or an angiomyolipoma, both of which have a predilection for bleeding. Other causes of spontaneous perinephric hemorrhage include complicated renal cysts, vasculitis, renal infarction, and renal infection. Therefore, spontaneous perinephric hemorrhage alone should lead the clinician to carefully and thoroughly investigate an underlying cause. When CT scanning does not help identify a cause, angiography may be useful to detect underlying vascular lesions.

In this patient the cause of bleeding is obvious. There is a large cystic mass. It is ball shaped, without visible fat. It is not a simple cyst because there are numerous septa that enhance, and there is clearly a thick rind of tissue at the circumference of the mass. These features alone suggest a neoplasm, either renal cell carcinoma or multilocular cystic nephroma. In combination with the perirenal hemorrhage, the diagnosis of renal cell carcinoma is more likely. In either case this abnormality represents a surgical renal mass. It was resected and found to be a papillary renal cell carcinoma.

Notes

CASE 68

Kidney: Stage II Renal Cell Carcinoma

1. Renal cell carcinoma.

2. More echogenic.

3. Oncocytoma, angiomyolipoma (without visible fat), and metastasis.

4. Stage II.

Reference

Ergen FB, Hussain HK, Caoili EM, et al: MRI for preoperative staging of renal cell carcinoma using the 1997 TNM classification: comparison with surgical and pathologic staging, *Am J Roentgenol* 182:217–225, 2004.

Cross-Reference

Zagoria RJ, *Genitourinary Radiology: THE REQUISITES*, 2nd ed, pp 96–97, 99.

Comment

This sonogram demonstrates a solid, heterogeneous hyperechoic mass protruding from the right kidney. This finding is confirmed on the MRI scan. Renal cell carcinomas (RCCs) of the kidney generally grow by expansion, causing a ball-shaped mass that may appear hyperechogenic, isoechogenic, or hypoechogenic to normal renal parenchyma on sonography. An exophytic, solid mass arising from the kidney without visible fat is an RCC in approximately 90% of cases. Other possibilities are an isolated metastasis, including lymphoma; an oncocytoma; or an angiomyolipoma without adequate fat to be visible radiologically. In any case, unless a known primary tumor is present elsewhere, this finding should be considered a surgical renal mass, and beyond demonstrating extent of the tumor, further imaging is unlikely to lead to additional information.

Once the mass is detected sonographically, cross-sectional imaging is of crucial importance to exclude the presence of intratumoral fat, which would indicate a benign angiomyolipoma. In addition, staging of the tumor is best accomplished with CT or MRI, both of which are essentially equivalent for this purpose. The Robson classification is a simple staging system for RCC. Radiologically, stage I and stage II tumors are difficult to distinguish from one another, but this determination is of little therapeutic significance. Stage III indicates tumor spread to regional lymph nodes or venous extension. The gradient echo image shown demonstrates a widely patent right renal vein entering the inferior vena cava. No visible lymphadenopathy is present. These findings indicate a stage I or II RCC. Stage IV indicates direct invasion of adjacent organs other than the ipsilateral adrenal gland, or distant metastases.

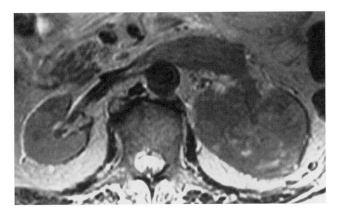 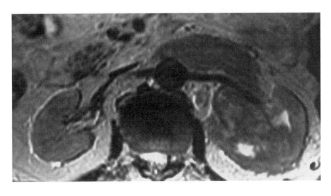

1. What is the most likely cause of this venous abnormality?

2. What are the main differential causes of renal vein thrombosis?

3. Using the Robson classification system, what stage is shown in these illustrations?

4. When there is extension into the vein, what venous landmarks are important for surgical planning?

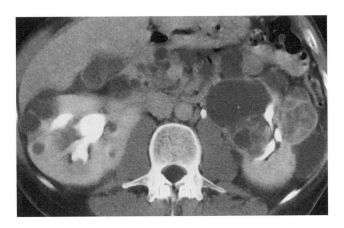

1. What is the most likely diagnosis?

2. What conditions are associated with the development of renal cysts and solid renal masses?

3. What type of central nervous system lesion is associated with this condition?

4. Are pancreatic cysts more commonly seen with autosomal-dominant polycystic kidney disease or von Hippel-Lindau disease?

Kidney: Renal Cell Carcinoma with Extension into the Left Renal Vein

1. Renal cell carcinoma extension.

2. Renal cell carcinoma extension, hypercoagulable states, glomerulonephritis, and dehydration.

3. Stage III.

4. If there is extension into the inferior vena cava, it is important to determine whether it is above or below the level where the hepatic veins drain into the inferior vena cava.

Reference

Ergen FB, Hussain HK, Caoili EM, et al: MRI for preoperative staging of renal cell carcinoma using the 1997 TNM classification: comparison with surgical and pathologic staging, *Am J Roentgenol* 182:217–225, 2004.

Cross-Reference

Zagoria RJ, *Genitourinary Radiology: THE REQUISITES*, 2nd ed, pp 96–97, 99.

Comment

This case demonstrates a soft tissue mass in the left renal vein. This finding indicates renal vein thrombosis. In addition, the left renal vein is markedly enlarged, suggesting that it is not just a simple blood clot but rather a neoplasm. The most common cause of renal vein thrombosis in adults is extension of a renal cell carcinoma into the renal vein. Rarely, other renal tumors, including transitional cell carcinoma, squamous cell carcinoma, oncocytoma, and angiomyolipoma, extend into the vein. Extension of the tumor into the vein is important clinically. It indicates an advanced stage of the disease, at least Robson classification stage III. Interestingly, venous extension without lymph node or distant metastases is associated with a better prognosis, similar to that for stage I or II disease. A tumor thrombus usually is found within the vein lumen but does not invade the vein wall. Once tumor extension has been detected, the length of extension into the venous system should be delineated for surgical planning. It should be noted whether the tumor extends into the inferior vena cava. If it does, the radiologist should determine the cephalad extent of the tumor. When the tumor does not extend above the level of the hepatic veins, it can usually be resected from an abdominal incision. Resection of more cephalad tumors usually requires combined thoracoabdominal incisions and possibly intraoperative cardiopulmonary bypass.

Notes

Kidney: von Hippel-Lindau Disease

1. Von Hippel-Lindau disease.

2. Von Hippel-Lindau disease, tuberous sclerosis, and long-term dialysis.

3. Cerebellar hemangioblastoma.

4. Von Hippel-Lindau disease.

References

Choyke PL, Filling-Katz MR, Shawker TH, et al: von Hippel-Lindau disease: radiologic screening for visceral manifestations, *Radiology* 174:805–810, 1990.

Choyke PL, Glenn GM, Walther MM, et al: Hereditary renal cancers, *Radiology* 226:33–46, 2003.

Cross-Reference

Zagoria RJ, *Genitourinary Radiology: THE REQUISITES*, 2nd ed, pp 111–112, 122, 146.

Comment

Von Hippel-Lindau disease is a genetic disorder inherited with an autosomal-dominant pattern. The common manifestations include retinal angiomas, central nervous system hemangioblastomas, and abdominal abnormalities. Renal cysts are seen in up to 90% of patients with von Hippel-Lindau disease. Renal cell carcinomas, the clear cell variety, develop in approximately 40% of these patients, and in the majority of patients the lesions are multiple and bilateral. In this case there are two solid, enhancing masses that represent renal cell carcinomas in the left kidney. Even the simple-appearing cysts in the kidneys of these patients are often dysplastic and may develop into neoplasms. The second most common intraabdominal organ involved in these patients is the pancreas, which often contains multiple cysts or cystic neoplasms. This finding helps to distinguish the abdominal pattern of this disease from autosomal-dominant polycystic kidney disease, which is not associated with an increased risk for renal cell carcinoma and rarely involves the pancreas. The most common cause of death in patients with von Hippel-Lindau disease relates to metastatic spread of the renal cell carcinomas.

Notes

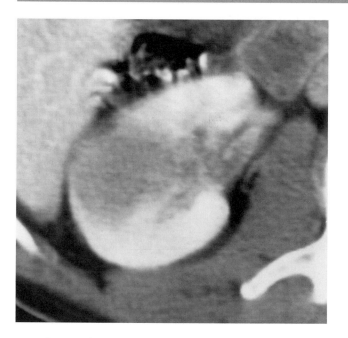 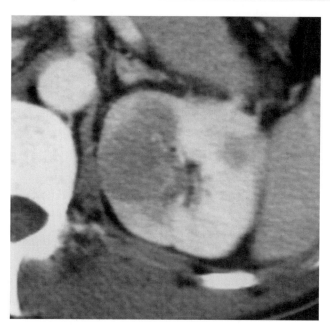

1. What is the most likely diagnosis for these bilateral renal lesions?

2. What are the common causes of solid renal masses occurring in both kidneys?

3. What neoplasms grow in the kidney in an infiltrative pattern?

4. Is the center of these lesions within the renal sinus or the renal parenchyma?

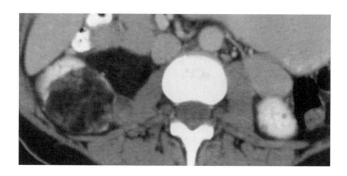 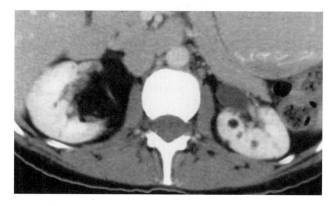

1. What is the diagnosis of the mass in the upper pole of the right kidney?

2. What syndrome does this patient probably have?

3. Besides the mass in the right kidney, what is another common renal manifestation of this syndrome?

4. What are some of the common extrarenal manifestations of this syndrome?

CASE 71

Kidney: Renal Lymphoma

1. Metastatic disease, including lymphoma.

2. Metastases, including lymphoma, and multifocal renal cell carcinomas, angiomyolipomas, and oncocytomas.

3. Urothelial tumors; some metastases, including lymphoma; and infiltrative renal cell carcinomas.

4. Renal parenchyma.

References

Davidson AJ, Hartman DS, Davis CJ Jr, et al: Infiltrative renal lesions: CT-sonographic-pathologic correlation, *Am J Roentgenol* 150:1061–1064, 1988.

Sheeran SR, Sussman SK: Renal lymphoma: spectrum of CT findings and potential mimics, *Am J Roentgenol* 171:1067–1072, 1998.

Cross-Reference

Zagoria RJ, *Genitourinary Radiology: THE REQUISITES*, 2nd ed, pp 104–106, 115–121.

Comment

This patient has bilateral solid renal lesions with a geographic, non-contour-deforming pattern. This finding indicates infiltrative growth. Infiltrative renal lesions fall into three main categories: inflammatory, infarction, and infiltrative neoplasm. The lesions shown are irregularly marginated, with generally rounded shapes. The center of these lesions is within the renal parenchyma, indicating that it is unlikely that they arose from the urothelium. No rim nephrogram is visible. The lesions are homogeneous.

These features suggest a diagnosis of metastatic disease. Metastases to the kidneys can lead to expansile, ball-shaped masses or infiltrative lesions. Infiltrative metastases usually result from primary squamous cell carcinomas or lymphoma. Patients usually have a known primary neoplasm, and renal metastases are typically seen late in the course of the disease. On CT, multifocal renal lymphoma cannot be distinguished from other infiltrative metastases. Sometimes the sonographic pattern is suggestive of lymphoma. Renal lymphoma is usually homogeneously low in echogenicity without significant through-transmission. The internal echogenicity of renal lymphoma may mimic that of a simple cyst, lacking only the through-transmission seen in fluid-containing masses.

Notes

CASE 72

Kidney: Tuberous Sclerosis

1. Angiomyolipoma.

2. Tuberous sclerosis.

3. Renal cysts.

4. Central nervous system hamartomas, facial adenoma sebaceum, pulmonary lymphangioleiomyomatosis, cardiac rhabdomyomas, and cutaneous shagreen patches.

References

Choyke PL, Glenn GM, Walther MM, et al: Hereditary renal cancers, *Radiology* 226:33–46, 2003.

Wagner BJ, Won-You-Cheong JJ, Davis CJ: Adult renal hamartomas, *Radiographics* 17:155–169, 1997.

Cross-Reference

Zagoria RJ, *Genitourinary Radiology: THE REQUISITES*, 2nd ed, pp 83, 113–114, 146.

Comment

Renal tumors that contain fat can be diagnosed as angiomyolipomas (AMLs) with near certainty. These tumors usually are isolated findings in middle-aged or older adults. Of patients with tuberous sclerosis, 80% develop AMLs. Patients with tuberous sclerosis usually develop AMLs earlier in life and develop larger and more numerous masses than in patients without this syndrome. There is a slightly increased risk for renal cell carcinoma development in these patients. This patient demonstrates multiple bilateral AMLs, with two large AMLs in the right kidney, one of which extends into the renal sinus and perirenal space. Tuberous sclerosis is an autosomal-dominant hereditary disorder characterized by the triad of facial adenoma sebaceum, periventricular hamartomas in the brain, and mental retardation. The extent of penetrance of each of these symptoms varies among patients with tuberous sclerosis. Approximately 20% of patients with tuberous sclerosis also develop renal cysts.

Notes

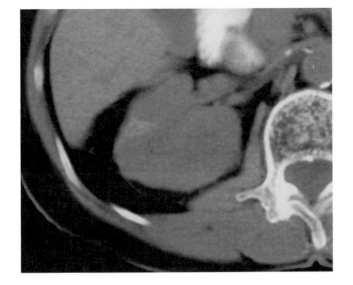

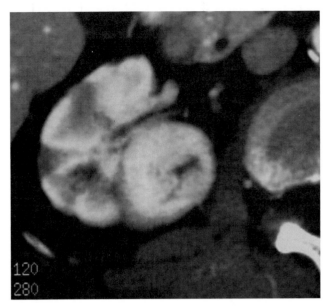

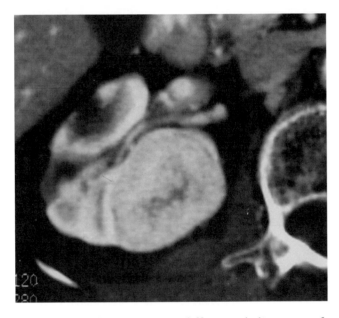

1. What are the two main differential diagnoses for this right renal mass?

2. What feature suggests that this mass may be benign?

3. What angiographic feature helps support the diagnosis of a benign mass?

4. Whether this mass is benign or malignant, what is the conventional management?

Kidney: Renal Oncocytoma

1. Oncocytoma and renal cell carcinoma.

2. Central, stellate low-attenuation area.

3. "Spoke wheel" pattern of feeding arteries.

4. Nephrectomy, radical or partial. If the mass is benign, partial nephrectomy is probably favorable.

Reference

Harrison RB, Dyer RB: Benign space-occupying conditions of the kidneys, *Semin Roentgenol* 22:275–283, 1987.

Cross-Reference

Zagoria RJ, *Genitourinary Radiology: THE REQUISITES*, 2nd ed, p 100.

Comment

Of solitary solid, ball-shaped renal masses with no visible fat, 90% are renal cell carcinomas (RCCs). However, certain features suggest an alternative diagnosis. One of these features is a central stellate scar in an otherwise homogeneous solid renal mass. This feature is suggestive but not diagnostic of oncocytoma. There are no absolute diagnostic imaging features of oncocytoma. It is best to consider this a surgical renal mass, and if there is no evidence of spread beyond the kidney and if the mass has a favorable location, the surgeon may attempt partial nephrectomy. RCCs may contain oncocytic components, and therefore it has been felt that preoperative percutaneous biopsy does not help the physician make management decisions. More recently, negative staining of biopsy samples with Hale's colloidal iron stain has been show to distinguish chromophobe RCCs from oncocytomas. Biopsy results indicating oncocytoma have not been universally accepted. If partial nephrectomy is being contemplated, renal arteriography (CT-angiography or MR-angiography) may help to delineate the number and distribution of renal arteries supplying the kidney and the tumor. Oncocytomas typically have a characteristic angiographic pattern, described as a "spoke wheel" configuration. Unfortunately, this appearance is not diagnostic of oncocytoma and may be seen with RCCs.

Therefore, a solitary renal mass containing a central stellate scar should be considered a surgical renal mass. The surgeon should be alerted that the tumor may be benign, and he or she may elect to attempt renal-sparing surgery if the mass's location is amenable.

Notes

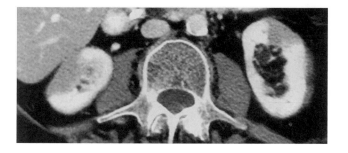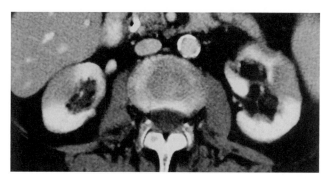

1. Which abnormalities commonly cause bilateral renal lesions with this radiologic pattern?

2. What lesions typically cause bilateral exophytic renal masses?

3. What nephrographic pattern would be diagnostic of infarction, if present?

4. What is the most common pattern of renal involvement with lymphoma?

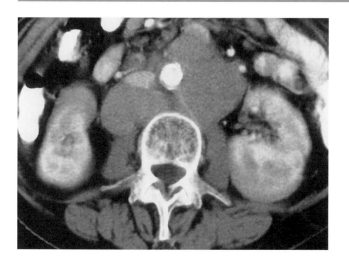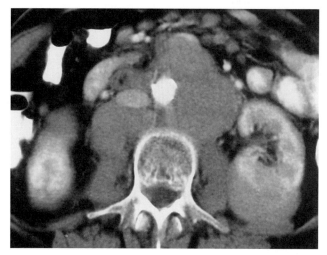

1. What is the most likely diagnosis in this patient?

2. What feature of the retroperitoneal mass makes the diagnosis of retroperitoneal fibrosis unlikely?

3. When bilateral solid renal masses are present, what are the major differential diagnoses?

4. Which type of lymphoma involves the kidneys?

CASE 74

Kidney: Renal Lymphoma

1. Renal infarcts; infiltrative renal neoplasms, including lymphoma; and renal infections.

2. Renal cysts, bilateral renal cell carcinoma, angiomyolipomas, Wilms' tumors, and renal metastases.

3. Rim nephrogram, which is absent in this case.

4. Multiple renal parenchymal masses.

References

Gash JR, Zagoria RJ, Dyer RB: Imaging features of infiltrating renal lesions, *Crit Rev Diagn Imaging* 33: 293–310, 1992.

Sheeran SR, Sussman SK: Renal lymphoma: spectrum of CT findings and potential mimics, *Am J Roentgenol* 171:1067–1072, 1998.

Cross-Reference

Zagoria RJ, *Genitourinary Radiology: THE REQUISITES*, 2nd ed, pp 104–106, 115, 118, 121.

Comment

This patient has bilateral, homogeneous renal masses with an infiltrative growth pattern. The cortical rim sign is absent. The cause of bilateral infiltrative renal lesions is usually renal metastases, lymphoma, renal infarcts, or bilateral pyelonephritis. The lack of the nephrographic rim sign and the homogeneous, nonstriated nature of the lesions make renal infarcts and pyelonephritis less likely. The homogeneous appearance of these infiltrative lesions suggests lymphoma. Renal lymphoma is usually a late finding in the course of systemic lymphoma. As in this patient, non-Hodgkin's lymphoma is the usual cell type when the kidneys are involved.

Renal lymphoma can occur with several different patterns. The most common pattern, which is illustrated in this case, is multifocal renal parenchymal lesions. These lesions usually have an infiltrative growth pattern and are homogeneous, with some contrast enhancement. On sonography, lymphoma typically has a homogeneous hypoechoic pattern. Other patterns of renal involvement with lymphoma include diffuse infiltration of one or both of the kidneys and a solitary renal mass. Additionally, renal lymphoma may result from direct spread of lymphoma from the retroperitoneal lymphatics to the renal sinus and perinephric space, with subsequent parenchymal invasion.

Notes

CASE 75

Kidney: Perirenal Lymphoma

1. Lymphoma.

2. Extensive soft tissue between the vertebra and the aorta and lateral ureteral deviation.

3. Metastases, including renal lymphoma, and renal cell carcinoma.

4. Non-Hodgkin's lymphoma.

References

Davidson AJ, Hartman DS, Davis CJ Jr, et al: Infiltrative renal lesions: CT-sonographic-pathologic correlation, *Am J Roentgenol* 150:1061–1064, 1988.

Sheeran SR, Sussman SK: Renal lymphoma: spectrum of CT findings and potential mimics, *Am J Roentgenol* 171:1067–1072, 1998.

Cross-Reference

Zagoria RJ, *Genitourinary Radiology: THE REQUISITES*, 2nd ed, pp 104–106, 115, 118, 121.

Comment

This patient has massive retroperitoneal lymphadenopathy with enlarged lymph nodes surrounding both the inferior vena cava and the aorta. The aorta is pushed anteriorly away from the spine by the lymphadenopathy. There also are bilateral perirenal masses. These features strongly suggest lymphoma. Lymphoma involving the kidneys can present in several different patterns. There can be direct spread from the retroperitoneum along the lymphatics into the renal sinus and eventually the kidney. Multifocal infiltrative renal masses, diffuse infiltration of one or both of the kidneys, or a solitary renal mass mimicking primary renal neoplasm may occur. Unlike most other neoplasms, lymphoma also has a predilection for involvement of the perirenal space, as illustrated by this case. Perirenal soft tissue masses are uncommon; their presence suggests lymphoma. Alternative diagnoses include metastases from other tumors, such as melanoma, amyloid, extramedullary hematopoiesis, and, if the mass is solitary, a primary retroperitoneal sarcoma, such as malignant fibrous histiocytoma.

Renal involvement by lymphoma, the most common site of extranodal disease, usually occurs with non-Hodgkin's lymphoma. Burkitt's lymphoma also has a predilection for extranodal disease, but it is uncommon in North America.

Notes

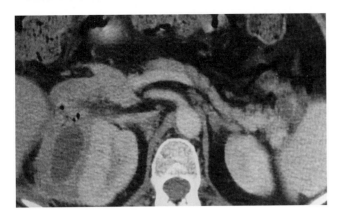
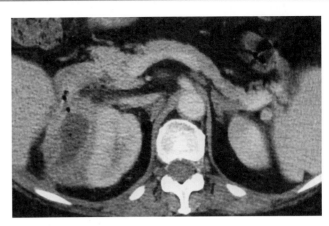

1. What finding is evident?

2. Which spaces of the retroperitoneum are involved?

3. What is the differential diagnosis?

4. What is the significance of the normal renal cortical enhancement?

Kidney: Perinephric Abscess Caused by Perforated Duodenal Ulcer

1. A perinephric fluid collection that exerts mass effect on the right kidney.

2. Anterior pararenal space and perirenal space.

3. Perinephric abscess, necrotic renal tumor, and perforated duodenal ulcer.

4. Normal cortical enhancement is unusual in pyelonephritis.

References

Dalla Palma L, Pozzi-Mucelli F, Ene V: Medical treatment of renal and perirenal abscesses: CT evaluation, *Clin Radiol* 54:792–797, 1999.

Lowe LH, Zagoria RJ, Baumgartner BR, et al: Role of imaging and intervention in complex infections of the urinary tract, *Am J Roentgenol* 163:363–367, 1994.

Papanicolaou N, Pfister RC: Acute renal infections, *Radiol Clin North Am* 34:965–995, 1996.

Cross-Reference

Zagoria RJ, *Genitourinary Radiology: THE REQUISITES*, 2nd ed, pp 136–139, 399–400.

Comment

This patient had fever, leukocytosis, and pyuria and an abdominal CT was performed to determine the source of infection. This case is an example of a perinephric abscess. The most common cause of an abscess in this area is spread from a renal infection (e.g., pyelonephritis). Pyelonephritis has typical imaging findings evident on CT, including unilateral renal enlargement, heterogeneous enhancement with wedge-shaped areas of decreased perfusion and enhancement (striated nephrogram), and perinephric inflammation. Pyelonephritis can be diffuse or focal.

Treatment of renal infections depends on the patient's clinical condition, underlying diseases, and extent of infection. Patients with pyelonephritis are treated with antibiotics. Patients with a focal perinephric collection can be treated with intravenous antibiotics and percutaneous drainage. Patients with emphysematous pyelonephritis require intravenous antibiotics and either percutaneous drainage or, in rare severe cases, nephrectomy. Percutaneous drainage is preferable if the gas collection is localized. In patients treated with percutaneous drainage, the radiologist should be certain that the ipsilateral collecting system is not obstructed by a calculus or tumor. If there is ureteral obstruction, the obstructed collecting system should be drained by a ureteral stent or percutaneous nephrostomy.

The illustrated case is a perinephric abscess resulting from a perforated duodenal ulcer that extended posteriorly into the perirenal or perinephric space. Clues to the correct diagnosis include the following: (1) the renal enhancement is normal, (2) there is no ureteral obstruction, (3) the fluid collection is contiguous with the decompressed duodenum, and (4) there are bubbles of air between the duodenum and the perinephric collection. This patient was treated with CT-guided percutaneous abscess drainage, placement of an nasogastric tube, intravenous antibiotic therapy, and antiulcer therapy and improved.

Notes

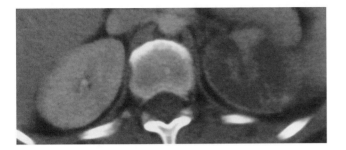
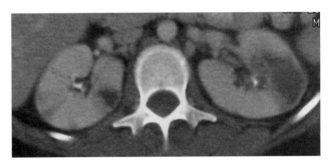

1. What term describes the nephrographic pattern shown in the area of the multiple renal abnormalities?

2. What artery is supplying the outer cortex of these kidneys?

3. What pathologic conditions should be considered when bilateral renal lesions with this shape are present?

4. What is the most likely diagnosis in this patient?

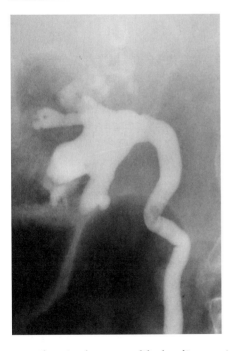
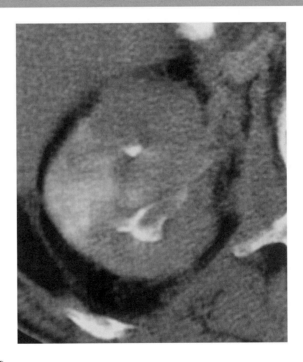

1. What is the most likely diagnosis?

2. What is the likely cause of the filling defect seen in the posterior calyx?

3. What name is used to describe the appearance of solid soft tissue replacing the normal renal sinus fat?

4. Which neoplasms involve the kidney with an infiltrative pattern, as illustrated in this case?

Kidney: Renal Infarction

1. Rim nephrogram.

2. Renal capsular artery.

3. Renal infarctions; metastases, including lymphoma; and renal infections.

4. Bilateral renal infarctions caused by emboli or vasculitis.

References

Gash JR, Zagoria RJ, Dyer RB: Imaging features of infiltrating renal lesions, *Crit Rev Diagn Imaging* 33: 293–310, 1992.

Saunders HS, Dyer RB, Shifrin RY, et al: The CT nephrogram: implications for evaluation of urinary tract disease, *Radiographics* 15:1069–1085, 1995.

Cross-Reference

Zagoria RJ, *Genitourinary Radiology: THE REQUISITES,* 2nd ed, pp 120–121.

Comment

The abnormal low-attenuation lesions present in both kidneys preserve the normal shape of the kidney without significant mass effect. There is decreased perfusion to the involved areas, with a rim of normally enhancing parenchyma at the peripheral edge of the abnormal areas. This pattern is typical of renal infarction, with the cortical rim nephrogram being diagnostic of this entity. The rim nephrogram results from the occlusion of segmental renal arteries leading to renal infarction with maintenance of flow to the capsular artery, which branches proximally from the main renal artery. The renal capsular artery maintains perfusion to the outermost renal cortex in the area of infarction. Unfortunately, the rim nephrogram sign is present in only one half of renal infarctions. Abnormalities that cause infiltrative renal lesions include infiltrative neoplasms, such as transitional cell carcinoma and some metastases; renal infarctions (as shown here); and some inflammatory renal lesions, including pyelonephritis and xanthogranulomatous pyelonephritis. Of these abnormalities, only renal infarctions, bacterial pyelonephritis, and infiltrative metastases to the kidney commonly cause bilateral lesions. The presence of the rim sign is diagnostic of renal infarction.

Renal infarction may result from numerous causes of renal vascular occlusion, including embolus, dissection, thrombosis, and vasculitis. Bilateral renal infarctions suggest systemic emboli or a vasculitis. The patient shown had subacute bacterial endocarditis with multiple systemic emboli.

Notes

Kidney: Transitional Cell Carcinoma of the Kidney: the Faceless Kidney

1. Transitional cell carcinoma.

2. Blood clot.

3. "Faceless" kidney.

4. Urothelial tumors (transitional and squamous cell carcinomas); some metastases, including lymphoma; and the uncommon infiltrative renal cell carcinoma.

References

Gash JR, Zagoria RJ, Dyer RB: Imaging features of infiltrating renal lesions, *Crit Rev Diagn Imaging* 33: 293–310, 1992.

Wong-You-Cheong JJ, Wagner BJ, Davis CJ Jr: Transitional cell carcinoma of the urinary tract: radiologic-pathologic correlation, *Radiographics* 18: 123–142, 1998.

Cross-Reference

Zagoria RJ, *Genitourinary Radiology: THE REQUISITES,* 2nd ed, pp 115–118.

Comment

This case demonstrates a typical appearance of transitional cell carcinoma of the pyelocalyceal system called the "faceless" kidney. This term describes a solid mass proliferating in the renal sinus and obliterating the normal renal sinus fat. In this case the mass has infiltrated the renal parenchyma, causing decreased contrast enhancement. The area of marked enhancement represents unaffected normal renal parenchyma. The appearance of a faceless kidney strongly suggests the diagnosis of transitional cell carcinoma. However, squamous cell carcinoma, which is much less common, can have an identical appearance. Approximately one fourth of transitional cell carcinomas arising in the renal pelvis or calyx invade the renal parenchyma. When invasion of the renal parenchyma occurs, it has an infiltrative pattern radiologically, meaning there is maintenance of the normal shape of the kidney (without formation of a ball-shaped mass) and an ill-defined interface between the normal kidney and the lesion. This pattern, in combination with extensive soft tissue in the renal sinus, strongly suggests transitional cell carcinoma. Renal tuberculosis, which is a much less common diagnosis in North America, can have an identical appearance. Definitive diagnosis requires histologic or bacteriologic studies.

The intraluminal filling defect in the posterior calyx has an appearance typical of a blood clot or infectious debris. It has conformed to the shape of the calyx, suggesting soft, pliable material. This blood clot is most likely secondary to the primary transitional cell carcinoma in this patient.

Notes

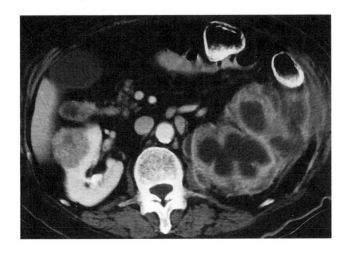
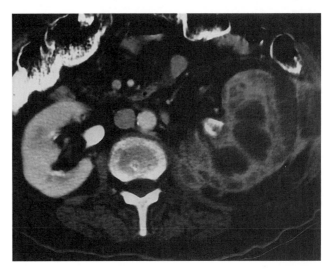

1. What is the diagnosis? What is the presumed pathophysiology of the disease involving the left kidney?

2. What organisms are most commonly involved?

3. What is the treatment for this disease process?

4. What are the findings on the image of the right kidney? Is there an association between these two entities? How should this patient be treated?

Kidney: Xanthogranulomatous Pyelonephritis and Renal Cell Carcinoma

1. Diffuse xanthogranulomatous pyelonephritis. Recurrent upper tract infection and calculus formation cause obstruction and renal inflammation, with lipid-laden histiocytes.

2. *Escherichia coli* and *Proteus* species.

3. Nephrectomy.

4. Solid enhancing renal mass consistent with renal cell carcinoma (RCC). There is no association between RCC and xanthogranulomatous pyelonephritis. The patient should be treated with right renal-sparing surgery.

Reference

Hayes WS, Hartman DS, Sesterhenn IA: Xanthogranulomatous pyelonephritis, *Radiographics* 11:485–498, 1991.

Cross-Reference

Zagoria RJ, *Genitourinary Radiology: THE REQUISITES,* 2nd ed, pp 89–100, 118–121, 139–141.

Comment

Xanthogranulomatous pyelonephritis (XGP) is a rare condition that has two variant forms: diffuse and focal. XGP is believed to occur secondary to chronic urinary tract infection (most commonly with *Escherichia coli* or *Proteus* species), which predisposes the patient to calculus formation. Of patients with XGP, 80% have a coexisting renal calculus. The presence of calculi and recurrent infections incites an inflammatory response in which lipid-laden macrophages destroy and replace normal renal parenchyma. The process causes enlargement of the kidney, and the infection can spread outside the kidney. Typical symptoms are pain, fever, and weight loss. The disease most often afflicts middle-aged women and those with diabetes.

Focal XGP is a more localized area of inflammation and is also associated with renal calculus disease. It may be difficult to differentiate from a solid renal mass caused by a neoplasm. There are no specific imaging findings to differentiate focal XGP from a neoplasm.

This patient had diffuse XGP of the left kidney and a right renal cell carcinoma (RCC); however, there is no reported association between these two diseases. The treatment of choice in this case is left nephrectomy and right partial nephrectomy. A newer technique for treating RCCs is image-guided thermal ablation, which might be considered in this case for treatment of the RCC.

Notes

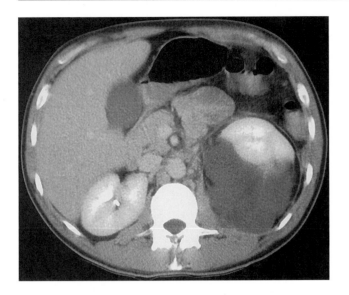

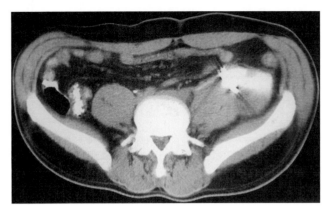

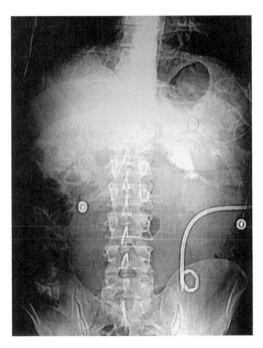

1. This patient was involved in a serious motor vehicle accident and had a partial ureteropelvic junction tear but refused treatment. At the time of this scan the patient complained of severe left flank pain and was hypertensive. What is the left perirenal mass?

2. Is this mass located in the perirenal or the posterior pararenal space?

3. What is causing hypertension in this patient?

4. Is percutaneous drainage of this mass adequate treatment?

Kidney: Perinephric Urinoma

1. Urinoma.

2. Urine is contained in the perinephric space, which is surrounded by Gerota's fascia. Some of this urine is in a subcapsular location, causing deformation of the normal renal shape.

3. Hypoperfusion of the left kidney caused by the subcapsular urinoma (Page kidney).

4. No. Percutaneous drainage may result in temporary resolution of the urinoma, but ureteral stenting or percutaneous nephrostomy drainage is required to allow the ureteral laceration to heal.

References

McCune TR, Stone WJ, Breyer JA: Page kidney: case report and review of the literature, *Am J Kidney Dis* 18:593–599, 1991.

Titton RL, Gervais DA, Hahn PF, et al: Urine leaks and urinomas: diagnosis and imaging-guided intervention, *Radiographics* 23:1133–1147, 2003.

Cross-Reference

Zagoria RJ, *Genitourinary Radiology: THE REQUISITES,* 2nd ed, p 77.

Comment

This patient developed a urinoma as a result of a ureteral laceration at the ureteropelvic junction. This segment of ureter is most commonly damaged in serious deceleration injuries that lead to complete or partial avulsion of the ureter from the renal pelvis. Urinoma development is a possible consequence of this injury. When fluid, either urine or blood, collects in a subcapsular location, it can compress the renal parenchyma. This compression leads to relative underperfusion and ischemia of the involved renal parenchyma. The kidney responds by oversecreting renin, leading to renovascular hypertension. This condition has been called the Page kidney and is one of two models of renovascular hypertension. The other, called the Goldblatt kidney, is renovascular hypertension caused by renal artery stenosis or occlusion.

Although urinomas can be easily evacuated with a percutaneously placed drain, as shown in the second and third figures in this case, other treatments may be necessary. In this case, the ureteropelvic junction laceration required ureteral stenting. In addition, the formation of a urinoma greatly increases the patient's risk for developing a stricture of the damaged segment of ureter. Therefore prompt evacuation of the urinoma and stenting are recommended for proper treatment of ureteral injuries resulting in urinomas.

Notes

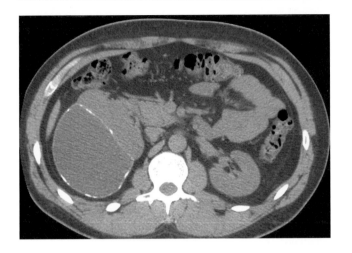
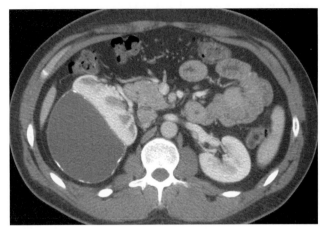
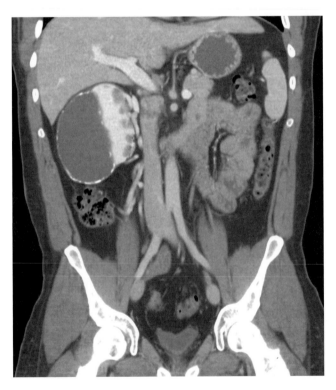

1. In what space is the low-attenuation material near the right kidney?

2. How can subcapsular fluid be distinguished from perirenal, extracapsular fluid?

3. What are common causes of fluid in this location?

4. What name is given to the ischemic kidney caused by fluid in this location?

Kidney: Renal Subcapsular Hematoma

1. Subcapsular space.

2. Subcapsular fluid leads to deformation of the renal shape, and there is no fat plane between the kidney and the fluid.

3. Traumatic injury (including iatrogenic injury resulting from renal biopsy or percutaneous nephrostomy), vasculitis, and rupture of a vascular formation.

4. Page kidney.

References

Kawashima A, Sandler CM, Corl FM, et al: Imaging of renal trauma: a comprehensive review, *Radiographics* 21:557–574, 2001.

Pollack HM, Wein AJ: Imaging of renal trauma, *Radiology* 172:297–308, 1989.

Cross-Reference

Zagoria RJ, *Genitourinary Radiology: THE REQUISITES*, 2nd ed, p 132.

Comment

In this case there is a fluid collection compressing the right kidney. This patient was involved in a motor vehicle accident, and this fluid was diagnosed as a subcapsular hematoma. Blunt trauma is the most common cause of subcapsular hematoma. This finding usually indicates injury to a peripheral renal artery branch, with arterial hemorrhage into the subcapsular space. Because the capsule is a rigid fibrous layer of tissue, the enlarging hematoma compresses and deforms the renal parenchyma. Venous bleeding is not usually of sufficient pressure to cause significant subcapsular hematomas.

This entity has clinical significance because there is compression of the renal parenchyma. This compression leads to ischemia of the kidney, which may cause increased excretion of renin and the development of hypertension. When this chain of events occurs, usually within 6 months of the development of the subcapsular hematoma, the resulting kidney is described as a Page kidney. Compression of the renal parenchyma leading to increased renin secretion is one model of renal vascular hypertension. In the other model, called the Goldblatt kidney, increased renin secretion caused by underperfusion is seen in patients with renal artery stenosis.

A subcapsular hematoma may be successfully treated with percutaneous evacuation.

Notes

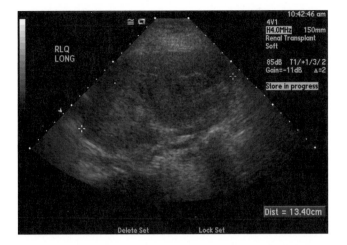

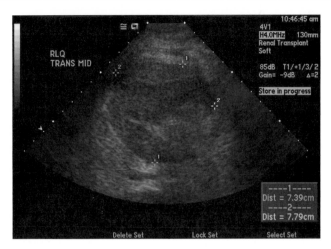

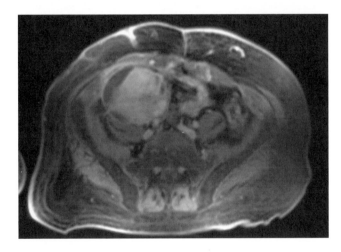

1. What complications can occur with a percutaneous biopsy?

2. True or false: Postbiopsy hemorrhage is more common in patients with uncontrolled hypertension.

3. What are some causes of high signal on the T1-weighted image?

4. What is a Page kidney?

Kidney: Perinephric Hematoma of Transplanted Kidney

1. Arteriovenous fistula, hemorrhage, hematuria, abscess, and sepsis.

2. True.

3. Fat, protein, melanin, methemoglobin, and gadolinium.

4. A subcapsular hematoma compresses the kidney and decreases its blood flow, triggering the renin-angiotensin-aldosterone system and causing hypertension.

Reference

Balci NC, Sirvanci M, Tufek I, et al: Spontaneous retroperitoneal hemorrhage secondary to subcapsular renal hematoma: MRI findings, *Magn Reson Imaging* 19: 1145–1148, 2001.

Cross-Reference

Zagoria RJ, *Genitourinary Radiology: THE REQUISITES*, 2nd ed, pp 390–391.

Comment

Percutaneous renal biopsy is useful in the diagnosis of acute or chronic rejection in the setting of renal transplantation and is important in guiding treatment. In most studies, the complication rate ranges from 7% to 15%. Ninety-eight percent of complications are discovered in the first 12 to 24 hours after the procedure. Minor complications are defined as those requiring minimal or no treatment and include macroscopic hematuria or a small subcapsular hematoma that resolves spontaneously. Major complications are those that require treatment and include bleeding requiring a transfusion, abscess, sepsis, or arteriovenous fistula or pseudoaneurysm requiring embolization. Complications are less common when smaller needles are used. Use of spring-loaded biopsy devices has also led to a decrease in the number of postbiopsy complications. Patients with uncontrolled severe hypertension and coagulopathies are more likely to suffer complications.

On ultrasound examination acute hematomas are usually echogenic. As the hematoma breaks down over the course of several days, it becomes more hypoechoic and may appear as a complex cystic structure with internal echoes and septations. On a non-contrast-enhanced CT scan, an acute hematoma is higher in attenuation than the renal parenchyma. Hematomas may become chronic, and over time become lower in attenuation. Chronic hematomas may also calcify. On MRI examination, an acute hematoma is low in signal on T1- and T2-weighted images because the deoxyhemoglobin in the erythrocytes is paramagnetic and causes T2 shortening. As shown here, in the early subacute phase, intracellular methemoglobin causes marked T1 shortening, which results in high signal intensity in T1-weighted images, but low signal on T2-weighted images. In the late subacute phase, the erythrocytes lyse and the extracellular methemoglobin results in high T1 and T2 signal. In chronic hematomas, hemosiderin causes T2 shortening, so the signal is dark on both T1- and T2-weighted images.

Notes

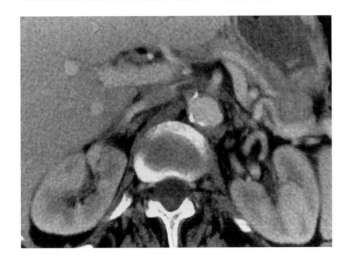 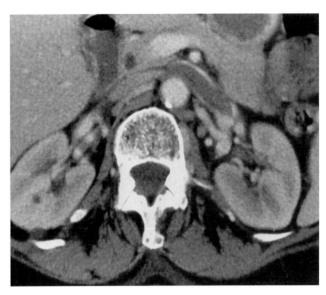

1. What radiologic findings are present?

2. Name three causes of this condition.

3. What might an MRI show?

4. Name three complications of this condition.

Kidney: Renal Vein Thrombosis

1. Enhanced CT demonstrates an enlarged left renal vein that contains a filling defect. Perivenous inflammation is visible. The left kidney is swollen and poorly perfused.

2. Renal cell carcinoma, dehydration, and hypercoagulable state.

3. A T1-bright defect in the left renal vein.

4. About one third of patients with renal vein thrombosis develop pulmonary embolism. Other complications include renal atrophy and papillary necrosis.

References

Kawamoto S, Lawler LP, Fishman EK: Evaluation of the renal venous system on late arterial and venous phase images with MDCT angiography in potential living laparoscopic renal donors, *Am J Roentgenol* 184:539–545, 2005.

Kawashima A, Sandler CM, Ernst RD, et al: CT evaluation of renovascular disease, *Radiographics* 20:1321–1340, 2000.

Cross-Reference

Zagoria RJ, *Genitourinary Radiology: THE REQUISITES,* 2nd ed, pp 95, 130, 140, 141.

Comment

The cause of renal vein thrombosis (RVT) is multifactorial and depends on the age of the patient and the existence of any comorbid disease. Primary RVT occurs because of a hypercoagulable state. In children, RVT is often the result of dehydration, and in adults, nephrotic syndrome is a frequent cause. Other less common causes include sickle cell disease, vasculitis, amyloidosis, and systemic lupus erythematosus. Causes of secondary RVT include renal or extrarenal tumors that either grow into or compress the renal vein, infection (e.g., acute pyelonephritis, abscess, tuberculosis, sepsis), trauma (accidental and iatrogenic), and extension of caval thrombus. RVT constitutes 5% of all renal transplant complications.

RVT has variable imaging findings, depending on the age of the thrombus. In acute RVT the kidney is enlarged with delayed excretion. In long-standing RVT there is characteristic ureteral notching caused by the development of periureteral venous collaterals. Late in the course of the disease, the kidney is small with decreased function. CT may demonstrate an enlarged renal vein containing a central filling defect, poor parenchymal perfusion, and delayed contrast material excretion. Similarly, MRI can directly demonstrate the thrombus. In the acute phase of the disease, ultrasonography may demonstrate an enlarged kidney, absence of the venous Doppler signal, and a high-resistance arterial waveform with reversal of diastolic flow. Multidetector row CT has increased the accuracy of detecting vascular disease by improved spatial and temporal resolution when compared with single detector CT.

Notes

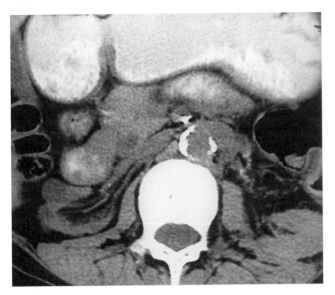 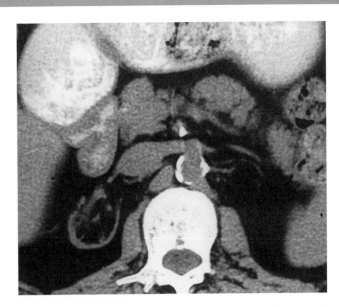

1. On the image on the left, given the appearance of the kidneys, what may have caused the right renal cyst to form?

2. What treatments may have been performed after the first and before the second CT scan?

3. True or false: Patients on hemodialysis have an increased risk for renal cell carcinoma.

4. True or false: Dialysis is a contraindication to the use of iodinated contrast media for CT.

Kidney: Renal Cystic Disease Secondary to Hemodialysis

1. Cyst is either idiopathic in nature or the result of dialysis.

2. Left nephrectomy and renal transplantation.

3. True. Of patients on long-term hemodialysis, 7% develop renal cell carcinoma.

4. False.

References

Choyke PL: Acquired cystic kidney disease, *Eur Radiol* 10:1716–1721, 2000.

Heinz-Peer G, Schoder M, Rand T, et al: Prevalence of acquired cystic kidney disease and tumors in native kidneys of renal transplant recipients: a prospective US study, *Radiology* 195(3):667–671, 1995.

Cross-Reference

Zagoria RJ, *Genitourinary Radiology: THE REQUISITES,* 2nd ed, pp 87–89, 112, 113.

Comment

Renal cysts are common and increase in prevalence with age. Half of all individuals older than 50 years have a renal cyst. The etiology of the cyst is believed to be obstruction of a renal tubule and subsequent dilation of the more proximal tubule with serous fluid. Cysts most often occur in the renal cortex and do not communicate with the collecting system. On ultrasonography a cyst is anechoic and has increased through-transmission of sound posterior to the cyst. No mural or central enhancement is visible on intravenous urography or CT. Fluid in a simple renal cortical cyst is isodense with water and should measure less than 15 Hounsfield units on noncontrast CT.

This patient had end-stage renal disease secondary to diabetic nephropathy. A right renal cortical cyst developed while the patient was on hemodialysis, and this cyst resolved after renal transplantation. Multiple renal cysts are common in patients on long-term dialysis. The number of cysts increases with the duration of hemodialysis or peritoneal dialysis. After 3 years of dialysis, 10% to 20% of patients develop renal cysts. Up to 90% of patients acquire renal cysts after 5 to 10 years of dialysis. The mechanism is not known, but one theory implicates the accumulation of nephrotoxins to cyst formation. Dysplasia may develop in the epithelial wall of these cysts, and 7% of patients on long-term dialysis develop a solid renal neoplasm (i.e., adenoma, oncocytoma, or adenocarcinoma). Renal adenocarcinoma that develops in the patient on dialysis tends to be less aggressive and metastasizes less frequently than conventional renal carcinoma. The treatment is nephrectomy or image-guided tumor ablation treatments such as radiofrequency ablation.

Iodinated contrast can be administered to patients on dialysis who produce no urine or who have been on dialysis for longer than 6 months. Nephrotoxicity is not an issue because damage to the renal parenchyma has already occurred.

Notes

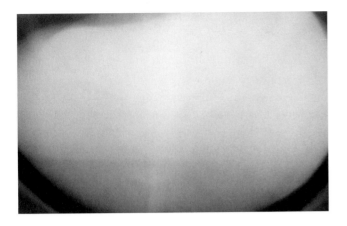

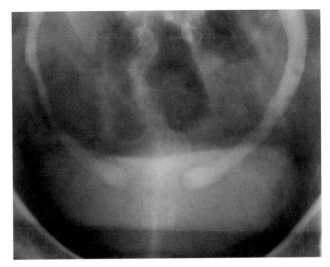

1. What is the diagnosis in this case?

2. What causes the lucent line around the bulbous segment of the ureter in the bladder?

3. What complications can be caused by the abnormality shown?

4. Failed resorption of what structure is the proposed cause of this abnormality?

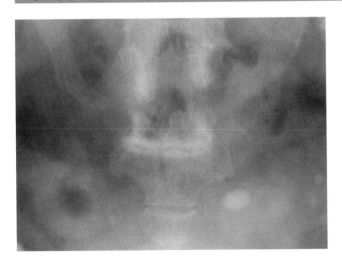

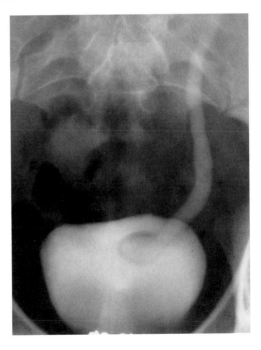

1. What name describes the bulbous portion of the lower left ureter in this case?

2. What causes this abnormality to occur?

3. What processes usually cause this abnormality?

4. To make the diagnosis of an orthotopic ureterocele, what is the maximum thickness of the radiolucent halo?

CASE 85

Pelvicalices and Ureter: Orthotopic Ureterocele

1. Bilateral orthotopic ureteroceles.

2. Bladder mucosa and ureteral wall herniating into the bladder.

3. Ureteral obstruction, urolithiasis, and urinary tract infection.

4. Chwalla's membrane.

Reference

Davidson AJ, Hartman DS, eds: *Radiology of the Kidney and Urinary Tract,* 2nd ed, Philadelphia, 1994, Saunders, pp 521–528.

Cross-Reference

Zagoria RJ, *Genitourinary Radiology: THE REQUISITES,* 2nd ed, pp 163–165.

Comment

This case demonstrates bilateral orthotopic ureteroceles, also known as adult-type ureteroceles. These ureteroceles are rarely seen in children; they usually do not cause symptoms and are an incidental finding. As shown in this case, bilateral orthotopic ureteroceles are easier to see when the bladder is only partially filled and may be difficult to see when the bladder is completely filled with opacified urine. Orthotopic ureteroceles, unlike ectopic ureteroceles, are not associated with other urinary tract anomalies. Specifically they are not related to ectopic ureters. The proposed mechanism for development of orthotopic ureteroceles is incomplete resorption of Chwalla's membrane during recanalization of the fetal ureter. This incomplete resorption causes minimal stenosis of the ureteral orifice and eventual prolapse of the bulbous ureterovesical junction into the bladder. Orthotopic ureteroceles can become quite large, and the larger ones are more likely to be associated with complications. When ureteroceles are more than 2 cm in diameter, the risk for significant urinary tract stasis, with obstruction, stone formation, or infection, is increased. In addition, the appearance of a simple ureterocele must be carefully evaluated. The lucent line around the bulbous segment of the ureter is characteristic. It should be regular, smooth, and no more than 1 to 2 mm in diameter. If this outline is more than 2 mm in diameter, a pseudoureterocele (caused by an underlying pathologic condition, such as a stone or tumor) should be suspected.

Notes

CASE 86

Pelvicalices and Ureter: Pseudoureterocele

1. Pseudoureterocele.

2. Partial obstruction of the ureteral orifice.

3. Ureteral stone, ureteral edema from recent passage of a stone, manipulation of the ureterovesical junction, and bladder neoplasm impinging on the ureteral orifice.

4. 2 mm.

Reference

Chen MYM, Zagoria RJ, Dyer RB: Interureteric ridge edema: incidence and etiology, *Abdom Imaging* 20:368–370, 1995.

Cross-Reference

Zagoria RJ, *Genitourinary Radiology: THE REQUISITES,* 2nd ed, pp 164, 166.

Comment

This patient has a small stone lodged in the left ureterovesical junction, causing ureteral obstruction and the appearance of a pseudoureterocele. This is described as a "pseudoureterocele" because the radiologic appearance is similar to that of an orthotopic ureterocele, but the appearance is caused by an underlying pathologic condition. In this case the pathology, a stone, is visible on the scout radiograph. A pseudoureterocele is caused by partial obstruction of the ureterovesical junction with marked dilation of the lower ureteral segment and bulging of this segment into the bladder lumen. This bulging is usually accompanied by surrounding edema, which causes thickening of the "halo" of lucency around the caudal end of the ureter. As illustrated in this case, the lucent segment is considerably thickened above the pseudoureterocele. In a simple or orthotopic ureterocele the lucent line is uniform and 2 mm or less in diameter. Irregularity or thickening of the halo suggests an underlying pathologic problem, such as a stone, edema resulting from recent stone passage or manipulation, or tumor encroachment and infiltration. When the diagnosis is not apparent with urography, it may be confirmed with endoscopy. Another important finding seen in association with a pseudoureterocele is hydronephrosis. Orthotopic ureteroceles are not often associated with any significant obstruction, and therefore hydronephrosis is absent. The combination of a ureterocele-like abnormality and obstruction suggests a pseudoureterocele and an underlying pathologic problem.

Notes

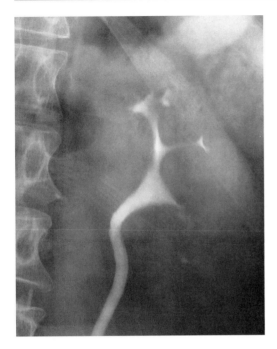

1. What abnormalities are visible on this intravenous urogram?

2. What are the main differential diagnostic considerations for this pattern of abnormality?

3. What is the best diagnostic test for confirming the diagnosis of this entity?

4. What causes the radiologic appearance of the lower pole calyx in this case?

Pelvicalices and Ureter: Calyceal Transitional Cell Carcinoma—Urogram

1. Irregularity and minimal filling of lower pole calyces.

2. Transitional cell carcinoma and tuberculosis.

3. Urine cytology and bacteriology.

4. Either infiltration by tumor or inflammation of the lower pole calyx and its infundibulum.

Reference

Wong-You-Cheong JJ, Wagner BJ, Davis CJ Jr: Transitional cell carcinoma of the urinary tract: radiologic-pathologic correlation, *Radiographics* 18: 123–142, 1998.

Cross-Reference

Zagoria RJ, *Genitourinary Radiology: THE REQUISITES,* 2nd ed, pp 84, 116, 122.

Comment

This intravenous urogram demonstrates the appearance of an "amputated" calyx. There is minimal opacification of the lower pole calyces and an apparent abrupt cut-off of the infundibulum, which should be draining these calyces. This finding almost always indicates the diagnosis of an infiltrative process involving the urothelium. The two main diagnostic considerations for this appearance are tuberculosis and transitional cell carcinoma. It is impossible radiologically to distinguish between these two entities in this type of situation. An exact diagnosis must be made after microscopic examination of tissue or urine. Once a diagnosis is made, cross-sectional imaging may help to better define the extent (i.e., stage) of the abnormality.

Transitional cell carcinoma can be either papillary or nonpapillary. The papillary variety tends to grow into polypoid masses and accounts for approximately two thirds of all cases of transitional cell carcinoma. The nonpapillary variety is infiltrating and leads to malignant strictures when it involves the upper tracts of the urinary system. Nonpapillary transitional cell carcinoma tends to invade through the mucosa at an earlier phase of the disease, but it is usually unifocal in the urinary tract. Papillary tumors are less invasive but more commonly multifocal.

Notes

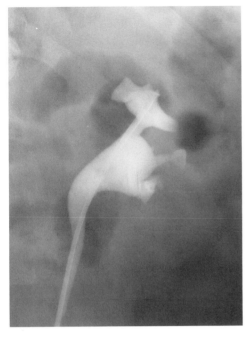
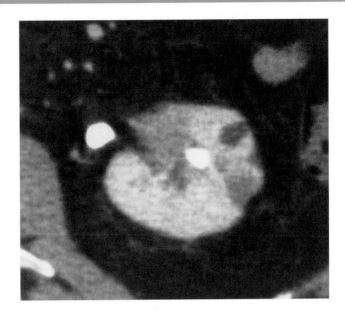

1. What are the two main diagnoses that should be considered in this patient with an abnormal left kidney?

2. What is the name of the line that connects the lateral edges of the laterally oriented calyces?

3. What causes calyceal amputation?

4. What percentage of patients with calyceal transitional cell carcinoma develop synchronous or metachronous tumors?

Pelvicalices and Ureter: Calyceal Transitional Cell Carcinoma—Retrograde Pyelogram and CT

1. TCC and tuberculosis.

2. Interpapillary line.

3. Obstruction of a major calyx, usually resulting from infiltration by tumor or from inflammation.

4. 25%.

Reference

Wong-You-Cheong JJ, Wagner BJ, Davis CJ Jr: Transitional cell carcinoma of the urinary tract: radiologic-pathologic correlation, *Radiographics* 18: 123–142, 1998.

Cross-Reference

Zagoria RJ, *Genitourinary Radiology: THE REQUISITES,* 2nd ed, p 86.

Comment

This case demonstrates calyceal amputation. Notice on the retrograde pyelogram that the calyces subtending the lower pole of the left kidney are not filling. The interpapillary line that connects the most lateral aspects of the marginal calyces should parallel the peripheral margin of the renal contour. Also, every lobe of the kidney should be drained by a calyx, with a similar distance from the marginal calyces to the edge of the kidney in all regions, which clearly is not so in this case. The CT scan demonstrates a soft tissue mass filling the renal sinus and invading the renal parenchyma. There is also a small incidental simple cyst adjacent to this mass. These findings strongly suggest the diagnosis of either transitional cell carcinoma (TCC) or tuberculosis. Other much less common causes include squamous cell carcinoma and infiltrative renal cell carcinoma. It is unlikely that this mass represents a renal parenchymal process because it is clearly centered in the renal sinus and there is infiltration of the major calyx. Renal tuberculosis and TCC cannot be reliably distinguished from one another with imaging, and definitive diagnosis should be based on histologic or bacteriologic studies. However, radiology can be used, as in this case, to demonstrate the abnormality, suggest the correct diagnosis, and delineate the extent of the disease. Calyceal TCC accounts for approximately 9% of urinary tract TCCs, and 90% of them occur within the bladder. Presence of an upper tract TCC indicates a high risk for multifocal TCC.

Notes

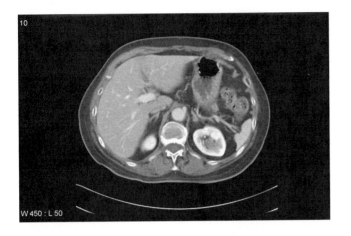

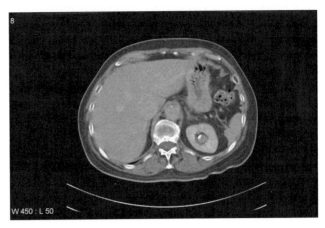

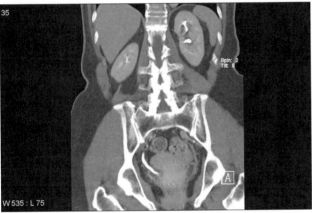

Upper right and lower left images reprinted with permission
from Lee JKT, Sagel SS, Stanley RJ, Heiken P, *Computed Body
Tomography with MRI Correlation*, ed 4, Philadelphia: Lippincott
Williams and Wilkins, 2006.

1. What is the most likely explanation for the soft tissue mass involving the left upper pole calyx?

2. What is the most important risk factor for this finding?

3. What is the most common clinical presentation for the above finding?

4. What is the risk of a synchronous bladder transitional cell carcinoma with the above finding?

Pelvicalices and Ureter: Transitional Cell Carcinoma of the Left Renal Pelvis

1. Transitional cell carcinoma.

2. Smoking.

3. Hematuria in 72% of cases, dull flank pain in 22% of cases, and rarely acute renal colic due to obstruction.

4. 39%.

References

Wong-You-Cheong JJ, Wagner BJ, Davis CJ Jr: Transitional cell carcinoma of the urinary tract: radiologic-pathologic correlation, *Radiographics* 18: 123–142, 1998.

Yousem DM, Gatewood OM, Goldman SM, Marshall FF: Synchronous and metachronous transitional cell carcinoma of the urinary tract: prevalence, incidence, and radiographic detection, *Radiology* 167:613–618, 1988.

Cross-Reference

Zagoria RJ, *Genitourinary Radiology: THE REQUISITES*, 2nd ed, pp 180–181.

Comment

Transitional cell carcinoma (TCC) of the urinary bladder comprises approximately 90% of all primary bladder tumors. TCC of the renal pelvis and ureter is less common, comprising only 5% of the total number of tumors of the urinary tract diagnosed yearly. TCC is most often diagnosed in older men, with a male-to-female ratio of approximately 3:1 and a mean age at diagnosis of 64 years. The most common clinical presentation of patients diagnosed with TCC is hematuria. Smoking is the single most important risk factor. Synchronous bladder TCCs are reported in approximately 39% of patients with ureteral TCC, and thus complete evaluation of the urinary tract is required.

Excretory urography has historically been the primary diagnostic tool for evaluation of upper tract TCC. Filling defects seen within the upper tracts on excretory urography have a relatively broad differential, including urothelial neoplasms, calculi, metastases, inflammatory lesions, fibroepithelial polyps, blood clots, and endometriosis. CT has proven useful in further characterizing filling defects within the intrarenal collecting system and ureter as it allows differentiation of calculi from solid masses. Intrarenal TCC generally presents as an intraluminal soft tissue mass or as thickening of the wall. The mass generally enlarges to fill and dilate the calyx and infundibulum. CT also provides advantages in diagnosis of extrarenal extension and regional lymphadenopathy, both of which are important in staging and surgical planning. Therapy usually consists of a nephroureterectomy. Interim follow-up at 3- to 6-month intervals is carried out with cystoscopy and either intravenous urography or CT-urography.

Notes

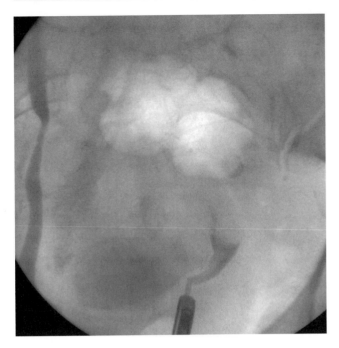

1. What is the diagnosis in this case?

2. How should the ureteral dilation in the ureter below the filling defect be described?

3. What causes this ureteral dilation?

4. Which subtype of tumor is this?

C A S E   9 0

Pelvicalices and Ureter: Transitional Cell Carcinoma with the "Goblet" Sign

1. Transitional cell carcinoma.

2. The "goblet" sign.

3. Long-standing, slowly growing polypoid mass in the ureter is repeatedly pushed into the ureter just caudal to it by peristalsis.

4. Papillary transitional cell carcinoma.

Reference

Bergman H, Friedenberg RM, Sayegh V: New roentgenologic signs of carcinoma of the ureter, *Am J Roentgenol* 86:707–717, 1961.

Cross-Reference

Zagoria RJ, *Genitourinary Radiology: THE REQUISITES,* 2nd ed, pp 166, 174, 180.

Comment

Transitional cell carcinomas (TCCs) grow in either a papillary or nonpapillary form. The papillary variety tends to grow into a polypoid mass that protrudes into the lumen of the urinary tract. When this occurs in the ureter, a "goblet" sign may ensue. The term *goblet sign* describes ureteral dilation below a radiolucent filling defect. The meniscus of contrast material in the upper extent of the dilated segment outlines the inferior side of the mass and is analogous to fluid in the goblet. This sign is significant because it is nearly pathognomonic for the diagnosis of TCC. Its presence excludes nonneoplastic filling defects, such as stones, blood, or infectious debris, and indicates a long-standing, slowly growing polypoid mass, almost always a TCC. Nonneoplastic filling defects do not lead to dilation inferior to the obstruction.

A related sign is known as *Bergman's coiled catheter sign*. This sign was described by a urologist who noted that passage of a ureteral catheter in a retrograde direction sometimes led to coiling of the catheter within a dilated segment of ureter below an obstructing tumor. Neither of these signs occurs in association with nonpapillary TCC, which accounts for approximately one third of all TCCs.

Notes

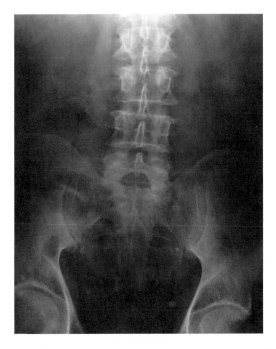 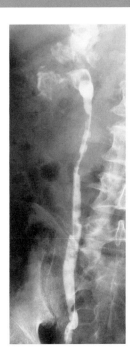

1. What are the most common causes of multiple radiolucent filling defects in the ureter?

2. Are the lesions shown more likely to be intraluminal, mucosal, or submucosal?

3. Of what substance are most radiolucent urinary tract calculi composed?

4. What is the incidence of multiple synchronous lesions in association with a papillary transitional cell carcinoma?

Pelvicalices and Ureter: Multifocal Transitional Cell Carcinoma

1. Radiolucent stones, air bubbles, multifocal transitional cell carcinoma, blood clots, infectious debris, and sloughed papillae.

2. Mucosal.

3. Uric acid.

4. One third of patients have multifocal disease.

References

Williamson B Jr, Hartman GW, Hattery RR: Multiple and diffuse ureteral filling defects, *Semin Roentgenol* 21: 214–223, 1986.

Wong-You-Cheong JJ, Wagner BJ, Davis CJ Jr: Transitional cell carcinoma of the urinary tract: radiologic-pathologic correlation, *Radiographics* 18: 123–142, 1998.

Cross-Reference

Zagoria RJ, *Genitourinary Radiology: THE REQUISITES,* 2nd ed, p 181.

Comment

The right retrograde pyelogram demonstrates multiple radiolucent filling defects in the right ureter and pyelocalyceal system. The lesions in the ureter appear to be attached to or to arise from the ureteral wall. They have acute angle margins with the ureteral wall, indicating that they are mucosal lesions rather than intraluminal or submucosal lesions. Intraluminal lesions are usually completely surrounded by contrast material, whereas submucosal lesions form obtuse angle margins with the ureteral wall. The presence of mucosal lesions strongly favors the diagnosis of transitional cell carcinoma. Other mucosal lesions include inflammatory lesions, such as forms of ureteritis, leukoplakia, and malacoplakia, and uncommon urothelial tumors, such as squamous cell carcinoma and adenocarcinoma.

Transitional cell carcinomas may grow in either a papillary or a nonpapillary form. Two thirds of transitional cell carcinomas are papillary, and one third are nonpapillary, or infiltrative. The papillary variety tends to be superficial and noninvasive but has a predilection for multifocality. One third of papillary transitional cell carcinomas, including lesions in all sites of the urinary tract, even the bladder, are multifocal. The presence of transitional cell carcinoma in the ureter increases the likelihood of synchronous or metachronous tumors to approximately 40%.

Notes

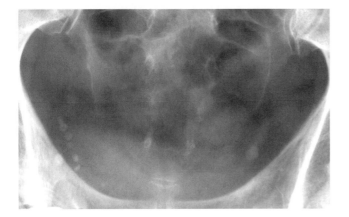

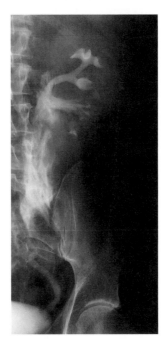

1. In which space is the contrast material located adjacent to the L4–5 region of the spine?

2. What is the underlying cause of this contrast material extravasation?

3. At what site does the extravasation usually originate?

4. What is the cause of hydronephrosis?

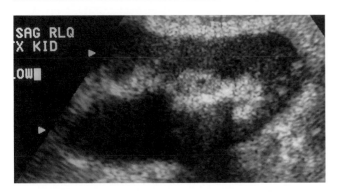

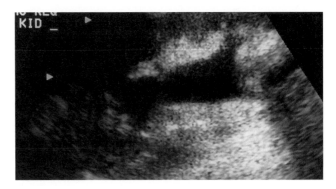

1. Sagittal sonograms of a renal transplant were performed in the perioperative period. What is the finding? What are the possible causes?

2. What normal structure can mimic the dilated collecting system, and how can the two be distinguished from one another?

3. What is the initial treatment for obstructive hydronephrosis in a recently transplanted kidney?

4. True or false: In the transplanted kidney, hydronephrosis caused by obstruction is usually painless.

Pelvicalices and Ureter: Ureteral Obstruction with Perirenal Contrast Material Extravasation

1. In the perirenal space.

2. Ureteral obstruction.

3. The fornix of a calyx.

4. An impacted stone at the ureterovesical junction.

Reference

Chapman JP, Gonzalez J, Diokno AC: Significance of urinary extravasation during renal colic, *Urology* 6: 541–545, 1987.

Cross-Reference

Zagoria RJ, *Genitourinary Radiology: THE REQUISITES,* 2nd ed, pp 135–136, 192.

Comment

This patient has a 5-mm-diameter stone obstructing the ureter at the left ureterovesical junction. The resulting hydroureteronephrosis has led to spontaneous rupture of a calyceal fornix and contrast material extravasation. Some contrast material is visible in the renal sinus (a part of the perirenal space), superimposed on the lower pole calyces, with most of the contrast material tracking within the perirenal space around the ureter.

Spontaneous forniceal rupture secondary to ureteral obstruction is not a rare phenomenon. However, it must be recognized as the totally benign entity that it is. It should not be confused with significant pathologic problems. This rupture likely represents a physiologic "pop-off" valve that opens when pyelocalyceal pressures reach very high levels. With ureteral obstruction, pyelocalyceal pressures can rise from near 0 to more than 70 mm Hg in a short time. This rise leads to hydroureteronephrosis and severe renal colic. When a fornix ruptures, the pressure reduces rapidly and there is a sudden relief of symptoms, which clinically may mimic the symptoms of stone passage. Forniceal rupture is of no clinical significance as long as the high-grade obstruction does not persist for a prolonged period. Urinoma formation after spontaneous forniceal rupture caused by ureteral obstruction is uncommon. Interestingly, it is quite common to see gallbladder opacification caused by vicarious contrast material excretion hours or days after perirenal extravasation of contrast material. This finding also is of no clinical significance.

Notes

Pelvicalices and Ureter: Obstructive Hydronephrosis in a Transplanted Kidney

1. Hydronephrosis. Ureteral edema, blood clot, anastomotic stricture, or peritransplant fluid collection.

2. Enlarged, branching veins in the renal sinus can be differentiated from the collecting system on color Doppler ultrasonography.

3. Percutaneous nephrostomy or placement of a nephrovesical stent.

4. True.

Reference

Reinberg Y, Bumgardner GL, Aliabadi H: Urological aspects of renal transplantation, *J Urol* 143:1087–1092, 1990.

Cross-Reference

Zagoria RJ, *Genitourinary Radiology: THE REQUISITES,* 2nd ed, pp 17, 152.

Comment

The management of end-stage renal disease was changed forever with the advent of renal transplantation in the 1950s. Although graft rejection remains of paramount importance, transplanted kidneys are subject to many urologic complications. For the evaluation of these potential complications, ultrasonography is the primary imaging modality. The complete ultrasound evaluation includes gray scale imaging and Doppler sonography. Gray scale imaging assesses parenchymal echogenicity, the size of the collecting system and its contents (e.g., calculus, clot, fungus balls), surrounding soft tissues, and fluid collections (e.g., hematoma, urinoma, lymphocele, abscess [HULA]). Color Doppler ultrasonography can assess graft perfusion and vascular anatomy and permits differentiation of vascular structures from pelvocaliectasis.

Hydronephrosis is common in the postoperative period and may have many causes. Calculi are a relatively uncommon cause, accounting for less than 2% of the cases of transplant hydronephrosis. Anastomotic edema, urinomas, blood clots, lymphoceles, and ureteral sloughing are common causes of perioperative transplant hydronephrosis. Because transplanted organs are denervated, hydronephrosis is usually painless and worsening graft function is the presenting sign. Of the 18% of transplanted kidneys that have a dilated collecting system, only 9% are truly obstructed. If ultrasound findings of dilation are confined to the renal pelvis, the likelihood of obstruction is low. If dilation involves the calyces, the chance of obstruction is as high as 67%. In most cases the exact level of obstruction cannot be identified on ultrasonography.

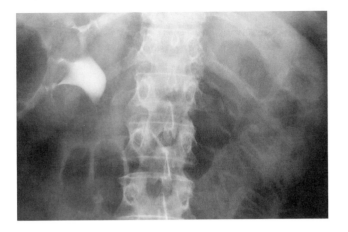
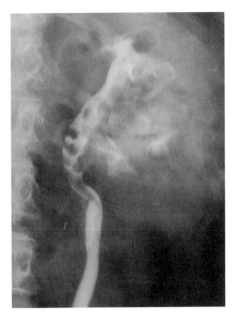

1. An intravenous urogram and a retrograde pyelogram are shown. What is the most likely cause of the ureteral obstruction in this patient?

2. In this patient with gross hematuria, what are likely underlying causes of the bleeding?

3. What are the most common causes of radiolucent filling defects that are visible on contrast studies of the pyelocalyceal system?

4. What enzyme in urine leads to rapid change of pyelocalyceal blood clots?

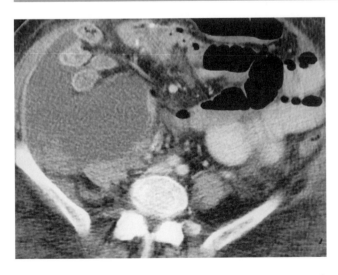
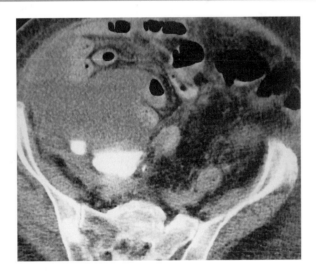

1. Two images, performed 5 minutes apart, are shown from an intravenous contrast-enhanced CT examination in a patient with a history of recent gynecologic surgery. What is the most likely diagnosis, and what is the most common cause of this lesion?

2. What is the most appropriate imaging technique when this diagnosis is suspected?

3. What is the diagnostic significance of the radiodensity of the material in the fluid collection?

4. True or false: For this lesion, surgery performed early is the treatment of choice.

Pelvicalices and Ureter: Pyelocalyceal Blood Clot

1. Blood clot, infectious debris, or fungal material.

2. Transitional cell carcinoma, renal cell carcinoma, or vascular malformation.

3. In order of descending frequency, radiolucent stones, urothelial neoplasms, blood clots, infectious debris, sloughed papilla, and fungal material.

4. Urokinase.

References

Fein AB, McClennan BL: Solitary filling defects of the ureter, *Semin Roentgenol* 21:201–213, 1986.

Williamson J Jr, Hartman GW, Hattery RR: Multiple and diffuse ureteral filling defects, *Semin Roentgenol* 21: 214–223, 1986.

Cross-Reference

Zagoria RJ, *Genitourinary Radiology: THE REQUISITES,* 2nd ed, pp 194–197.

Comment

There are numerous causes of radiolucent filling defects in the urinary tract. The most common of these causes are solid lesions, including uric acid stones and neoplasms, which are noncompliant. Alternatively, other causes of radiolucent filling defects, such as blood clot, infectious debris, and fungal material, are compliant and tend to conform to the shape of their container, in this case the pyelocalyceal system. In this case the intravenous urogram demonstrates unilateral nephromegaly and evidence of ureteral obstruction with delayed pyelogram. The retrograde study shows a large amount of radiolucent material, some of which is linear, that conforms to the shape of the ureter. This finding indicates a liquid or semisolid material in the pyelocalyceal system, making the diagnosis of blood clot the most likely in this patient with gross hematuria. Unfortunately, blood clots obscure the pyelocalyceal system, making diagnosis of an underlying lesion difficult. When gross hematuria is present, a search for the source of the bleeding is relevant. Sometimes the cause of intermittent gross hematuria remains occult, but common causes include urothelial neoplasm, renal cell carcinoma, vascular malformation, and traumatic injury.

In this case a follow-up retrograde study performed 1 week later demonstrated complete resolution of the filling defect and a normal-appearing pyelocalyceal system with no evidence of urothelial neoplasm. As is typical of clots in the urinary tract, it evolved and changed rapidly because of urokinase in the urine. Large clots can be completely lysed within a few days. This rapid change, when seen on sequential studies, helps to confirm the diagnosis of blood clot as the cause of radiolucent filling defects.

Notes

Pelvicalices and Ureter: Traumatic Injury of the Ureter

1. Ureteral disruption, which is most commonly iatrogenic in nature (i.e., caused by surgery). A less common cause is traumatic injury (blunt or penetrating).

2. CT after intravenous contrast administration (but without oral contrast enhancement); both early and delayed images should be performed.

3. Very dense contrast, as shown in this case, has been concentrated by the kidney and therefore is more radiodense than intravascular contrast.

4. False.

Reference

Lask D, Abarbanel J, Luttwak Z, et al: Changing trends in the management of iatrogenic ureteral injuries, *J Urol* 154:1693–1695, 1995.

Cross-Reference

Zagoria RJ, *Genitourinary Radiology: THE REQUISITES,* 2nd ed, pp 197–199.

Comment

Ureteral injury accounts for 3% to 5% of all traumatic injuries of the urinary tract. The majority of cases are the result of iatrogenic injury. Although gynecologic surgery leads the list, abdominal-perineal resection, cystectomy, vascular surgery, and spinal fusion all have been implicated. The ureter is well protected, and therefore traumatic injury is rare; penetrating trauma is much more likely than blunt trauma to cause injury.

Typical CT findings in ureteral disruption include normal renal enhancement, medial perirenal contrast extravasation, and nonopacification of the ipsilateral distal ureter. Extrarenal contrast has been concentrated by the kidney and is more radiodense than intravascular or oral contrast material. When there is a question of ureteral injury, early imaging, followed by delayed imaging (5 minutes after intravenous contrast administration), is suggested.

Antegrade pyelography can be performed to diagnose the ureteral tear and may be followed by interventions such as percutaneous nephrostomy or nephroureteral stent placement, and percutaneous urinoma drainage. One study of 44 patients with ureteral injury compared treatment with surgery to that with percutaneous nephrostomy alone. Those patients treated with percutaneous nephrostomy had significantly fewer secondary operations, had lower morbidity, and had spontaneous repair of the damaged ureter in the majority of cases.

Notes

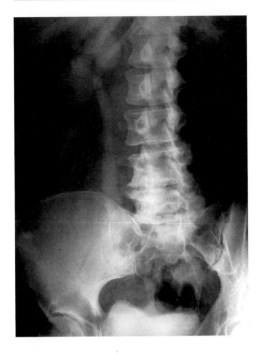 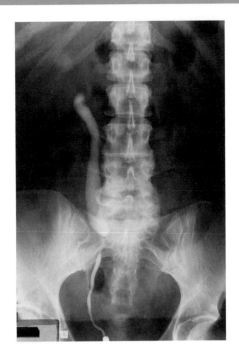

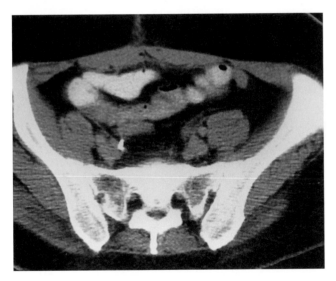

1. This patient has a history of cervical cancer treated with hysterectomy, lymph node dissection, and radiation therapy. Name the three studies that were performed.

2. What is the differential diagnosis?

3. What are the treatment options for this patient?

4. In this case, what is the indication for retrograde pyelography?

Pelvicalices and Ureter: Ureteral Stricture Resulting from Retroperitoneal Surgery

1. Intravenous urogram, retrograde pyelogram, and CT with oral contrast only.

2. Extrinsic ureteral compression by tumor, iatrogenic stricture, ureteral infection (tuberculosis or schistosomiasis), periureteral inflammation (endometriosis, inflammatory bowel disease, appendicitis, or diverticulitis), and radiation-induced stricture.

3. Stent placement, balloon dilation, and surgical resection of the stricture.

4. To further evaluate the obstructed right ureter, particularly the distal ureter, which is not visible on the excretory urogram.

References

Ghersin E, Brook OR, Meretik S, et al: Antegrade MDCT pyelography for the evaluation of patients with obstructed urinary tract, *Am J Roentgenol* 183: 1691–1696, 2004.

O'Malley ME, Hahn PF, Yoder IC, et al: Comparison of excretory phase, helical computed tomography with intravenous urography in patients with painless hematuria, *Clin Radiol* 58:294–300, 2003.

Cross-Reference

Zagoria RJ, *Genitourinary Radiology: THE REQUISITES,* 2nd ed, pp 179–186, 388–395.

Comment

This patient had a history of cervical carcinoma and had a hysterectomy with pelvic lymph node dissection and pelvic radiation 2 months before these imaging studies. She had no evidence of hydronephrosis before the surgical procedure. The intravenous urogram demonstrated right hydronephrosis and hydroureter extending down to the pelvis. The distal ureter could not be visualized on the intravenous urogram. The retrograde pyelogram demonstrated a short stricture and a normal distal ureter. The contrast-enhanced pelvic CT demonstrated enhancement of the right ureter but no adjacent soft tissue mass. The etiology of this stricture is believed to be iatrogenic (i.e., secondary to a right pelvic lymph node dissection with postoperative scarring adjacent to the ureter).

Ureteral narrowing has many different etiologies. As with most tubular structures, the causes of obstruction can be classified as intrinsic or extrinsic. Intrinsic causes of ureteral obstruction, such as a transitional cell carcinoma, tend to cause mucosal irregularity, which is not present in this case. Extrinsic causes of ureteral stricture occur from adjacent tumor (e.g., prostate cancer, cervical carcinoma, or lymphoma) or extrinsic masses (e.g., retroperitoneal fibrosis, endometriosis, inflammatory bowel disease, appendicitis). Extrinsic causes of ureteral obstruction are best demonstrated with cross-sectional imaging studies, such as CT. CT was helpful in this case because it demonstrated a normally opacified ureter but no mass adjacent to the stricture. Even though this patient received radiation therapy, a radiogenic stricture is unlikely because they typically develop 12 months or more after therapy.

Patients with strictures soon after surgery tend to respond well when treated with balloon dilation and stent placement. These patients have a better than 50% chance of complete resolution of the stricture. Long-standing strictures or those from malignant etiologies do not respond as well and may require other therapies. The ureteral stricture in this case was successfully treated with balloon dilation and stent placement.

Notes

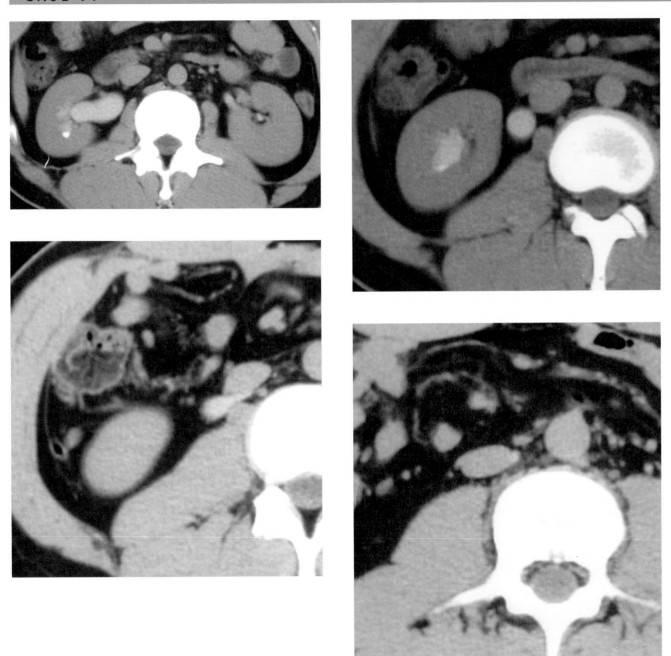

1. What is the cause of the right hydronephrosis and hydroureter of the proximal ureter seen above?

2. Abnormal development of which structure results in the above findings?

3. What is the differential diagnosis for medial displacement of the ureter in the lumbar region?

Pelvicalices and Ureter: Retrocaval Ureter

1. The right hydronephrosis and proximal hydroureter is caused by an abnormal course of the ureter posterior to the inferior vena cava known as a retrocaval (or circumcaval) ureter.

2. Retrocaval ureter is the result of anomalous embryologic development of the inferior vena cava.

3. Retroperitoneal fibrosis, retroperitoneal mass, previous surgery, and retrocaval ureter.

Reference

Lautin EM, Haramati N, Frager D, et al: CT diagnosis of circumcaval ureter, *Am J Roentgenol* 150:591–594, 1988.

Cross-Reference

Zagoria RJ, *Genitourinary Radiology: THE REQUISITES,* 2nd ed, p 166.

Comment

Retrocaval ureter results from anomalous development of the inferior vena cava and not from the ureter. Retrocaval ureter is a relatively rare condition with a reported autopsy prevalence of 0.9 in 1000 and a male-to-female ratio of approximately 3:1. The anomalous development of the inferior vena cava (IVC) results in the right ureter taking a course posterior to the IVC. The ureter then courses medially and anteriorly to resume its normal position. Symptoms when present from a retrocaval ureter are the result of obstructive symptoms related to the abnormal course.

Contrast-enhanced CT is the modality of choice for the diagnosis of retrocaval ureter because it allows visualization of the ureter and IVC simultaneously. Conventional intravenous urography (IVU) can demonstrate findings suggestive of retrocaval ureter, but is not diagnostic. These findings include medial displacement of the ureter relative to the pedicle of L3 and L4; however, this displacement can also be seen in retroperitoneal fibrosis, retroperitoneal mass, previous surgery, and retrocaval ureter.

Two types of retrocaval ureter have been defined radiologically. The more common form is type 1 in which the ureter courses behind the inferior vena cava at the level of the third lumbar vertebra and has an "S" or "fish-hook" deformity of the proximal ureter at the point of obstruction, usually resulting in moderate to severe hydronephrosis. In type 2, the hydronephrosis is usually less severe and the ureter crosses behind the IVC at the level of the renal pelvis.

Notes

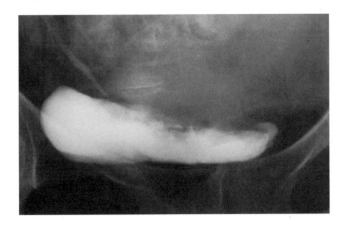
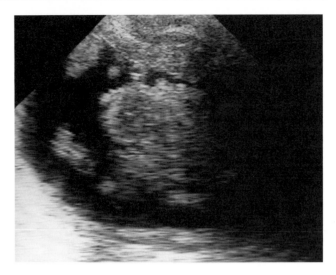

1. This patient has gross hematuria. Is it a clot or a tumor?

2. Within the bladder, what is the most common location of bladder carcinomas?

3. What is an important prognostic factor for bladder carcinoma?

4. What are the treatment options for patients with bladder carcinoma?

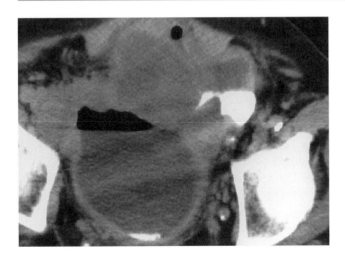

1. What is the most likely diagnosis?

2. True or false: The perivesical fat is normal.

3. Name four complications of bladder diverticula.

4. What is the most accurate cross-sectional imaging test for staging this disease?

Bladder: Bladder Carcinoma on Urography and Ultrasonography

1. Tumor.

2. Posterolateral wall near the trigone.

3. Depth of bladder wall invasion.

4. Cystoscopic fulguration, cystectomy, and chemotherapy.

Reference

Kundra V, Silverman PM: Imaging in the diagnosis, staging, and follow-up of cancer of the urinary bladder, *Am J Roentgenol* 180:1045–1054, 2003.

Cross-Reference

Zagoria RJ, *Genitourinary Radiology: THE REQUISITES,* 2nd ed, pp 206–207.

Comment

The filling defect demonstrated on the urogram shown here is typical for a carcinoma. Of bladder neoplasms, 95% are carcinomas, and of bladder carcinomas, 90% are transitional cell carcinomas. Risk factors are industrial carcinogen exposure, smoking, and analgesic abuse. Squamous cell carcinomas account for 5% of malignant neoplasms and are seen with increased frequency in patients with schistosomiasis. Squamous cell carcinoma is also more common in patients with a neurogenic bladder or a chronic indwelling Foley catheter and in the patient who has had multiple episodes of cystitis. Adenocarcinomas represent 2% of bladder carcinomas, are more frequently seen in urachal remnants, and usually affect patients with the rare condition of bladder exstrophy.

Depth of bladder wall invasion continues to be one of the most important prognostic factors. Five-year survival rates for patients with tumors invading the deep muscularis of the bladder are significantly worse than for those with noninvasive and superficial tumors. Superficial tumors (T1) are usually resected transurethrally, but the recurrence rate is high (50% to 90% within 2 years). Patients with deeper invasion of the bladder musculature (T2 or T3) are treated by cystectomy. Patients with metastatic disease or unresectable local spread (T4), are typically treated with chemotherapy.

Notes

Bladder: Stage IV Bladder Carcinoma Arising from a Diverticulum

1. Locally advanced bladder carcinoma arising in a bladder diverticulum.

2. False.

3. Infection, stone formation, neoplasm, and ureteral obstruction.

4. Enhanced MRI.

References

Kim JK, Park SY, Ahn HJ, et al: Bladder cancer: analysis of multi-detector row helical CT enhancement pattern and accuracy in tumor detection and perivesical staging, *Radiology* 231:725–731, 2004.

Tekes A, Kamel I, Imam K, et al: Dynamic MRI of bladder cancer: evaluation of staging accuracy, *Am J Roentgenol* 184:121–127, 2005.

Cross-Reference

Zagoria RJ, *Genitourinary Radiology: THE REQUISITES,* 2nd ed, pp 206–210, 219–220.

Comment

This case of locally advanced transitional cell carcinoma of the bladder arose from a bladder diverticulum. Bladder diverticula are usually acquired secondary to bladder outlet obstruction and increased intravesical pressure. Diverticula are common, increase in incidence with age, and are associated with a higher risk (2%–8%) of lower urinary tract infection, calculi, and neoplasm. These complications are presumably due to chronic irritation caused by urinary stasis.

The most sensitive technique for staging bladder carcinoma is enhanced MRI with dedicated surface coils. The accuracy for bladder staging ranges from 80% to 90% depending on the study. Notably, the accuracy of MRI in staging bladder carcinoma is highly technique-, operator-, and machine-dependent; institutions with extensive experience have reported the most accurate results. Multidetector row CT is accurate for detecting enlarged lymph nodes and direct invasion of the pelvic organs but is less accurate for predicting the depth of wall invasion because the carcinoma is isodense with the bladder wall.

The diagnosis of bladder carcinoma is usually made by cystoscopy and biopsy. Cystoscopic biopsy is important to establish the diagnosis and assess the depth of tumor invasion into the bladder wall. Depth of invasion determines tumor stage and treatment options. Surveillance cystoscopy is also used to assess for tumor recurrence in patients with previously diagnosed bladder neoplasms.

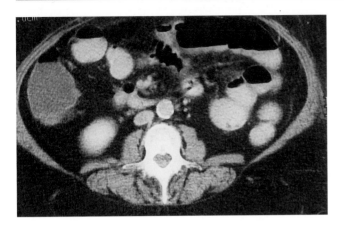 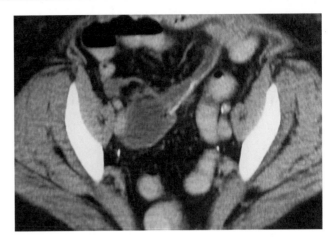

1. What procedure has been performed on this patient?

2. What are the indications for this procedure?

3. What are the advantages of this procedure over the traditional ileal loop?

4. What is an appropriate CT protocol for evaluating this type of patient?

Bladder: Indiana Pouch

1. Urinary diversion with an Indiana pouch formed from cecum and distal terminal ileum.

2. Prior cystectomy to treat carcinoma, a neurogenic bladder, or incapacitating urinary incontinence.

3. Larger reservoir, decreased reflux, and a continent ostomy.

4. Give either oral contrast alone or intravenous contrast alone. In this way the diversion can be separated reliably from the gastrointestinal tract.

References

Amis ES, Newhouse JH, Olsson CA: Continent urinary diversions: review of current surgical procedures and radiologic imaging, *Radiology* 168:395–401, 1998.

Nabi G, Yong SM, Ong E, et al: Is orthotopic bladder replacement the new gold standard? Evidence from a systematic review, *J Urol* 174:21–28, 2005.

Siegel C: Imaging of the various continent urinary diversions after cystectomy, *J Urol* 173:148, 2005.

Cross-Reference

Zagoria RJ, *Genitourinary Radiology: THE REQUISITES,* 2nd ed, pp 242–243.

Comment

In the past two decades, multiple new surgical procedures have been developed for the creation of continent urinary diversions. With continent diversions, the conduit is made of either small bowel alone or a combination of a terminal ileum and cecum. Egress from these loops can be to the skin through a continent ostomy or, if the sphincter and urethra are intact, to the proximal urethra. The latter procedure is called a bladder replacement or orthotopic diversion. To undergo an orthotopic diversion, patients must have unifocal bladder cancer with no involvement of the prostatic urethra. The goal of continent urinary diversions is to prevent reflux and to provide urinary continence. This technique obviates the need for an ostomy bag and provides sufficient capacity (0.5–1 liter) so that self-catheterization is required only every 3 to 6 hours.

The various types of continent diversions use different portions of the bowel and different types of anastomoses. For the Camey and Kock pouches, small bowel is used exclusively. Continent ostomy devices also can be created from terminal ileum and cecum (e.g., the Indiana, Mainz, Penn, and King techniques). For these procedures the cecum acts as a reservoir.

Postoperative complications of this procedure include extravasation of urine, infection, stone or fistula formation, and obstruction. Radiologic studies for the evaluation of continent urinary diversions include a loopogram to assess for leakage at the anastomosis site and an intravenous urogram to evaluate for urinary tract obstruction. CT is the study of choice to evaluate for abscess. In these patients it is usually preferable to use either oral or intravenous contrast material but not both. In this way the loop can be differentiated reliably from the bowel.

The most common long-term complications of urinary diversions are pyelonephritis from reflux (10%–30% of patients), nephrolithiasis (5%) and metachronous urothelial cancer (up to 33%) in patients with a history of bladder cancer.

Notes

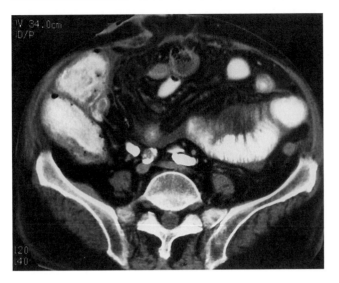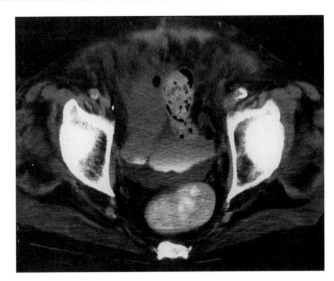

1. This patient had abdominal pain after creation of a Koch pouch. What is a Koch pouch?

2. What complication should be diagnosed in this case?

3. Name late complications of the Koch pouch.

4. Why do some patients with a Koch pouch develop megaloblastic anemia?

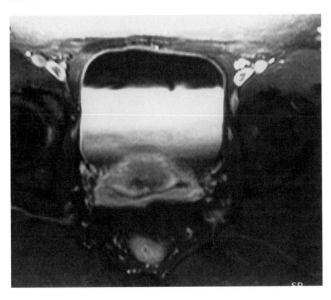

1. This is a T1W fat saturated image of the pelvis after administration of gadolinium-diethylene triamine pentaacetic acid (Gd-DTPA). True or false: Gd-DTPA is eliminated primarily in the urine.

2. True or false: After the intravenous administration of Gd-DTPA, the trilaminar appearance of urine in the bladder is visible on T1W images but not on T2W images.

3. At 1.5 T, what is the ratio of T1:T2 relaxation times for most tissues?

4. What is the ratio of T1:T2 when very high concentrations of Gd-DTPA are found in the urinary bladder?

CASE 101

Bladder: Urinary Leak from Koch Pouch

1. Continent cutaneous urinary diversion created from detubularized ileum.

2. Urinary leak.

3. Pouch stones, afferent nipple stenosis, ureteral reflux, incisional hernia, and anterior urethral stricture (in patients with hemi-Koch neobladder).

4. If more than 50 cm of terminal ileum is used to create this reservoir, diminished absorption of vitamin B_{12} may occur.

Reference

Nieh PT: The Koch pouch urinary reservoir, *Urol Clin North Am* 24:755–772, 1997.

Cross-Reference

Zagoria RJ, *Genitourinary Radiology: THE REQUISITES*, 2nd ed, pp 231–234.

Comment

The Koch pouch is a continent cutaneous urinary reservoir created from an 80-cm segment of ileum that has been detubularized (split longitudinally). The proximal end of ileum is intussuscepted to create a long, nonrefluxing nipple valve, and spatulated distal ureters are attached to this afferent limb. An efferent continent nipple valve is formed for the stoma, sited on the lower abdominal wall. Long-term exposure of the ileal mucosa to urine results in diminished prominence of the villi and production of mucus. A modification of this procedure is the hemi-Koch neobladder in which the most dependent portion of the pouch is anastomosed to the urethra.

Koch reservoirs are most often created for patients undergoing total cystectomy to treat bladder cancer; other situations in which these reservoirs are used include salvage prostatectomy to treat prostate cancer, refractory interstitial cystitis, neurogenic bladder, radiation cystitis, and conversion from other types of urinary diversions.

Early and late complications occur in approximately 15% of patients. The major early complications related to the pouch include anastomotic urine leak (2.5%), dehydration (2%), and urosepsis (1.7%). In this case urinary leak was suspected when a large amount of "free fluid" was noted on noncontrast CT. Anastomotic leak was confirmed on enhanced CT that demonstrated extravasated contrast pooling in the pelvis. Major late complications include struvite pouch stones (4%), afferent nipple stenosis (3%), and reflux (2%). Tumor may recur in the reservoir or upper urinary tracts.

Notes

CASE 102

Bladder: The Parfait Sign: MRI of the Bladder after Intravenous Gadopentetate Administration

1. True.

2. False.

3. Ranges from 5 to 10.

4. Approximately 1.3.

Reference

Elster AD, Sobol WT, Hinson WH: Pseudolayering of Gd-DTPA in the urinary bladder, *Radiology* 174:379–381, 1990.

Cross-Reference

Zagoria RJ, *Genitourinary Radiology: THE REQUISITES*, 2nd ed, pp 29–35.

Comment

Many radiologists have noticed the trilaminar appearance of urine in the bladder on MRI after contrast administration. Why is there no gradual change in signal intensity similar to the density change shown on enhanced CT? The signal of an MRI relates to the T1, T2, and number of protons (or proton density) of the tissue. T1 and T2 are physical properties of matter that describe how it behaves when placed in a magnetic field. MRI sequences can accentuate the T1 value of tissue (T1W images), the T2 value of tissue (T2W images) or the number of protons within tissue (proton density images). The T1 and T2 relaxation times of urine are approximately 7 seconds and 900 ms, respectively. With increasing concentrations of gadopentetate, the T1 and T2 relaxation times of urine-gadopentetate mixtures decrease.

There is a gradual increase in the concentration of gadopentetate in the dependent bladder of a supine patient, but three distinct "pseudolayers" are visible. The top layer represents pure urine with long T1 and is thus dark on the T1W image. The bottom layer of fluid represents urine with a high concentration of Gd-DTPA. The T2 value of the gadopentetate-urine mixture is very short, which accounts for the dark signal on T2W images. On T1W images the lowest layer has low signal intensity because the short T2 value (decreased signal intensity) predominates over the short T1 (increased signal intensity). The middle layer is hyperintense on T1W images because the T1 value of the mixture is relatively short and the T2 values are very long compared with the echo time.

Notes

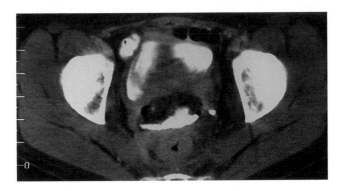 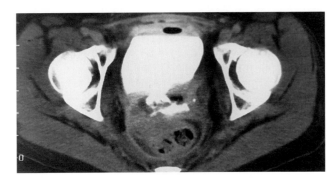

1. What is the most likely diagnosis in this case? What is the most common cause of this lesion in the United States?

2. What is the most common cause of this lesion worldwide?

3. What technical modifications of the CT protocol may improve detection of this lesion?

4. True or false: When this lesion is identified in the patient with cancer, viable tumor is always present.

CASE 103

Bladder: Vesicovaginal Fistula after Radiation Therapy for Cervical Cancer

1. Fistula from vagina to bladder. Radiation therapy for cervical carcinoma.

2. Obstetric trauma.

3. Administration of intravenous contrast only, thin-section imaging through the bladder and vagina, and delayed imaging.

4. False.

Reference

Kuhlman JE, Fishman EK: CT evaluation of enterovaginal and vesicovaginal fistulas, *J Comput Assist Tomogr* 14: 390–394, 1990.

Cross-Reference

Zagoria RJ, *Genitourinary Radiology: THE REQUISITES,* 2nd ed, pp 222–224.

Comment

Vaginal fistulas to the urinary or gastrointestinal tract reportedly occur in 1% to 10% of patients with cervical cancer who are treated with radiation therapy. Although vesicovaginal or ureterovaginal fistulas occur in patients who have not received radiation treatment, this presentation is uncommon. Some of the risk factors for the development of vaginal fistulas include extensive disease, the addition of hysterectomy to irradiation, and a high cumulative dose of radiation.

Many patients with vesicovaginal fistulas experience the classic symptom of passing urine via the vagina. Urography, cystography, vaginography, cystoscopy, and vaginoscopy have been used to evaluate vaginal fistulas to the urinary tract with variable results. Contrast radiologic studies may not demonstrate the fistula tract, particularly if the fistula is small or if its course is oblique or tortuous. Kuhlman and Fishman report that carefully performed enhanced CT detected 60% of vaginal fistulas to the bladder and bowel, whereas other radiologic and endoscopic studies provided false-negative results in 72% of cases. To detect vesicovaginal fistulas, their recommendations for optimal CT technique include (1) administration of intravenous contrast medium but no oral or rectal contrast and (2) additional delayed imaging 5 to 15 minutes later if the initial images show intravesical contrast but no contrast in the vagina. Thin-section (3–5 mm) images through the bladder and vagina may detect a small fistula. An additional advantage of CT is that it can provide insight regarding the cause of a vaginal fistula. For instance, in this case note the thickened rectal wall and the stranding of the perirectal fat resulting from radiotherapy.

Notes

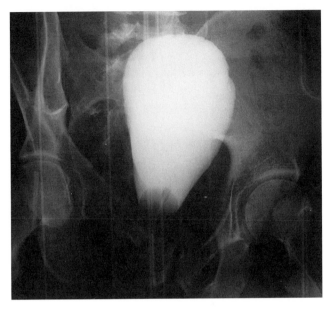
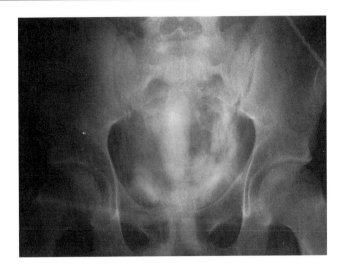

1. What is the most likely cause of the pear-shaped bladder in this case?

2. Name three other causes of pear-shaped bladder.

3. What disease causes increased pelvic radiolucency and a pear-shaped bladder?

4. What disease causes ureteral notching and a pear-shaped bladder?

CASE 104

Bladder: Pear-Shaped Bladder

1. Pelvic hematoma and urinoma.

2. Lipomatosis, inferior vena cava obstruction, lymphadenopathy, and lymphocysts.

3. Pelvic lipomatosis.

4. Venous collaterals that form after inferior vena cava obstruction.

Reference

Ambos MA, Bosniak MA, Lefleur RS, Madayag MA: The pear-shaped bladder, *Radiology* 122:85–88, 1977.

Cross-Reference

Zagoria RJ, *Genitourinary Radiology: THE REQUISITES*, 2nd ed, pp 170–171, 233.

Comment

In 1950 Prather and Kaiser used the term *teardrop* to describe the bladder deformity observed after pelvic fracture and hematoma formation. Nearly 50 years later, pelvic hematoma is still the most common cause of the pear-shaped, gourd-like, or inverted tear-shaped bladder. Pelvic hematoma (resulting from fractures, traumatized muscles, or torn branches of hypogastric arteries or pelvic veins), extraperitoneal urinoma, or both may cause the symmetric bladder compression and elevation that typifies this abnormal shape of the urinary bladder.

Of course, there is a differential diagnosis. Pelvic lipomatosis is caused by the deposition of large amounts of benign adipose and fibrous tissue in the perivesical and perirectal space. Symmetric compression and elevation by excessive pelvic fat cause the bladder to become gourd shaped; the rectum and lower ureters also have a characteristic compressive deformity. Lipomatosis is really the only disease that compresses the bladder bilaterally and causes increased radiolucency in the pelvis. Obstruction of the inferior vena cava may also cause a pear-shaped bladder. This diagnosis should be suspected when there is bilateral peripheral edema or venous collateral vessels visible on the lower abdominal wall. Bladder distortion is the result of compression by pelvic venous collateral vessels and edema. On urography, the ureters may be notched and displaced anteriorly and medially. Rarely, massive bilateral pelvic lymphadenopathy (caused by lymphoma or leukemia) or extensive lymphocyst formation (after extensive pelvic nodal dissections) may cause the bladder to assume a pear shape.

Notes

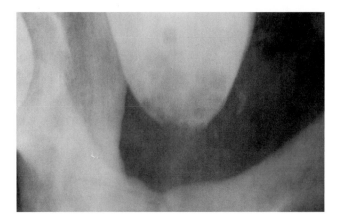

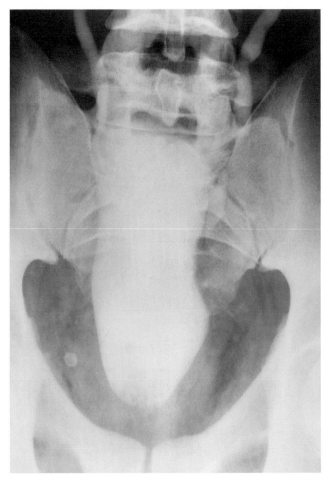

1. Two images of the bladder from an excretory urogram are shown. What is the differential diagnosis for the abnormal shape of the bladder?

2. On a barium enema examination (not shown), the rectosigmoid colon was elongated, straightened, and narrowed. What is the most likely diagnosis in this case?

3. What is the most likely cause of the lobulated filling defects in the urinary bladder?

4. True or false: In this disease, significant urinary obstruction is treated with excision of abnormal tissue around the bladder or ureters.

Bladder: Pelvic Lipomatosis with Cystitis Glandularis

1. The differential diagnosis for a pear- or gourd-shaped bladder includes perivesical hematoma, urinoma, abscess; iliopsoas hypertrophy; pelvic lipomatosis; lymphadenopathy; and inferior vena cava obstruction.

2. Pelvic lipomatosis.

3. Proliferative cystitis.

4. False. The massive amount of fat, its adherence to the pelvic viscera, and the ill-defined fascial planes make surgery difficult. When treatment of urinary obstruction is necessary, supravesical urinary diversion or ureteroneocystostomy can be performed.

Reference

Heyns CF, de Kock MLS, Kirsten PH, van Velden DJJ: Pelvic lipomatosis associated with cystitis glandularis and adenocarcinoma of the bladder, *J Urol* 145:364–366, 1991.

Cross-Reference

Zagoria RJ, *Genitourinary Radiology: THE REQUISITES*, 2nd ed, pp 170–171, 212.

Comment

Pelvic lipomatosis is a rare and poorly understood disease typified by the proliferation of mature adipose tissue, fibrous tissue, and chronic inflammatory cells in the pelvis. There is a marked gender and racial predominance; 94% of patients are men, and two thirds of them are African-American. Many patients have systemic hypertension and are obese. Obstruction of the urinary tract, rectum, iliac veins, and inferior vena cava may occur. Although usually confined to the pelvis, fibrofatty proliferation may extend cephalad to involve the perinephric space, omentum, and small bowel mesentery.

Findings that suggest this diagnosis include anterosuperior elevation and symmetric compression of the urinary bladder (i.e., pear- or gourd-shaped bladder). The lower third of the ureters may be deviated medially, and there can be hydroureteronephrosis.

Heyns and co-workers reported proliferative cystitis (i.e., cystitis cystica or cystitis glandularis) in 78% of patients with pelvic lipomatosis. Several other diseases have been associated with pelvic lipomatosis, including chronic urinary tract infection, superficial thrombophlebitis, retroperitoneal fibrosis, nontropical chyluria, and the Proteus syndrome (lipomatosis, cutaneous and visceral vascular malformations, hemihypertrophy, and exostoses).

Notes

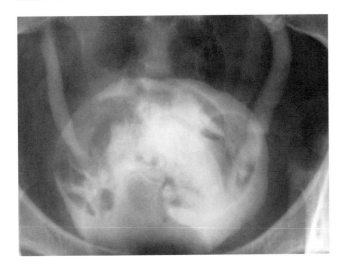
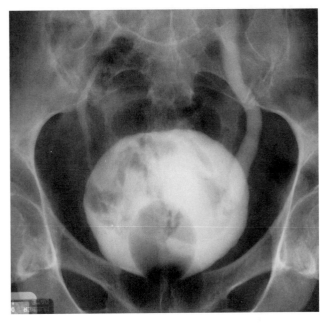

1. This patient has atraumatic, fulminant, gross hematuria. What is the most likely cause of the large filling defects in the bladder?

2. Name three causes of this disease.

3. True or false: The association of penicillin use with hemorrhagic cystitis has been linked to a urotoxic metabolite.

4. Diffuse vesical bleeding may be the initial sign of what disease? (Hint: This disease may occur in patients with long-standing rheumatoid arthritis.)

Bladder: Hemorrhagic Cystitis

1. Blood clots.

2. Consumption of urotoxins, radiation therapy, and viral infection.

3. False.

4. Amyloidosis.

Reference

deVries CR, Freiha FS: Hemorrhagic cystitis: a review, *J Urol* 143:1–9, 1990.

Cross-Reference

Zagoria RJ, *Genitourinary Radiology: THE REQUISITES,* 2nd ed, p 212.

Comment

Hemorrhagic cystitis (HC) is defined as diffuse vesical bleeding and can be either acute or insidious. The major causes of HC are (1) chemical toxins, (2) radiation therapy, (3) immune-mediated injury, and (4) idiopathic disease. Most cases of severe vesical hemorrhage are caused by radiotherapy or chemotherapeutic agents. Of the latter, oxazaphosphorine alkylating agents (e.g., cyclophosphamide and ifosfamide) are most commonly linked to HC, but busulfan and thiotepa also have been implicated. Cyclophosphamide cystitis is discussed more completely in Case 107, but an important point is that its urotoxic effects are mediated by acrolein, the aldehyde by-product of cyclophosphamide metabolism. In contrast, other drugs may cause HC through an immune-mediated mechanism that is the proposed etiology of bladder mucosal injury associated with the use of penicillin and danazol.

Radiation cystitis most commonly presents after treatment for prostate or cervical cancer and less commonly after treatment for rectal or bladder cancers. Approximately 20% of patients treated with pelvic radiation have symptoms referable to the bladder, and in one study, 9% of patients treated with full-dose radiation therapy developed HC. Hematuria may occur months to years after treatment and begins with mucosal edema, telangiectasia, and submucosal hemorrhage. Over the long term an obliterative endarteritis of the detrusor may manifest as a shrunken, fibrotic bladder.

In the middle of the 1970s, irritative voiding symptoms and gross hematuria were reported in children during several outbreaks of adenovirus type 11. Subsequently, HC has been observed in bone marrow transplant recipients, presumably as a result of reactivation of a latent form of this virus. Other viruses implicated in HC include adenovirus type 21, polyoma, and influenza A.

Notes

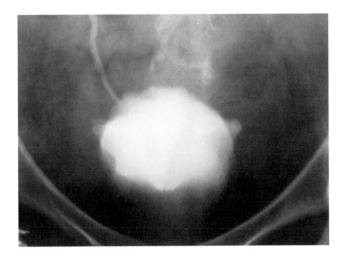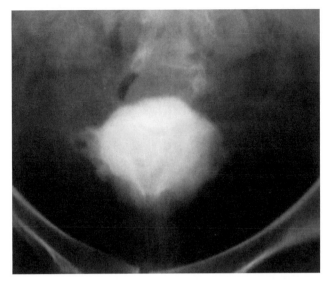

1. This patient was treated with multiple, high doses of cyclophosphamide. True or false: Cystitis secondary to cyclophosphamide administration usually occurs during or immediately after treatment is begun.

2. True or false: The prophylactic administration of mesna is effective in reducing bladder toxicity caused by the oxazaphosphorine alkylating agents (cyclophosphamide and ifosfamide) because it binds directly to the drugs.

3. What is the first-line treatment for hemorrhagic cystitis associated with cyclophosphamide toxicity?

4. True or false: The risk for invasive urothelial bladder cancer is increased in patients who have undergone prolonged cyclophosphamide treatment.

Bladder: Cyclophosphamide Cystitis

1. True.

2. False.

3. Forced diuresis, bladder irrigations, and mesna.

4. True.

Reference

Bramble FJ, Morley R: Drug-induced cystitis: the need for vigilance, *Br J Urol* 79:3–7, 1997.

Cross-Reference

Zagoria RJ, *Genitourinary Radiology: THE REQUISITES,* 2nd ed, p 212.

Comment

Shortly after it was introduced for clinical use in 1958, cyclophosphamide was noted to cause frequency, urgency, dysuria, and hematuria in some patients. The reported incidence of cyclophosphamide cystitis is 2% to 4%; hemorrhagic cystitis occurs commonly and more often in patients on cyclophosphamide than in patients on other drugs that cause cystitis. Ifosfamide is a structural isomer of cyclophosphamide and has even greater urotoxicity. Symptoms usually begin during or just after treatment, and delayed hemorrhage occurs only in patients on long-term therapy. In the short term, bladder injury is manifested as mucosal erythema, inflammation, ulceration, necrosis, and oozing from small vessels. Marked bladder contraction (caused by fibrosis) and invasive bladder tumors take much longer to develop, appearing months to years after cessation of therapy. There is a 45-fold increased risk for and a 5% incidence of invasive transitional cell carcinoma after prolonged cyclophosphamide use.

Urotoxicity is mediated by an aldehyde metabolite of the oxazaphosphorine alkylating agent acrolein. Mesna (2-mercaptoethane sulfonate) was developed specifically to bind acrolein and, when prophylactically administered, can reduce the bladder toxicity but not the therapeutic effects of cyclophosphamide.

The treatment of hemorrhagic cystitis secondary to cyclophosphamide or ifosfamide begins with saline bladder irrigations, diuresis, and mesna administration. If these measures are not successful, cystoscopy and diathermy of bleeding points can be performed. Chemical cautery by intravesical administration of formalin, phenol, silver nitrate, or alum also has been advocated. If hemorrhage is life threatening, embolization or ligation of the internal iliac arteries and even cystectomy have been performed.

Notes

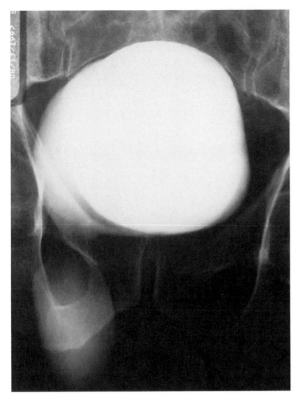
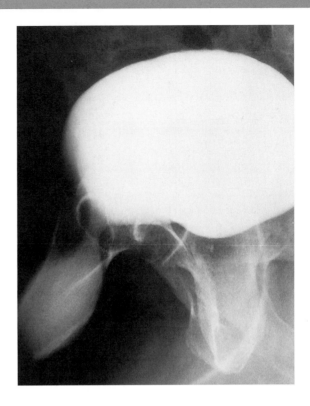

1. Through which canal is the bladder herniating?

2. What is the classic clinical voiding pattern associated with bladder hernia?

3. An indirect inguinal hernia lies lateral to which artery?

4. Name three complications of bladder hernia.

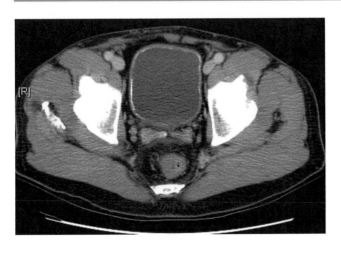
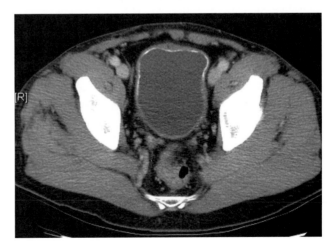

1. What is the finding and differential diagnosis?

2. What is the next step in diagnostic workup?

3. What is the most frequent worldwide cause of bladder wall calcification?

4. What additional imaging features would be suspicious for malignancy?

Bladder: Inguinal Herniation of the Bladder

1. Inguinal canal.

2. Two-stage voiding.

3. Deep inferior epigastric artery.

4. Hydronephrosis, strangulation, stone formation, vesicoureteral reflux, tumor, and inadvertent perforation during surgery.

Reference

Bacigalupo LE, Bertolotto M, Barbiera F, et al: Imaging of urinary bladder hernias, *Am J Roentgenol* 184:546–551, 2005.

Cross-Reference

Zagoria RJ, *Genitourinary Radiology: THE REQUISITES,* 2nd ed, pp 221–222.

Comment

Herniations of the bladder are usually found at herniorrhaphy and are rarely discovered clinically. Large herniations may present with two-stage voiding; the patient empties the normotopic bladder initially but voids again after manually decompressing the hernia. Almost three fourths of all hernias occur through the inguinal canal and predominantly affect men. Femoral hernias are more common in women. With respect to the relationship of the hernia to the peritoneal space, the paraperitoneal hernia is most common; part of the parietal peritoneum herniates lateral to the bladder hernia, which remains extraperitoneal. Rarely the bladder can herniate into the obturator canal, ventral abdominal wall, or other abdominopelvic openings. Conditions that predispose individuals to bladder herniation include structural defects in the abdominal wall, atrophy of inguinal supportive tissues, and bladder outlet obstruction.

The radiologist should suspect herniation of the bladder when there is lateral displacement of the pelvic ureter or hydronephrosis (caused by traction on the trigone), an asymmetric and small bladder, and when the bladder base is not completely visible or is drawn to one side. Supine and prone radiographs are successful in demonstrating only 30% and 50% of bladder hernias, respectively. Only the erect view is uniformly successful in showing the abnormality. The herniated bladder is clearly demonstrated on cystography, whereas the hernial opening may be overlooked on cystoscopy.

Inguinal or scrotal ultrasonography or CT may show the bladder herniation, although the differential diagnosis for a scrotal fluid collection includes hydrocele, varicocele, spermatocele, epididymal cyst, intestinal hernia, and ectopic ureterocele.

Notes

Bladder: Bladder Schistosomiasis

1. Mural bladder calcification. The differential diagnosis includes schistosomiasis, tuberculous cystitis, radiation cystitis, alkaline-encrusted cystitis, intravesicular chemotherapy, and neoplasm.

2. Cystoscopy and biopsy.

3. Schistosomiasis.

4. Associated bladder mass and disruption of mural calcifications.

References

Jorulf T, Lindstedt E: Urogenital schistosomiasis: CT evaluation, *Radiology* 157:745–749, 1985.

Thoumas D, Darmallaicq C, Pfister C, et al: Imaging characteristics of alkaline-encrusted cystitis and pyelitis, *Am J Roentgenol* 178:389–392, 2002.

Cross-Reference

Zagoria RJ, *Genitourinary Radiology: THE REQUISITES,* 2nd ed, pp 227–228.

Comment

Schistosomiasis is the most common worldwide cause of bladder wall calcification. *Schistosoma haematobium* liver flukes travel from the lungs to reside in the portomesenteric veins, and then migrate to the lower urinary tract, prostate, and lower gastrointestinal tract. Female schistosomes deposit eggs in the venules of the bladder wall, resulting in granuloma formation, obliterative end-arteritis, and fibrosis. The entire bladder is usually involved, but the calcification pattern is variable. Chronic schistosomiasis is a risk factor for all types of bladder carcinoma, most commonly squamous cell type. Calcification disruption should raise suspicion for malignant transformation. Cystoscopy is usually performed to confirm diagnosis and exclude malignancy. Schistosomiasis is usually treated with praziquantel.

Chronic tuberculous cystitis may be associated with bladder wall calcification. Tuberculous infection of the genitourinary tract usually begins in the kidney and descends, whereas schistosomiasis affects the prostate and bladder first and then ascends. In addition, tuberculous cystitis usually results in a fibrotic bladder with decreased volume while a bilharzial bladder is usually distensible. Alkaluria and inflammatory bladder wall lesions may result in dystrophic bladder wall calcifications known as alkaline encrustation cystitis. Urea-splitting bacteria such as *Proteus* and *Corynebacterium* lead to urine alkalinization, which leads to subsequent dystrophic calcification in regions of bladder wall necrosis.

Notes

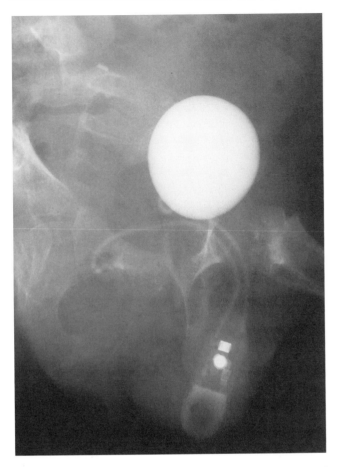

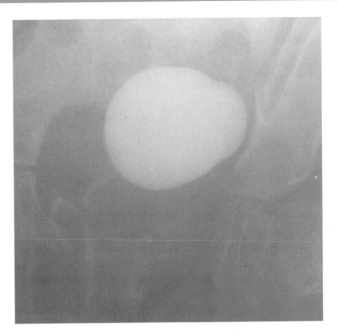

1. What device is shown in the radiograph on the left?

2. The radiograph on the right was taken 2 years later. What is the diagnosis?

3. What is the most common indication for the implantation of this device in children?

4. True or false: A normal upper urinary tract is considered a prerequisite for implanting this device.

Urethra: Artificial Urinary Sphincter

1. Artificial urinary sphincter.

2. Deformity suggests mechanical failure of the reservoir.

3. Incontinence as a result of spinal dysraphism.

4. True.

Reference

Simeoni J, Guys JM, Mollard P, et al: Artificial urinary sphincter implantation for neurogenic bladder: a multi-institutional study in 107 children, *Br J Urol* 78:287–293, 1996.

Cross-Reference

Zagoria RJ, *Genitourinary Radiology: THE REQUISITES,* 2nd ed, pp 232, 234.

Comment

The artificial urinary sphincter (AUS) was introduced in 1972 and has been used in the management of stress incontinence and postprostatectomy sphincter weakness and as a part of complex reconstructive surgery of the lower urinary tract. In the large series referenced above, the most common indication for implantation of the AUS in children was incontinence caused by spinal dysraphism.

The AUS consists of the following three tube-connected components: (1) a pressure-regulated reservoir in the abdomen, (2) a pump (in this case placed in the scrotum), and (3) a periurethral cuff. The reservoir, filled with dilute iodinated contrast, maintains a constant and pre-determined pressure in the periurethral cuff, which can be placed around the bladder neck or bulbar urethra. When squeezed, the scrotal pump shifts fluid out of the cuff and into the reservoir. This action decreases the urethral pressure to permit bladder emptying. Fluid then is automatically returned to the cuff by a resistor that is incorporated in the pump.

Despite achieving urinary continence in 77% of children, the AUS has a reported long-term complication rate of 59%. Complications include mechanical problems with the AUS, surgical complications, and long-term bladder adaptations. The most common mechanical problem is pump malfunction. A common surgical complication is erosion of the bulbous urethra or bladder neck caused by an improperly fitted cuff. Detrusor hyperreflexia and low bladder compliance are the most common changes in bladder function that occur with long-term use. There is a high incidence of secondary reflux in patients with neurogenic bladder that might be exacerbated by the AUS. Hence a normal upper urinary tract and, if necessary, surgical treatment of vesicoureteral reflux are necessary before implantation of the AUS.

Notes

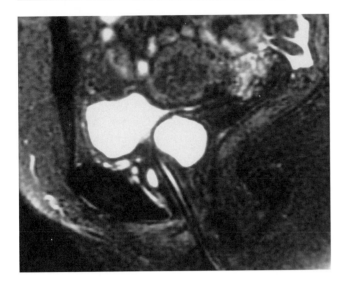 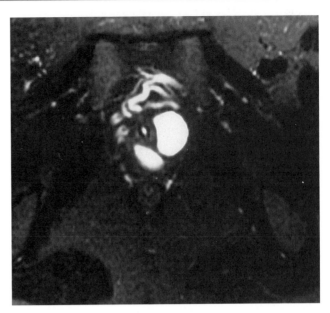

1. This patient has postvoid dribbling and dyspareunia. What is the differential diagnosis?

2. True or false: The congenital form of this lesion most often affects girls and may obstruct the urethra.

3. True or false: Urethral diverticula are much more common in African-American women.

4. True or false: Gartner's ducts are the remnants of the wolffian ducts left in the wall of the vagina, cervix, or broad ligament.

Urethra: MRI of Urethral Diverticulum

1. Diverticulum of either the urethra or the bladder.

2. False. 98% occur in boys.

3. True.

4. True.

Reference

Kim B, Hricak H, Tanagho EA: Diagnosis of urethral diverticula in women: value of MR imaging, *Am J Roentgenol* 161:809–815, 1993.

Cross-Reference

Zagoria RJ, *Genitourinary Radiology: THE REQUISITES,* 2nd ed, pp 250, 254.

Comment

Diverticula of the urethra are uncommon but often overlooked causes of dyspareunia, postvoid dribbling, irritative voiding symptoms, and urinary tract infections in women. They are estimated to occur in 1.4% to 4.7% of women and are about six times more common in the African-American population. The diverticulum is believed to form after obstruction of the paraurethral glands by traumatic injury or infection. Chronic inflammation leads to a cavity that may epithelialize, producing a diverticulum.

Although they can form anywhere along the length of the female urethra, diverticula are more commonly located dorsolaterally in the middle third (in 66% of cases) and are rarely located distally (in about 10% of cases). Conventional evaluation of a suspected urethral diverticulum includes urethroscopy and contrast urethrography. For the diagnosis of female urethral diverticulum, the following studies are specific but less sensitive: urethroscopy (70% sensitivity), voiding cystourethrography, (65% sensitivity), and double-balloon urethrography (85% sensitivity).

MRI may be used to evaluate periurethral masses, particularly when conventional diagnostic tests are inconclusive or discrepant. Diverticula appear as septated, horseshoe-shaped, fluid-filled periurethral masses on MRI; calculi and neoplasms arising from within the diverticulum also can be demonstrated. The displaced urethra can be separated from the diverticulum, and sagittal MRIs show the relationship of the mass to the vagina and bladder floor well. The size and extent of the diverticulum and the extent of periurethral inflammation can be more accurately assessed by cross-sectional imaging.

Notes

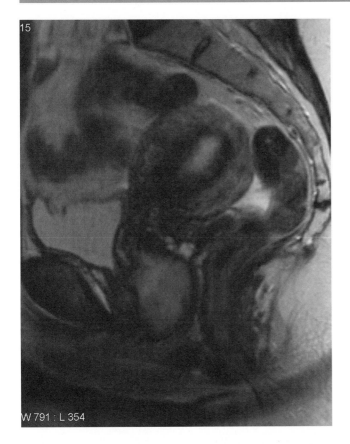

W 791 : L 354

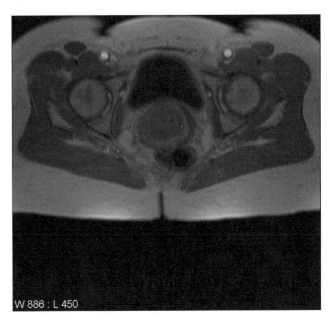

W 886 : L 450

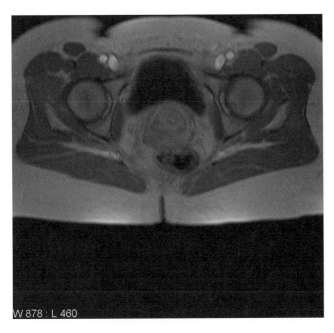

W 878 : L 460

1. On the T2-weighted sagittal image, where is the mass located?

2. On the axial T1-weighted images, what is the relevance of contrast administration?

3. What is the diagnosis?

4. What is the most common tumor cell type within a diverticulum?

Urethra: Urethral Diverticulum with Cancer

1. Between the vagina and urethra.

2. Demonstration of vascular neoplasm within the diverticulum; note that the bladder does not enhance.

3. Urethral diverticulum containing a malignant tumor.

4. Adenocarcinoma.

Reference

Siegelman E, Banner M, Ramchandani P, et al: Multicoil MR imaging of symptomatic female urethral and periurethral disease, *Radiographics* 17:349–365, 1997.

Cross-Reference

Zagoria RJ, *Genitourinary Radiology: THE REQUISITES*, 2nd ed, pp 248–249.

Comment

The walls of the female urethra are filled with glands, the greatest number posteriorly. Skene's glands arise from the lower urethra but drain on the vestibular surface on either side of the urethral meatus. Obstruction presents as a fluctuant mass extending inferiorly from the perineum. The obstruction of the smaller, secretory glands leads to the formation of a diverticulum. These outpouchings may be saccular, bilobed, or circumferential. Presentation is that of recurrent urinary dribbling or infection, and physical examination reveals a labial mass. It is important to identify the neck of the diverticulum with as great a degree of accuracy as possible because surgery is often technically difficult.

Multiple imaging tests can be used to diagnose urethral diverticula, the simplest being a voiding cystourethrogram. When this fails, transperineal ultrasonography and MRI should be considered. T2-weighted MRIs in the sagittal, axial, and coronal plane will show a well-circumscribed high-signal-intensity mass that abuts or encases the ureter. A debris level may be identified in the dependent portion of the diverticulum. When a tumor is suspected, contrast material must be administered intravenously to clearly delineate the presence of a vascular neoplasm. Unfortunately, because no muscle layer separates the diverticulum from adjacent tissues, tumor extension beyond the confines of the urethra is usually rapid and the prognosis is poor. Treatment usually consists of radiation and pelvic exenteration. Occasionally, a tumor arising from the vagina or other adjacent tissues will mimic a periurethral mass. Close review of the sagittal MRIs can be of particular help in identifying the organ of origin.

Notes

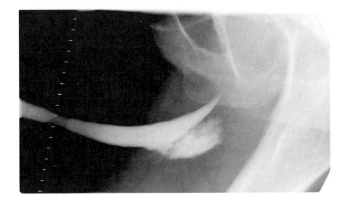
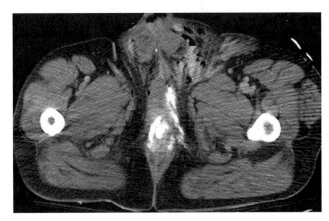

1. What is the diagnosis?

2. What are the four parts of the male urethra?

3. What is more common in the trauma setting, complete or partial urethral disruption? How do you differentiate these two entities on a retrograde urethrogram?

4. What is initial treatment?

Urethra: Urethral Injury

1. Traumatic urethral injury.

2. There are anterior and posterior portions, separated by the urogenital diaphragm. Each is made up of two parts: penile and bulbous in the anterior portion and membranous and prostatic in the posterior portion.

3. Complete disruption is twice as common as partial disruption. With complete disruption, there is no retrograde filling of contrast into the bladder.

4. Diversion of urinary stream via suprapubic catheter.

Reference

Goldman SM, Sandler CM, Corriere JN Jr, McGuire EJ: Blunt urethral trauma: a unified anatomical mechanical classification, *J Urol* 157:85–89, 1997.

Cross-Reference

Zagoria RJ, *Genitourinary Radiology: THE REQUISITES,* 2nd ed, pp 203–204, 243–248.

Comment

Urethral injury is seen most commonly in the setting of blunt trauma. Approximately 10% of major pelvic ring disruptions result in urethral injury. Males are four times more likely than females to have urethral injury due to increased length of the male urethra. The retrograde urethrogram remains the preferred radiologic test for diagnosing urethral injury. In the trauma setting, a patient who is unable to void, has a distended bladder on physical examination, or particularly has meatal blood should prompt performance of this procedure. Positive findings necessitate suprapubic catheter placement for 3 to 6 months.

Differentiation of partial from complete disruptions is important because complete disruptions (which are twice as common) have a much higher incidence of stricture formation.

The Colapinto-McCallum classification system for posterior urethral injury is based on retrograde urethrogram findings:

Type I: Elongated, but intact prostatic urethra. There is no extravasation of contrast on retrograde urethrogram.

Type II: Disrupted membranous urethra at the apex of the prostate proximal to an intact urogenital diaphragm. There is extravasation of contrast in the retropubic extraperitoneal space, but not extension of contrast into the perineum due to the intact urogenital diaphragm.

Type III: The most common injury (and demonstrated in this case); disrupted membranous and bulbous urethra with a disrupted urogenital diaphragm. There is extravasation of contrast into the perineum.

Anterior urethral injuries are less common than posterior injuries and the most frequent etiologies include iatrogenic instrumentation or straddle injuries. On retrograde urethrography there is extravasation of contrast from the penile or bulbous urethra into the corpus spongiosum or corpus cavernosum.

The diagnosis of urethral injury in the trauma patient is important to establish and prevent (1) misplacement of a Foley catheter through a urethral tear, (2) bladder outlet obstruction, and (3) long-term complications including stricture, incontinence, and impotence. Urethral strictures are estimated to occur in up to 97% of complete traumatic urethral disruptions but are much less common with partial lacerations. Strictures are treated with urethral dilatations or urethroplasty.

Notes

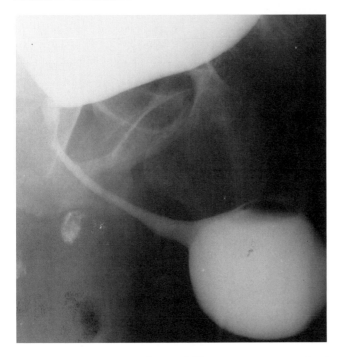 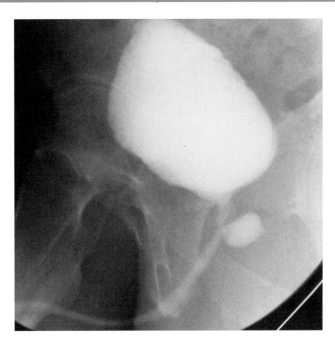

1. These images are from different patients with the same type of lesion. What is the diagnosis?

2. True or false: This lesion can be congenital or acquired.

3. Name two causes of the acquired form of this lesion.

4. Of utricular and müllerian cysts, which is usually identified in patients younger than 20 years of age?

C A S E   1 1 4

Urethra: Acquired Urethral Diverticulum

1. Urethral diverticulum in a male patient.

2. True.

3. Infection, trauma, and prolonged catheterization.

4. Utricular cysts.

Reference

Calenoff L, Foley MJ, Hendrix RW: Evaluation of the urethra in males with spinal cord injury, *Radiology* 142:71–76, 1982.

Cross-Reference

Zagoria RJ, *Genitourinary Radiology: THE REQUISITES,* 2nd ed, pp 250, 254.

Comment

These cases are examples of acquired urethral diverticula in men. The first image shows a giant anterior urethral diverticulum that developed in an incontinent, paraplegic man as a result of long-term use of a penile clamp. The second image shows a posterior urethral diverticulum with a narrow neck and an off-midline orifice. Recall that utricle and müllerian duct cysts are typically midline prostatic cysts.

Although occasionally discovered in men, acquired urethral diverticula are much more common in women. Diverticula may occur after urethral infection or trauma, as a result of prolonged use of an indwelling catheter, or after urethral surgery or use of other instrumentation. In some cases a periurethral abscess may drain into the urethra and thereby form a diverticulum; this process is the most common etiology of a posterior urethral diverticulum. Because of prolonged transurethral catheterization, paraplegics are particularly prone to developing urethritis and diverticula. Unlike congenital diverticula, acquired diverticula are not lined by epithelium. Although stones and carcinoma may form in diverticula of the female urethra, these complications are rare in men with acquired urethral diverticula.

When they occur after urethral instrumentation or catheterization, these focal dilations are located in areas of normal urethral narrowing (e.g., the membranous urethra and penoscrotal junction). A premonitory sign of a membranous urethral diverticulum on urethrography is the "spiral sign," a few rings of contrast material encircling the membranous urethra. This sign is usually the result of overdistention of the external sphincter during instrumentation.

Notes

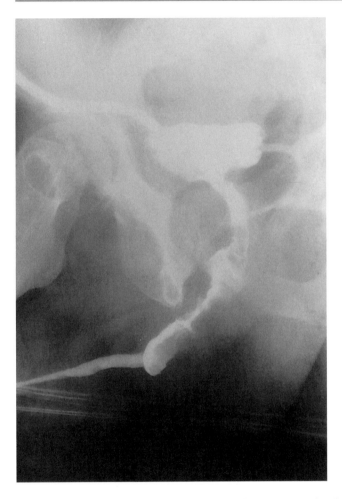

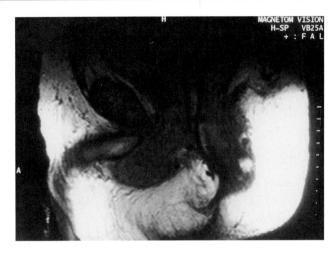

1. What is the differential diagnosis for this urethral lesion?

2. Name three benign urethral lesions that can mimic a urethral neoplasm.

3. What is the most commonly cited risk factor for squamous cell carcinoma of the urethra?

4. What findings should alert the clinician to the presence of urethral carcinoma after urethroplasty?

Urethra: Squamous Cell Carcinoma of the Male Urethra

1. Tumor and tumorlike conditions of the urethra. Malignant tumor is most likely.

2. Papillary urethritis, nephrogenic adenoma, and inflammatory polyp can mimic a benign urethral tumor. Condylomata acuminata, amyloidosis, sarcoidosis, and balanitis xerotica obliterans can mimic a more aggressive malignant tumor.

3. Chronic urethral stricture of any cause.

4. Recurrence of stricture or urethral obstruction, fistula or abscess formation, and induration or ulceration.

Reference

Hricak H, Marotti M, Gilbert TJ, et al: Normal penile anatomy and abnormal penile conditions: evaluation with MR imaging, *Radiology* 169:683–687, 1998.

Cross-Reference

Zagoria RJ, *Genitourinary Radiology: THE REQUISITES,* 2nd ed, p 248.

Comment

Carcinoma of the urethra is at least twice as common in women as in men. These uncommon tumors are discovered in men older than 50 years of age. Common clinical presentations include a palpable mass or induration in the perineum or urethra, obstructive voiding symptoms, a urethral fistula, and a periurethral abscess.

The major histologic types of urethral malignancy include squamous cell carcinoma (80%), transitional cell carcinoma (15%), adenocarcinoma (4%), and undifferentiated tumor (1%). The major risk factor for squamous cell carcinoma is chronic urethral irritation secondary to urethral stricture, and it has been suggested that urethroplasty reduces the risk for carcinoma associated with urethral stricture. Approximately 60% of urethral squamous cell carcinomas occur in the bulbomembranous urethra, and 34% arise in the distal bulbar or penile urethra. The prognosis for anterior urethral carcinoma is much better than that of the posterior urethra (5-year survival rate of 43% versus 14%, respectively).

Carcinoma should be suspected when a urethral stricture is associated with multiple, irregular filling defects. A stricture with ill-defined margins is suspicious. Diverticula, fistula, or perineal abscess formation may be associated. MRI may demonstrate the full extent of the stricture-associated mass, as well as local invasion of the corporal bodies or perineum and lymphatic metastases.

Notes

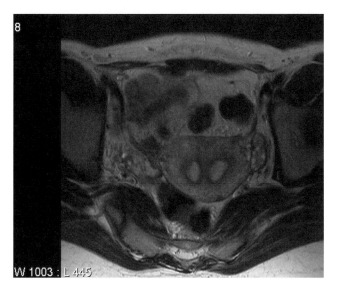
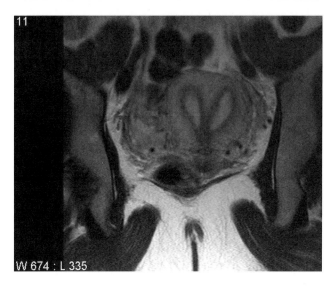

1. Based on the uterine fundal contour, what is the most likely diagnosis?

2. Based on the type of tissue between the uterine cornua, what is the most likely diagnosis?

3. From the perspective of treatment, why is it important to identify the type of dividing tissue in patients with uterine fusion anomalies?

4. True or false: Infertility is more common in patients with septate uterus than in those with bicornuate uterus.

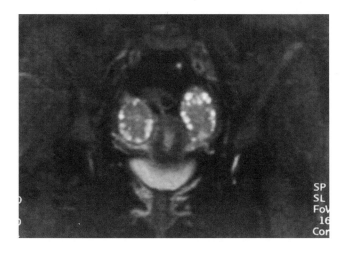
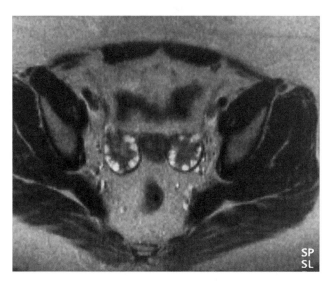

1. What are the significant findings on the T2W images in this case?

2. What is the likely clinical history in this case?

3. How is this disease diagnosed?

4. True or false: The appearance of the ovaries is pathognomonic for this disease.

Ob/Gyn: Septate Uterus on MRI

1. Septate uterus.

2. Bicornuate uterus.

3. Septate uterus containing a fibrous septum can be treated with hysteroscopic metroplasty; bicornuate uterus is usually treated with abdominal metroplasty.

4. True.

Reference

Troiano RN, McCarthy SM: Müllerian duct anomalies: imaging and clinical issues, *Radiology* 233:19–34, 2004.

Cross-Reference

Zagoria RJ, *Genitourinary Radiology: THE REQUISITES,* 2nd ed, pp 261–266.

Comment

Both bicornuate and septate uteri represent incomplete fusion of the two müllerian ducts. When corrective surgery is contemplated, the nature of the dividing tissue is important. When a thin (typically fibrous) septum separates the endometrial cavity, excision of the hypovascular septum may be accomplished using the hysteroscope. Hysteroscopic metroplasty may be performed as an outpatient procedure. However, if unification surgery is elected to correct a uterus divided by myometrial tissue, the vascularity of that tissue necessitates metroplasty by an abdominal approach. Abdominal resection usually requires a 5- to 10-day hospital stay. Although there are diagnostic criteria for both bicornuate and septate uteri on ultrasonography and hysterosalpingography, the nature of the dividing tissue is most accurately defined by MRI.

For the oral board examination it is prudent to be aware of the classic definitions of these two müllerian anomalies on MRI. However, many gynecologists believe that an accurate definition of the dividing tissue is more important than the diagnosis of bicornuate or septate uterus per se. In bicornuate uterus the fundus is typically more deeply concave, and the two horns are usually divergent. A distance of more than 4 cm separates the two horns, and the dividing tissue is isointense with outer myometrium on T2W images. However, Carrington and co-workers noted that this tissue may be hypointense at the level of the lower uterine segment in some cases. The fundal contour of the septate uterus is convex, flat, or minimally indented (less than 1 cm), and the intercornual distance is normal (2–4 cm). The septum has an intermediate to low signal intensity on both T1W and T2W images. More recent work has shown that some septate uteri may contain dividing tissue that is typical of outer myometrium (as in this case).

Notes

Ob/Gyn: Polycystic Ovary Disease

1. There are multiple small follicles along the periphery of both ovaries in this obese patient.

2. Infertility, hirsutism, obesity, and oligomenorrhea.

3. Through the combination of an appropriate clinical history and an elevated luteinizing hormone/follicle-stimulating hormone (LH:FSH) ratio. Characteristically the LH:FSH ratio is greater than 2.

4. False.

Reference

Kimura I, Togashi K, Kawakami S, et al: Polycystic ovaries: implications of diagnosis with MR imaging, *Radiology* 201:549–552, 1996.

Cross-Reference

Zagoria RJ, *Genitourinary Radiology: THE REQUISITES,* 2nd ed, p 282.

Comment

Polycystic ovary disease (PCOD), or Stein-Leventhal syndrome, was originally described as an X-linked autosomal-dominant disease. The fundamental pathophysiologic characteristic of this disease is chronic anovulation in the setting of acyclic estrogen production. The ovaries were originally described as being enlarged, with multiple small follicles located peripherally in the gland, but the ovary is normal in size in as many as 30% of patients. The primary abnormality in PCOD is increased production of androgens (initially from the adrenal glands and in later stages from the ovary) and its peripheral conversion to estrogen in subcutaneous fat. This conversion is facilitated in obese patients. The elevated serum estrogen level causes suppression of follicle-stimulating hormone (FSH) and elevation of luteinizing hormone (LH) by the pituitary gland. An increased level of LH increases production of androgens by the ovarian stroma and perpetuates this cycle. The decreased level of FSH prevents ovulation and results in oligomenorrhea.

Current treatment is directed toward interrupting the cycle of excess ovarian androgen production through the use of oral contraceptives or wedge resection of the ovary. Other treatments include weight loss (to decrease the conversion of androgens to estrogens) and use of medications that promote FSH secretion (e.g., clomiphene, human menopausal gonadotropin, luteinizing hormone–releasing hormone, and purified FSH).

On ultrasonography or MRI, enlarged ovaries with multiple small peripheral follicles, the so-called "string of pearls" sign, may be visible. The ovary also has been described as echogenic because of the prominent ovarian stroma.

Notes

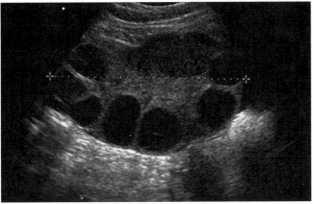

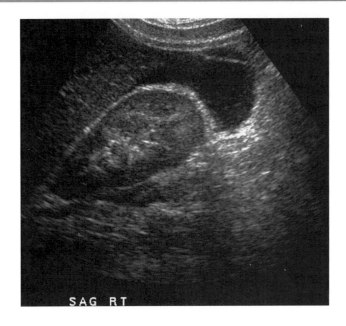

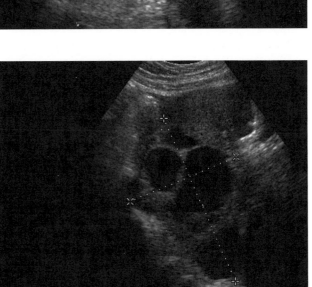

1. Ultrasound images of both adnexa and the right upper quadrant are shown. In what setting do these findings occur?

2. Which patients are at increased risk for developing this syndrome?

3. What other findings on ultrasonography would support this diagnosis?

4. What other early pregnancy complication are patients undergoing in vitro fertilization at risk for?

Ob/Gyn: Ovarian Hyperstimulation Syndrome

1. Patients undergoing assisted fertility with controlled ovarian stimulation cycles.

2. Young patients with low body weight, patients exposed to higher does of exogenous gonadotropins, patients with high serum estradiol levels, and patients with polycystic ovary syndrome or prior episodes of ovarian hyperstimulation syndrome.

3. Pleural effusions, pericardial effusion, and ascites.

4. Ectopic pregnancy.

Reference

Whelan JG, Vlahos NF: The ovarian hyperstimulation syndrome, *Fertil Steril* 73:883–896, 2000.

Cross-Reference

Zagoria RJ, *Genitourinary Radiology: THE REQUISITES*, 2nd ed, pp 292–298.

Comment

Ovarian hyperstimulation syndrome is a serious condition typically occurring in women who have undergone ovarian stimulation from exogenous gonadotropins. On very rare occasions it may also complicate spontaneous pregnancies. The syndrome consists of enlarged ovaries with multiple macroscopic luteinized follicular cysts and increased capillary permeability leading to third spacing of fluids. Ultrasonography is useful in documenting the enlarged ovaries and the presence of ascites, pleural effusions, and pericardial effusions.

Patients present with rapid weight gain from the accumulation of fluid, oliguria, and hemoconcentration. The syndrome is typically self-limited, with spontaneous regression occurring over 10 to 14 days. Regression is usually associated with declining levels of human chorionic gonadotropin, so pregnancy can worsen or lengthen the course of symptoms. Treatment is usually supportive in nature.

Complications of the syndrome include ovarian torsion, hemorrhagic rupture of cysts, deep venous thrombosis, and pulmonary embolism.

Notes

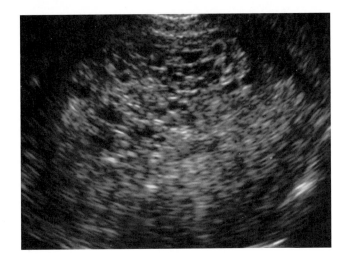

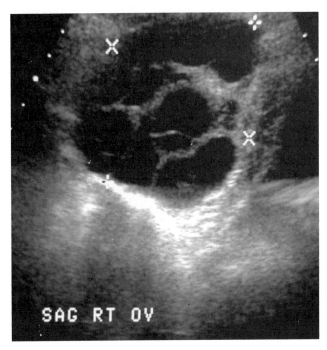

1. The figure on the left is a transvaginal ultrasound of the uterus. What is the classic term used to describe this finding in the endometrium?

2. What pathologic feature is responsible for this appearance?

3. What laboratory test could help confirm this entity?

4. What type of ovarian cysts are seen with this entity?

Ob/Gyn: Molar Pregnancy

1. "Snowstorm" appearance.

2. Hydropic placental villi in a complete molar pregnancy.

3. Markedly elevated human chorionic gonadotropin levels.

4. Theca lutein cysts.

Reference

Zhou Q, Lei XY, Xie Q, Cardoza JD: Sonographic and Doppler imaging in the diagnosis and treatment of gestational trophoblastic disease, *J Ultrasound Med* 24:15–24, 2005.

Cross-Reference

Zagoria RJ, *Genitourinary Radiology: THE REQUISITES*, 2nd ed, pp 302–303, 305.

Comment

This is a typical case of a complete hydatidiform mole in the early second trimester. Ultrasonography demonstrates the endometrium to be filled with abnormal hydropic placental tissue, which appears as solid and hyperechoic with tiny cystic components, yielding the classic "snowstorm" appearance. Gestational trophoblastic disease includes classic or complete hydatidiform mole, invasive hydatidiform mole, choriocarcinoma, partial hydatidiform mole, and placental site trophoblastic tumors. A partial hydatidiform mole can be differentiated by the concomitant presence of a fetus which typically carries a triploid karyotype.

Patients with molar pregnancies typically present with hyperemesis, vaginal bleeding, rapid uterine enlargement, and markedly elevated human chorionic gonadotropin (hCG) levels. The characteristic sonographic "snowstorm" appearance does not usually occur until the second trimester. In the first trimester, complete molar pregnancies can have a variety of appearances, most often that typical of a failed early pregnancy. Theca lutein cysts develop in the ovaries secondary to overstimulation by high levels of hCG. They are typically multilocular and expand the ovary.

Malignant forms of gestational trophoblastic disease can be suggested on sonography by the presence of myometrial invasion by spiral arteries with increased flow on Doppler studies. Patients with choriocarcinoma may also have local or distant metastatic disease at the time of diagnosis.

Notes

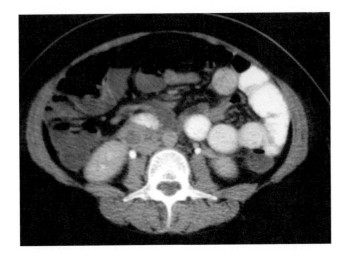
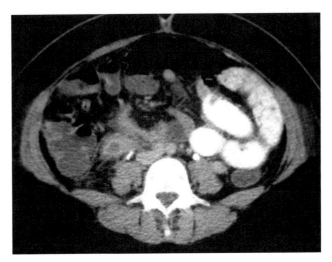
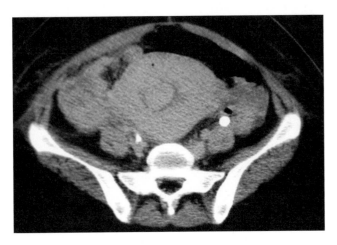

1. What is the most likely diagnosis?

2. What imaging features are used to establish this diagnosis on CT?

3. What imaging studies can be used to make this diagnosis?

4. What is the differential diagnosis for postpartum patients with fever and lower abdominal pain?

Ob/Gyn: Ovarian Vein Thrombosis

1. Right-sided ovarian vein thrombosis and endometrial debris from endometritis.

2. An unenhanced tubular structure (thrombus) with a surrounding enhancing wall extending from the right adnexa to the inferior vena cava.

3. Magnetic resonance angiography is close to 100% accurate in the diagnosis of ovarian vein thrombosis. Contrast-enhanced CT remains the favored imaging modality because of rapid access and lower cost. Duplex color Doppler ultrasonography may be diagnostic, but is less sensitive and specific.

4. Ovarian vein thrombosis, appendicitis, pyelonephritis, endometritis, tuboovarian abscess, and acute cholecystitis.

References

Bennett GL, Slywotzky CM, Giovanniello G: Gynecologic causes of acute pelvic pain: spectrum of CT findings, *Radiographics* 22:785–801, 2002.

Kubik-Huch RA, Hebisch G, Huch R, et al: Role of duplex color Doppler ultrasound, computed tomography, and MR angiography in the diagnosis of septic puerperal ovarian vein thrombosis, *Abdom Imaging* 24:85–91, 1999.

Cross-Reference

Zagoria RJ, *Genitourinary Radiology: THE REQUISITES*, 2nd ed, pp 36–37.

Comment

Patients with ovarian vein thrombosis usually present with fever and lower abdominal pain, which is usually right sided. Ovarian vein thrombosis usually occurs after delivery, but may also be seen in the setting of pelvic surgery, trauma, neoplasm, and pelvic inflammatory disease. Ovarian vein thrombosis often occurs concomitantly with endometritis, and a correct diagnosis is important because it requires administration of anticoagulants for proper treatment. Its predilection for the right ovarian vein is likely secondary to compression of the right ovarian vein during pregnancy by the gravid uterus and to the presence of retrograde flow in the left ovarian vein, which inhibits stasis and ascending infection. On CT, ovarian vein thrombosis appears as a dilated tubular structure with an enhancing wall and low-density lumen in the expected location of the ovarian vein anterior to the ureter. The diagnosis can be made on duplex color Doppler ultrasonography, but overlying bowel or obesity may obscure the diagnosis. CT is highly accurate in diagnosis and can also be helpful in distinguishing other pathology that may occur in the same clinical setting. Magnetic resonance angiography is useful for problematic cases.

Notes

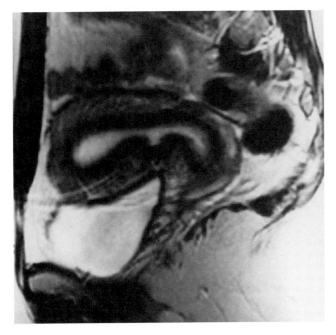

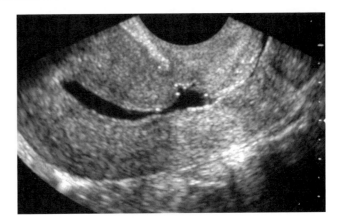

1. MRI and ultrasound images demonstrate the same entity in two different patients. What is the abnormality?

2. What pulse sequence was employed in these T2W images?

3. What is the name of the inner third of the myometrium?

4. What is the hypoechoic area in the uterus on the ultrasound image?

Ob/Gyn: Cesarean Section Scar

1. A focal disruption in the junctional zone along the ventral uterine corpus secondary to prior cesarean section.

2. Fast spin-echo or turbo spin-echo.

3. Junctional zone.

4. Saline instilled during a sonohysterogram.

References

Mayo-Smith WW, Lee MJ: MR imaging of the female pelvis, *Clin Radiol* 50:667–676, 1995.

Regnard C, Nosbusch M, Fellemans C, et al: Cesarean section scar evaluation by saline contrast sonohysterography, *Ultrasound Obstet Gynecol* 23:289–292, 2004.

Cross-Reference

Zagoria RJ, *Genitourinary Radiology: THE REQUISITES*, 2nd ed, pp 257–259.

Comment

The MRI is an "Aunt Minnie" of a uterine scar resulting from cesarean section several years earlier. There is thinning of the inner myometrium in the lower ventral uterus with focal outpouching of the endometrial cavity, which appears hyperintense on this T2W sequence. The dark band deep to the endometrium is called the junctional zone and represents the inner third of the myometrium. It is believed to be relatively hypointense because of an increased nuclear-to-cytoplasmic ratio or relative decrease in free water. Thickening of the junctional zone has been described in focal and diffuse adenomyosis. Invasive endometrial or cervical carcinoma, postoperative scarring, and leiomyomas may disrupt the junctional zone. Pelvic phased-array coils and faster imaging techniques such as fast (turbo) spin-echo and HASTE (*h*alf-Fourier *s*ingle-shot *t*urbo spin-*e*cho) have led to improved spatial resolution and faster imaging of the uterus.

Sonohysterography can also improve evaluation of the endometrium. A catheter is advanced through the cervix into the endometrial cavity, and a transvaginal ultrasound probe is inserted. The endometrial cavity is then distended with saline, allowing more detailed ultrasound evaluation of the endometrium. This sonohysterogram demonstrates hypoechoic saline in the uterine cavity with a small outpouching of fluid in the lower anterior uterine segment at the site of the prior hysterectomy. Anterior to the endometrial outpouching, the myometrium is thin compared with the myometrium of the uterine fundus.

Complications of cesarean section scars include ectopic pregnancies in the scar and placental abnormalities (placenta accreta, increta, or percreta). There is an approximately 0.4% risk for uterine rupture with vaginal births after cesarean section.

Notes

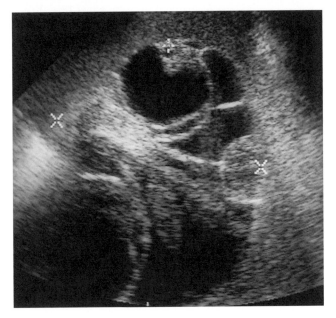
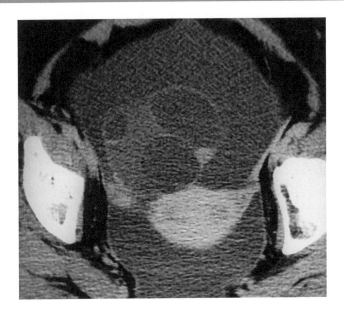

1. What is the most likely diagnosis? What findings on the ultrasound image support this diagnosis?

2. What role do serum markers play in screening for this disease?

3. Name a few risk factors for this disease.

4. Name four types of ovarian neoplasms.

Ob/Gyn: Epithelial Ovarian Carcinoma

1. Ovarian carcinoma. Ovarian mass, with multiple septations (several of which are abnormally thick) and solid peripheral nodules, and ascites.

2. Measuring CA-125 levels alone is not an effective screening test for ovarian cancer.

3. Early menarche, nulliparity, infertility, late menopause (all entities in which there is an increased incidence of ovulation), and family history.

4. Epithelial, germ cell, sex cord-stromal, metastases.

References

Jung SE, Lee JM, Rha SE, et al: CT and MR imaging of ovarian tumors with emphasis on differential diagnosis, *Radiographics* 22:1305–1325, 2002.

Woodward PJ, Hosseinzadeh K, Saenger JS: From the archives of the AFIP: radiologic staging of ovarian carcinoma with pathologic correlation, *Radiographics* 24:225–246, 2004.

Cross-Reference

Zagoria RJ, *Genitourinary Radiology: THE REQUISITES,* 2nd ed, pp 287–298.

Comment

Ovarian is the sixth most common neoplasm of female patients but is the most common cause of death of the gynecologic malignancies, mostly because it presents at a late stage. Because there is no effective screening test, the National Institutes of Health Consensus Conference has recommended against screening for ovarian cancer in members of the general population with no known risk factors for the disease. The tumor marker CA-125, a high-molecular-weight glycoprotein, is elevated in 80% of patients with epithelial neoplasms, but the marker is not specific for malignancy since it can be elevated in benign conditions such as uterine leiomyoma, endometriosis, and pelvic inflammatory disease, or during early pregnancy. The primary value of CA-125 is in monitoring for tumor recurrence in those with an elevated level at the time of diagnosis.

Ultrasonography is the initial imaging modality of choice for a suspected ovarian mass. If the ovarian mass is not a small, simple cyst, sonographic criteria that should raise the suspicion of ovarian malignancy include increased ovarian size (diameter greater than 7.5 cm); presence of a solid component, mural nodules, internal papillary projections, or thickened septations; lymphadenopathy; and ascites. Enhancement of the nodular component of an ovarian mass on CT, as in this case, or on MRI suggests malignancy. Enhanced CT and MRI can be used to detect pelvic and retroperitoneal adenopathy and to evaluate the lung and liver for metastatic disease but are not sensitive enough to detect the small peritoneal implants that are present in patients with stage III disease.

Four types of ovarian neoplasms are epithelial, germ cell, sex cord-stromal, and metastases. Epithelial cancers are derived from the peritoneal mesothelial cells and comprise 65% of ovarian neoplasms. The subtypes of epithelial ovarian neoplasms are serous, mucinous, and endometrioid. Sixty percent of epithelial neoplasms are benign, 15% are borderline, and 25% are malignant. Treatment is surgical resection.

Notes

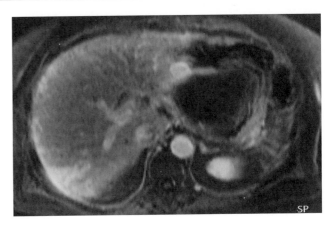

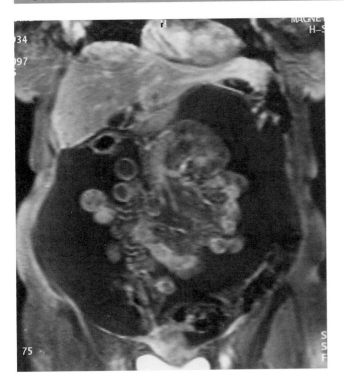

1. What is the most likely diagnosis?

2. What are the most common sites of peritoneal tumor implantation?

3. What technical options for MRI may improve detection of this disease?

4. What is pseudomyxoma peritonei?

Ob/Gyn: Peritoneal Carcinomatosis on MRI

1. Peritoneal carcinomatosis caused by epithelial carcinoma of the ovary.

2. Pouch of Douglas, ileocecal region, and right paracolic gutter.

3. Gadolinium enhancement, air distention of the bowel, and glucagon administration.

4. Accumulation of large amounts of gelatinous material in the peritoneal cavity caused by the transformation of peritoneal mesothelium to a mucin-secreting epithelium after perforation of a mucinous cystadenoma or cystadenocarcinoma.

References

Chou CK, Liu GC, Su JH, et al: MRI demonstration of peritoneal implants, *Abdom Imaging* 19:95–101, 1994.

Jeong Y-Y, Outwater EK, Kang HK: Imaging evaluation of ovarian masses, *Radiographics* 20:1445–1470, 2000.

Cross-Reference

Zagoria RJ, *Genitourinary Radiology: THE REQUISITES,* 2nd ed, pp 288, 289.

Comment

Epithelial carcinoma of the ovary is one of the classic neoplasms that can present with extensive peritoneal disease. There are two theories for this observed disease pattern. One theory is that cells exfoliate into the peritoneal cavity only after the tumor has grown locally and invaded the ovarian capsule and mesovarium. Another theory is that the entire coelomic epithelium of the peritoneum undergoes malignant transformation. This theory may explain primary peritoneal or surface papillary adenocarcinoma in which multifocal or diffuse peritoneal carcinoma occurs with minimal or no ovarian involvement. In the International Federation of Gynecology and Obstetrics (FIGO) staging system of ovarian carcinoma, histologically confirmed abdominopelvic peritoneal implants less than 2 cm in diameter are designated as stage IIIb disease, and those that exceed 2 cm in diameter are considered stage IIIc ovarian cancer. Retrospective studies have suggested that survival in patients with stage III disease is related to residual tumor after surgery; therefore, detection and surgical debulking of peritoneal carcinomatosis are essential.

Although enhanced CT remains the imaging test of choice for the detection of peritoneal carcinomatosis, MRI also has been used to stage ovarian carcinoma. Although most implants have higher signal intensity than ascites on T1W images, differentiation of implants from ascites is facilitated by intravenous administration of gadolinium contrast. In this case nodular implants can be identified along the surface of the liver and in the gastrosplenic ligament.

Notes

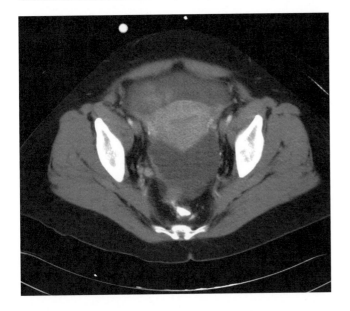

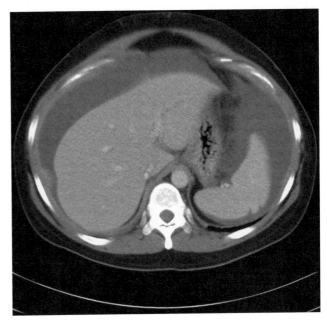

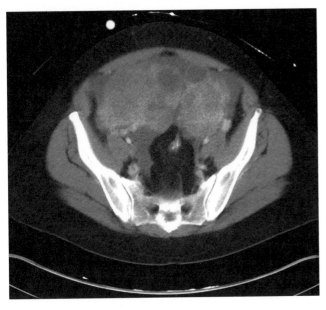

1. What are the salient abnormalities in the image on the left?

2. What is the differential diagnosis for the solid and cystic structure(s)?

3. What is the most common origin for metastatic tumors to the ovaries?

4. True or false: Signet-ring tumors only occur in the ovaries by metastatic infiltration.

Ob/Gyn: Krukenberg Metastasis

1. Bilateral solid and cystic ovarian masses with ascites.

2. Primary or metastatic ovarian tumors.

3. Gastrointestinal adenocarcinomas.

4. False. Although rare, primary signet-ring tumors do occur.

References

Brown DL, Zou KH, Tempany CMC, et al: Primary versus secondary ovarian malignancy: imaging findings of adnexal masses in the radiology diagnostic oncology group study, *Radiology* 219:213–218, 2001.

Krukenberg FE: Über das Fibrosarcoma ovarii mucocellulare (carcinomatodes), *Arch Gynäkol Berlin* 50: 287–321, 1896.

Cross-Reference

Zagoria RJ, *Genitourinary Radiology: THE REQUISITES,* 2nd ed, pp 290–301.

Comment

This eponymous tumor was originally described by Dr. F.E. Krukenberg in reference to a rare form of malignant primary ovarian signet-ring tumor and its difficult microscopic distinction from metastatic signet-ring tumors from the stomach. In modern radiology a similar difficulty exists in distinguishing metastatic tumors to the ovaries (Krukenberg metastases) from primary ovarian neoplasms.

The clinical importance of distinguishing primary from metastatic ovarian neoplasms is for treatment and prognosis. The rare, malignant primary ovarian signet-ring tumor is usually discovered in an early stage, occurs unilaterally and is easily resected. The more common primary ovarian neoplasms also usually occur unilaterally, but may be found in early, intermediate, or late stage. Krukenberg metastases always indicate a late stage of disease.

Krukenberg metastases are predominately from gastrointestinal adenocarcinomas (stomach or colon). Other primary sites of origin include the breast, uterus, pancreas biliary tract, and lymphomas.

Unfortunately, there are no accurate imaging criteria by ultrasonography, CT, or MRI that can reliably distinguish between primary and metastatic ovarian neoplasms. There are, however, a few imaging features that can frequently assist in their distinction. Primary ovarian neoplasms are often cystic, large (greater than 10 cm), unilateral, and in early stage of disease. In contrast, Krukenberg metastases tend to be solid, small (less than 10 cm), involve both ovaries, and present late. Krukenberg metastases are also more commonly found with other evidence of metastatic disease, such as adenopathy, ascites, and lung/liver/bone lesions.

Notes

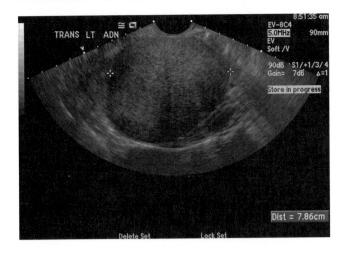

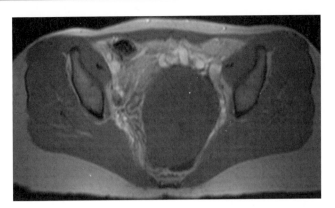

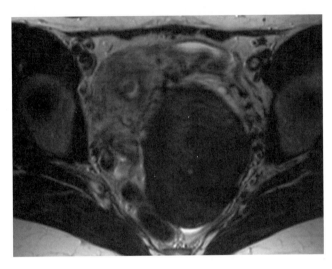

1. Give the two most likely diagnoses for the large pelvic mass shown above.

2. On the left image, high T2 signal within the mass is due to what processes?

3. What is Meigs' syndrome?

4. True or false: Ovarian fibromas secrete steroids.

Ob/Gyn: Ovarian Fibroma

1. Pedunculated uterine leiomyoma and ovarian fibroma.

2. Edema and cystic degeneration.

3. Ovarian fibroma, ascites, and hydrothorax.

4. False.

References

Schwartz RK, Levine D, Hatabu H, et al: Ovarian fibroma: findings by contrast-enhanced MRI, *Abdom Imaging* 22:535–537, 1997.

Troiano RN, Lazzarini KM, Scoutt LM, et al: Fibroma and fibrothecoma of the ovary: MR imaging findings, *Radiology* 204:795–798, 1997.

Cross-Reference

Zagoria RJ, *Genitourinary Radiology: THE REQUISITES,* 2nd ed, p 290.

Comment

Ovarian fibromas are gonadal stromal tumors that comprise 4% of all ovarian neoplasms. Ovarian fibromas most frequently occur in middle-aged women, with the average age 48 years. Rare cases of ovarian fibroma in pediatric patients as young as 7 months have been reported. Ovarian fibromas in younger patients may be associated with basal cell nevus syndrome (Gorlin's syndrome), which is characterized by basal cell carcinomas, jaw cysts, skeletal dysplasias, pitting of the hands and feet, and ectopic calcifications. Ovarian fibromas can also be associated with ovarian torsion and ascites. The triad of ovarian fibroma, ascites, and hydrothorax is known as Meigs' syndrome.

Ovarian fibromas may be difficult to distinguish from pedunculated uterine leiomyomas, as both entities appear as solid hypoechoic adnexal masses on ultrasonography. Visualization of a discrete pedicle extending from the uterus or identification of two normal ovaries infers uterine origin and the diagnosis of leiomyoma. Other rare solid ovarian tumors to consider in the differential include Brenner tumor and dysgerminoma.

MRI characteristics of ovarian fibroma, as shown here, have helpful distinguishing features. A well-circumscribed mass demonstrating homogeneous, low signal intensity similar to striated muscle is seen on T1-weighted MRIs. On T2-weighted MRIs, fibromas demonstrate mostly low signal intensity with variable high T2 signal in areas of edema or cystic degeneration. A pseudocapsule of compressed ovarian tissue seen as a band of T2 hypointensity separating the mass from the uterus is a useful sign and has been described. This is well illustrated in the T2-weighted image.

The MRI enhancement pattern of ovarian fibromas can be variable from minimal enhancement to marked heterogeneous enhancement. Marked heterogeneous gadolinium enhancement of ovarian fibromas when present can be a useful distinguishing feature. Nondegenerated uterine leiomyomas have low T1 and T2 signal but enhance only minimally. Degenerated or cellular leiomyomas often enhance significantly but demonstrate mostly high T2 signal in contrast to ovarian fibromas.

Although most ovarian fibromas are benign, rare cases of malignant potential have been described. Most ovarian fibromas are therefore surgically removed, whereas uterine leiomyomas can be medically managed or ignored if asymptomatic.

Notes

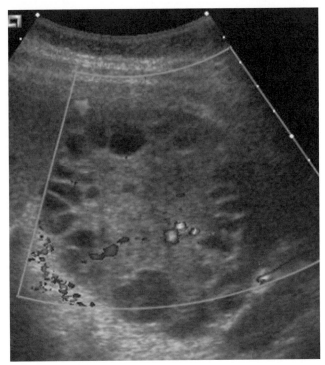
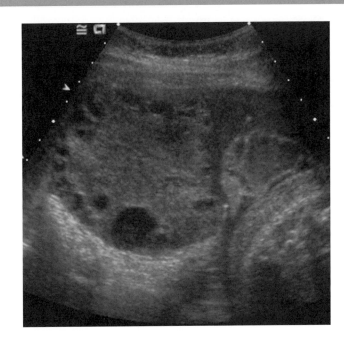

See also Color Plate

1. What is the most common predisposing condition for the above entity?

2. What are the CT findings for the same diagnosis?

3. Does blood flow within the ovary on color Doppler ultrasonography exclude this diagnosis?

4. True or false: This condition may occur in prepubertal girls with normal ovaries.

Ob/Gyn: Ovarian Torsion

1. Benign ovarian teratoma.

2. Soft tissue density adnexal mass often with adjacent inflammation and free fluid.

3. No, the ovary has dual blood supply and may torse intermittently.

4. True.

References

Lee EJ, Kwon HC, Joo HJ, et al: Diagnosis of ovarian torsion with color Doppler sonography: depiction of twisted vascular pedicle, *J Ultrasound Med*;17: 83–89, 1998.

Rha SE, Byun JY, Jung SE, et al: CT and MR imaging features of adnexal torsion, *Radiographics*;22: 283–294, 2002.

Cross-Reference

Zagoria RJ, *Genitourinary Radiology: THE REQUISITES*, 2nd ed, pp 274–276.

Comment

Ovarian torsion results from the ovary twisting on its vascular pedicle, thus compromising blood flow. An ipsilateral ovarian mass is present in as many as 50% to 80% of cases. A benign cystic teratoma is the most common predisposing mass. Torsion in the absence of a mass is unusual in postpubertal females. However, children may develop ovarian torsion without a predisposing mass. This is thought to be secondary to increased mobility of the adnexa in children.

Sonography remains the first-line imaging modality for the evaluation of acute female pelvic pain. The classic finding, as shown here, for ovarian torsion is a diffusely enlarged ovary with multiple peripheral cysts. However, the absence of this finding does not exclude ovarian torsion. Often, normal ovarian parenchyma cannot be identified with imaging. Other sonographic features of ovarian torsion include a complex, cystic or solid, mass; free intraperitoneal fluid; absent blood flow in the ovary; and/or visualization of the twisted vascular pedicle. Ovarian torsion should still be considered, even if blood flow to the ovary is preserved. Arterial blood flow may be preserved due to dual arterial supply from the ovarian artery and ovarian branches of the uterine artery. Arterial blood flow may also appear normal in early cases where venous thrombosis has occurred, producing symptoms, but the artery has not yet occluded.

Women with acute abdominal pain may have an abdomen and pelvis CT performed as the first diagnostic imaging examination. According to Rha and colleagues, the CT findings of ovarian torsion include thickening of the ipsilateral fallopian tube (84%), smooth wall thickening of the twisted ovarian cystic mass (76%), ascites (64%), uterine deviation to the twisted side (36%), tubal hemorrhage (16%), hemorrhage within the adnexal mass (8%), and hemoperitoneum (8%). CT also has the benefit of helping to characterize any associated ovarian masses. The presence of hemoperitoneum with ovarian torsion is highly concerning for hemorrhagic infarction, which can lead to peritonitis and death. Hemorrhagic ovarian cyst, endometriosis with rupture, and ectopic pregnancy more commonly lead to a hemorrhagic mass and hemoperitoneum, and therefore must be excluded.

Ovarian torsion is most commonly treated with adnexectomy, in order to prevent retorsion and thromboembolism from a thrombosed ovarian vein. However, conservative treatment with detorsing of the adnexa has been reported as an option for conserving ovarian viability and fertility in young females.

Notes

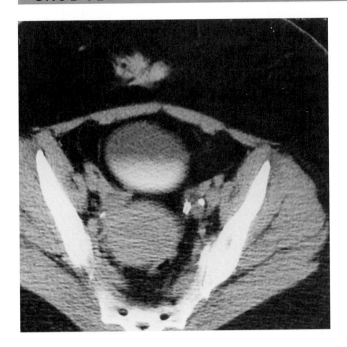 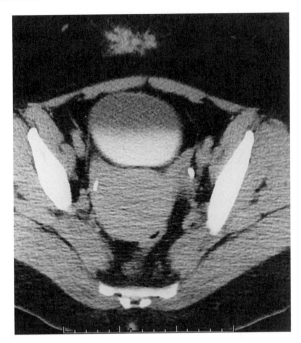

1. Two images from a CT examination performed to investigate severe, intermittent abdominal pain are shown. Where is the lesion located?

2. What is the radiologic differential diagnosis for the lesion?

3. On further questioning the patient describes cyclical pain that began after a cesarean section. Based on this information, should any other condition be added to the differential diagnosis?

4. Would MRI provide any new information? What might it show?

Ob/Gyn: Scar Endometrioma

1. Subcutaneous fat in the anterior abdominal wall.

2. Hematoma, surgical scar, metastasis, or abscess.

3. Yes, endometriosis.

4. Possibly. It might show characteristic findings of hemorrhage.

References

Amato M, Levitt R: Abdominal wall endometrioma: CT findings, *J Comput Assist Tomogr* 8:1213–1214, 1984.

Blanco RG, Parithivel VS, Shah AK, et al: Abdominal wall endometriomas, *Am J Surg* 185:596–598, 2003.

Matthes G, Zabel DD, Nastala CL, Shestak KC: Endometrioma of the abdominal wall following combined abdominoplasty and hysterectomy: case report and review of the literature, *Ann Plast Surg* 40: 672–675, 1998.

Cross-Reference

Zagoria RJ, *Genitourinary Radiology: THE REQUISITES*, 2nd ed, pp 267–270.

Comment

This unusual case of ectopic endometrial tissue in the subcutaneous fat occurred after cesarean section. The patient had severe, cyclical abdominal pain, and the correct diagnosis was made by the emergency room radiologist to the disbelief of the general surgeons.

Scar endometriosis reportedly occurs in up to 5% of patients who undergo cesarean section or hysterectomy. The pathogenesis is iatrogenic transplantation of endometrial tissue to the abdominal wall during surgery. Treatment is surgical excision. Biopsy should be avoided to prevent further seeding of the endometrial tissue along the biopsy tract. If the lesion is large, it may be reduced preoperatively by the administration of a gonadotropin-releasing hormone antagonist.

Notes

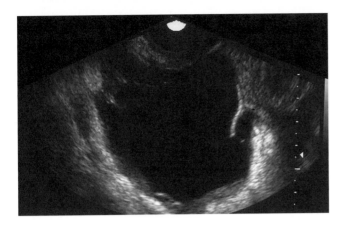 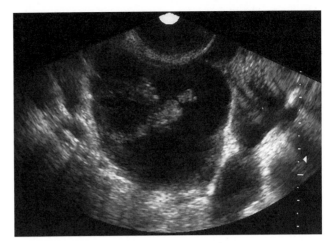

1. True or false: With respect to gray scale sonography, the presence and echogenicity of any solid element are the most important features for distinguishing between a benign and malignant ovarian mass.

2. True or false: With respect to the wall of an ovarian mass, a thickness of less than 3 mm is more typical of a benign mass.

3. True or false: With respect to Doppler sonography, the identification of flow within the wall of an ovarian mass suggests that it is malignant.

4. With respect to Doppler arterial flow patterns in an ovarian mass, define the pulsatility index (PI) and resistive index (RI).

Ob/Gyn: Ultrasound Evaluation of the Ovarian Mass

1. True.

2. True.

3. False.

4. PI = (peak systolic velocity − end-diastolic velocity) ÷ mean velocity

   RI = (peak systolic velocity − end-diastolic velocity) ÷ peak systolic velocity

Reference

Brown DL, Doubilet PM, Miller FH, et al: Benign and malignant ovarian masses: selection of the most discriminating gray-scale and Doppler sonographic features, *Radiology* 208:103–110, 1998.

Cross-Reference

Zagoria RJ, *Genitourinary Radiology: THE REQUISITES,* 2nd ed, p 294.

Comment

What sonographic features suggest that an ovarian mass is malignant? One of the better studies that attempts to answer this question is referenced above. Brown and co-workers used stepwise logistic regression to select gray scale and Doppler sonographic features that best discriminated between 28 malignant and 183 benign masses. Among several features, four were found most discriminant. By a factor of 10, the presence and nature of a solid component were most important. Masses without a solid component or with a markedly hyperechoic solid component (consistent with a teratoma) were benign. For masses with a nonhyperechoic solid component, the presence and location of flow were the next most valuable features. Sixty percent of malignant masses had flow in a septation or solid component, and only 9% had no flow or flow within the wall alone. Any free intraperitoneal fluid was considered abnormal in postmenopausal women, but in premenopausal women, free fluid was considered abnormal only when it filled the cul-de-sac or extended around the ovaries, above the uterus, into the paracolic gutters, or into the upper abdomen. Finally, the presence and thickness of any septation were considered important. The absence of any septation had a stronger association with malignancy than did the presence of a thin septation (3 mm in diameter); a thick septation had intermediate value.

In this retrospective study, other features, such as wall thickness, fluid echogenicity, and both average and lowest resistive and pulsatility indexes, were significantly associated with histopathologic findings but did not add to the discriminant value of the four aforementioned features. Also, this study excluded women beyond the tenth day of the menstrual cycle to avoid low resistance flow associated with the corpus luteum. By the way, the mass shown in this case was a chronic hematoma.

Notes

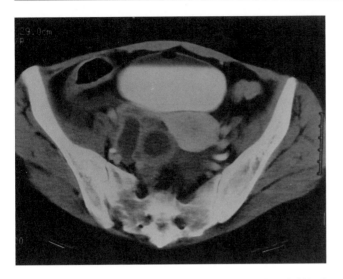
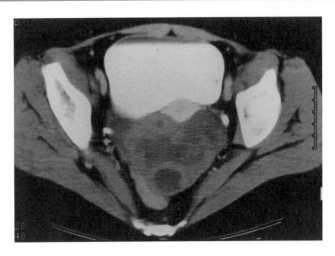

1. In the image on the left, what is the fluid-filled mass to the right of the uterus?

2. Name a cause of "massive ovarian edema."

3. What is the arterial supply of the ovary?

4. True or false: On Doppler sonography of the ovary, the presence of high-resistance flow excludes malignancy and ovarian torsion.

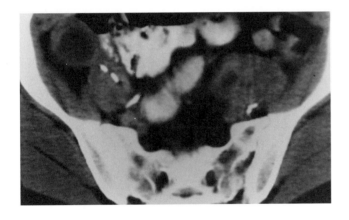
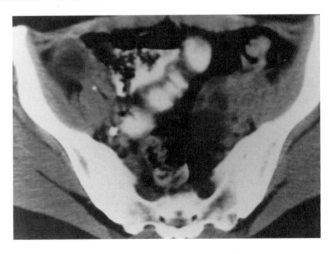

1. Images from a CT scan through the upper pelvis are shown. What are the bilateral low-density masses?

2. The patient underwent an operative procedure to move the gonads out of the lower pelvis. What is the name of this procedure?

3. Why was this operation performed?

4. What imaging procedure could be performed to confirm this anatomic finding?

CASE 129

Ob/Gyn: Ovarian Torsion

1. Dilated right fallopian tube with a thickened wall.

2. Partial or intermittent torsion of the ovary.

3. Ovarian artery (branch of the abdominal aorta) and uterine artery (branch of the anterior trunk of the internal iliac artery).

4. False.

Reference

Kimura I, Togashi K, Kawakami S, et al: Ovarian torsion: CT and MR imaging appearances, *Radiology* 190: 337–341, 1994.

Cross-Reference

Zagoria RJ, *Genitourinary Radiology: THE REQUISITES,* 2nd ed, pp 274–276.

Comment

Ovarian torsion can be challenging to diagnose, particularly when the clinical presentation is atypical (e.g., the course is intermittent because of incomplete torsion or cycles of torsion and detorsion). In many cases an underlying ovarian mass predisposes to adnexal torsion, but torsion also occurs in patients with normal adnexa. In prepubertal girls, ovarian torsion should be suspected when there is a large unilateral pelvic mass with multiple peripheral "cysts" representing cortical follicles. An enlarged ovary bearing multiple enlarged follicles (8–12 mm in diameter) is unexpected in this age group. Kimura and co-workers found that deviation of the uterus to the twisted side, engorgement of blood vessels, ascites, and obliteration of pelvic fat planes identified on pelvic CT and MRI suggested ovarian torsion. Other reported signs include an ipsilateral, dilated fallopian tube with a thickened wall; this finding is illustrated in this case. In adnexal torsion associated with an ovarian tumor, a marked change in the position of an identifiable tumor marker (e.g., calcified vegetation or Rokitansky protuberance on a dermoid tumor) on CT scans obtained before and after the onset of adnexal torsion has been reported. An atypical presentation of partial or intermittent ovarian torsion is massive ovarian edema.

Doppler sonography has limited usefulness for the diagnosis of adnexal torsion. Doppler flow may be absent in masses without torsion, and the identification of blood flow in a mass does not exclude this diagnosis. Arterial flow may be preserved in cases of torsion when only venous flow is compromised. Furthermore, the ovary is supplied by both the uterine artery and the ovarian artery, and therefore arterial flow to the adnexa may persist when arterial flow to the ovary is reduced.

Notes

CASE 130

Ob/Gyn: Ovarian Pexy

1. Ovaries.

2. Ovarian pexy.

3. To remove gonadal tissue from the therapeutic radiation field.

4. Transabdominal sonography or MRI.

Reference

Hricak H, Yu KK: Radiology in invasive cervical cancer, *Am J Roentgenol* 167:1101–1108, 1996.

Cross-Reference

Zagoria RJ, *Genitourinary Radiology: THE REQUISITES,* 2nd ed, pp 258–259.

Comment

This young woman with cervical carcinoma was treated with hysterectomy and postoperative radiation therapy. The ovaries were moved out of the pelvis and "pexed" along the superior pelvic sidewall so that they would not be included in the radiation field. Knowledge of this procedure is important so that the pexed ovary is not confused with adenopathy, particularly if one ovary has been removed. If necessary, appropriate imaging modalities, including transabdominal ultrasonography (the ovaries are usually too high to be seen with transvaginal sonography) or MRI, can confirm the location of a pexed ovary.

Patients with early invasive carcinoma (stages Ib and IIa) have a 10% to 15% risk for pelvic nodal spread of disease and a 5% risk for periaortic lymph node involvement. These patients usually require radical hysterectomy with lymphadenectomy, with or without radiation therapy. Because early cervical carcinoma rarely spreads to the ovaries, oophorectomy usually is not performed. Patients retain ovarian function; do not suffer from secondary complications of oophorectomy, such as osteoporosis; and do not require exogenous hormone supplementation. Pelvic radiation to the ovaries results in loss of ovarian function. This disadvantage favors surgical treatment of early cervical cancer over radiation and explains why ovarian pexy is performed in patients who may subsequently undergo radiation therapy.

Notes

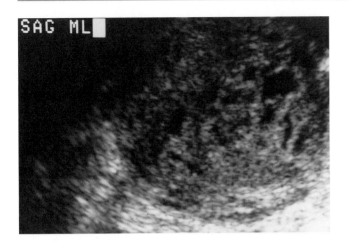

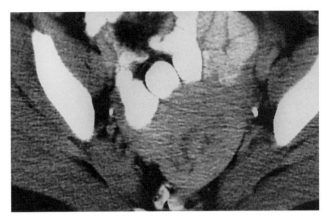

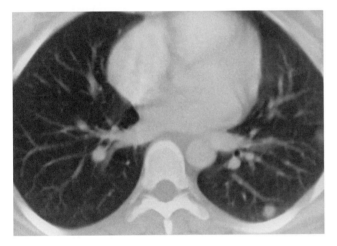

1. A sagittal transvaginal sonogram of the uterus and CT images of the upper pelvis and lower chest are shown. What is the most likely diagnosis?

2. What is the differential diagnosis based on the findings in the images of the uterus?

3. What are the clinical indications for staging this disease?

4. What is the abnormal karyotype of the diseased tissue?

Ob/Gyn: Gestational Trophoblastic Disease

1. Molar pregnancy.

2. Degenerated uterine leiomyoma, hydropic degeneration of the placenta, and endometrial proliferative disease, including carcinoma.

3. Sonographic evaluation is warranted when the uterus is too large for the fetus' gestational age, human chorionic gonadotropin titers are disproportionate to the gestational age, there is severe pregnancy-induced hypertension before 24 weeks' gestation, and there is vaginal bleeding. CT examination is performed when malignancy is suspected.

4. Ninety percent of complete moles have a karyotype, 10% 46XY, and likely develop when an egg with an absent nucleus is fertilized by a haploid sperm. Incomplete moles usually (80%) have a karyotype of XXY and present with a triploid dysmorphic fetus.

Reference

Jauniaux E: Ultrasound diagnosis and follow-up of gestational trophoblastic disease, *Ultrasound Obstet Gynecol* 11:367–377, 1998.

Cross-Reference

Zagoria RJ, *Genitourinary Radiology: THE REQUISITES,* 2nd ed, pp 302–305.

Comment

The term *gestational trophoblastic disease* (GTD) refers to a spectrum of gestational disease, ranging from the benign (complete [hydatidiform] or partial mole) to the overtly malignant (chorioadenoma destruens and choriocarcinoma). All of these diseases can produce human chorionic gonadotropin (hCG). Affected patients usually have painless vaginal bleeding in the first trimester of pregnancy. Less commonly, patients have severe pregnancy-induced hypertension or hyperemesis gravidarum. Treatment for a molar pregnancy is suction curettage of the endometrial cavity. Successful treatment is heralded by the return of serum hCG levels to normal in 12 weeks.

The sonographic appearance of molar pregnancy is characteristic. The uterus is enlarged, and hydropic degeneration of molar villi produces multiple small (3–10 mm in diameter) anechoic structures; this finding has been termed the cluster of grapes appearance. The myometrium appears normal. Frequently, accompanying areas of hemorrhage or necrosis present as irregular hypoechoic or anechoic areas. The presence of fetal membranes and parts suggests a partial molar pregnancy. This characteristic appearance may not be present in the first trimester, when the molar tissue may appear as a homogeneous echogenic endometrial mass. Myometrial invasion or abdominal metastatic disease confirms the diagnosis of the malignant form of GTD.

Notes

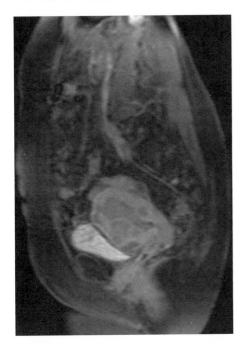
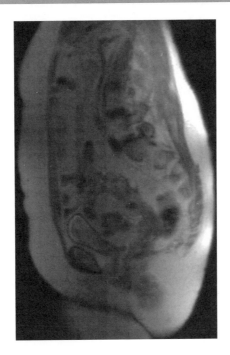
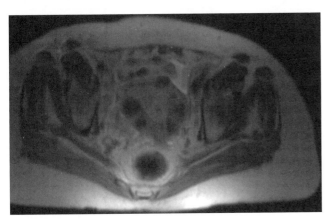

1. Name four causes of a thickened endometrium in a postmenopausal woman.

2. What are complications associated with a lesion obstructing the internal os?

3. True or false: As the depth of myometrial invasion increases, so does the likelihood of extrauterine disease.

4. True or false: Tamoxifen increases the risk of endometrial carcinoma.

Ob/Gyn: Endometrial Carcinoma Stage IA

1. Endometrial hyperplasia, polyps, carcinoma, and drugs (tamoxifen or estrogen replacement).

2. Pyometra and hematometra.

3. True. If the myometrium is not invaded, approximately 3% of patients will have pelvic nodal metastases. However, when invasion extends to the outer half of the myometrium, nodal metastases are present in about 40% of cases.

4. True.

References

Frei KA, Kinkel K, Bonél HH, Lu Y, et al: Prediction of deep myometrial invasion in patients with endometrial cancer: clinical utility of contrast-enhanced MR imaging, *Radiology* 216:444, 2000.

Kinkel K, Kaji Y, Yu KK, Segal MR, et al: Radiologic staging in patients with endometrial cancer: a meta-analysis, *Radiology* 212:711–718, 1999.

Cross-Reference

Zagoria RJ, *Genitourinary Radiology: THE REQUISITES,* 2nd ed, pp 298–302.

Comment

MRI scans shows thickening and enlargement of the endometrium and multiple uterine fibroids. The endometrial abnormalities do not extend into the myometrium. Endometrial carcinoma is the most common invasive malignancy of the female genital tract. Histologically, the vast majority of endometrial cancers are adenocarcinoma (70%). The prognosis is largely determined by histology, grade, and the stage of the tumor. Well-differentiated adenocarcinomas of the endometrium are often localized on initial presentation, unlike undifferentiated adenocarcinomas or rare endometrial sarcomas. As depth of myometrial invasion increases, so does the incidence of distant metastases. Direct local spread to the cervix, adnexa, broad ligament, and metastasis to the peritoneum and omentum can occur. The revised surgical International Federation of Gynecology and Obstetrics (FIGO) staging of endometrial carcinoma is as follows:

Stage 0: Carcinoma in situ
IA: Tumor limited to endometrium
IB: Tumor invasion limited to less than 50% thickness of myometrium
IC: Invasion of greater than 50% thickness of myometrium
IIA: Invasion of endocervix
IIB: Cervical stromal invasion
IIIA: Invasion of serosa and/or adnexal or positive peritoneal cytology
IIIB: Invasion of vagina
IIIC: Pelvic and/or paraaortic lymphadenopathy
IVA: Invasion of bladder or rectal mucosa
IVB: Distant metastasis (includes intraabdominal or inguinal lymphadenopathy)

Endometrial carcinoma has a variable MRI appearance. Most are isointense to uterus on T1-weighted images, with tumor nodules on T2 of intermediate signal between normal endometrium and myometrium. When discrete nodules are not visible, only expansion of the central high signal intensity area of the uterus is seen. To differentiate between mass and increased uterine secretions, postgadolinium T1 imaging is helpful. Most tumors enhance less than the myometrium, although early hyperenhancement or isointensity to myometrium also occurs. Since endometrial carcinoma occurs predominantly in postmenopausal women who normally have a thin (less than 5 mm) high signal endometrium on T2-weighted images, any expansion of this area should raise suspicion. In addition, on T2-weighted imaging, preservation of the low-signal intensity junctional zone implies the absence of myometrial invasion.

Notes

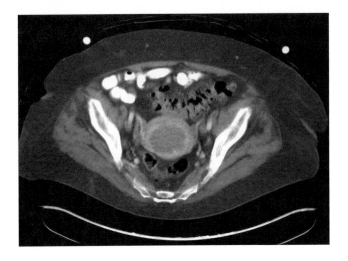 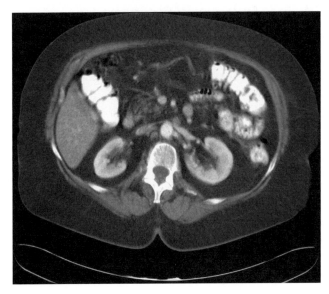

1. What is the most common clinical presentation of this disease?

2. Which radiologic test is preferred for initial evaluation of the endometrium?

3. Name three risk factors for this entity.

Ob/Gyn: Endometrial Carcinoma

1. With abnormal or postmenopausal uterine bleeding.

2. Transvaginal ultrasonography.

3. Risk factors include obesity, diabetes, nulliparity, unopposed estrogen, tamoxifen therapy, and history of breast and colon cancer.

References

Dubbins PA, Subba B: Screening for gynecological malignancy, *Semin Ultrasound CT MRI* 20:231–238, 1999.

Hardesty LA, Sumkin JH, Hakim C, et al: The ability of helical CT to preoperatively stage endometrial carcinoma, *Am J Roentgenol* 176:603–606, 2001.

Lim PS, Nazarian LN, Wechsler RJ, et al: The endometrium on routine contrast-enhanced CT in asymptomatic postmenopausal women. Avoiding errors in interpretation, *Clin Imaging* 26:325–329, 2002.

Cross-Reference

Zagoria RJ, *Genitourinary Radiology: THE REQUISITES,* 2nd ed, pp 300–302.

Comment

The images show massive enlargement at the endometrium with no evidence of extrauterine spread or ureteral obstruction. Endometrial carcinoma is the most common gynecologic malignancy in developed countries. Endometrial carcinoma occurs primarily during the postmenopausal years. Risk increases with age.

Peri- and postmenopausal patients who present with abnormal uterine bleeding (of which 15%–20% will be due to cancer) should undergo evaluation with transvaginal ultrasonography, the initial test of choice. This characterizes the endometrial thickness and morphology. Abnormalities (thickness greater than 5 mm or focal irregularities) require further evaluation, which can include hysterosonography (transvaginal ultrasonography with saline infusion into the endometrial cavity) or endometrial biopsy. However, endometrium thickness varies depending on menopausal status and use of hormone replacement. Also, abnormal thickening can be seen in a number of different entities, including hyperplasia, submucosal fibroids, and endometrial polyps.

Staging at the time of diagnosis is accomplished with a combination of imaging and surgery. MRI is currently the test of choice for preoperative staging due to its superiority in evaluating depth of myometrial invasion and extension to the cervix. Surgical lymph node dissection is indicated if myometrial invasion is greater than 50%. Endometrial carcinoma manifests on CT as enlargement of the uterus with thickened, ill-defined, or irregular endometrium. The tumor usually enhances less than the adjacent normal myometrium. Pyometra can be the presentation in a patient with long-standing occlusion of the lower uterine segment or cervix. Extension of disease can occur via direct extension, through the fallopian tubes into the adnexa and to lymph nodes in the pelvic side walls and retroperitoneum. Hematogenous spread leads primarily to liver metastases.

Notes

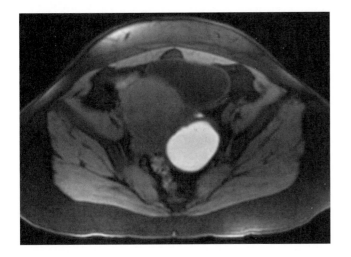
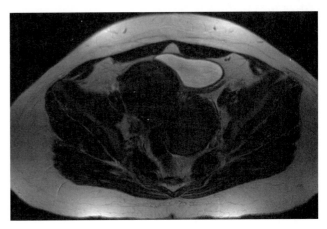

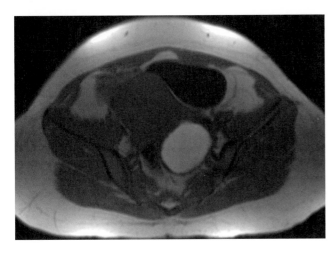

1. Name the most common sites of this disease process.

2. Name two unusual sites of disease outside of the abdomen and pelvis.

3. True or false: Ovarian torsion is a common complication of this disease process.

4. True or false: MRI is the test of choice for diagnosis of endometriosis.

Ob/Gyn: Endometrioma

1. Ovaries, uterine ligaments, cul-de-sac and pelvic peritoneum reflected over the uterus, fallopian tubes, rectosigmoid, and bladder.

2. Lungs (catamenial pneumothorax) and central nervous system.

3. False. Compared with other ovarian masses, endometriomas are less likely to undergo torsion due to associated adhesions.

4. False. Laparoscopy is used to diagnose and stage endometriosis. Either transvaginal ultrasonography or MRI may be used to diagnose endometrioma.

References

Gougoutas CA, Siegelman ES, Hunt J, Outwater EK: Pelvic endometriosis, various manifestations and MR imaging findings, *Am J Roentgenol* 175:353–358, 2000.

Jeong YY, Outwater EK, Kang HK: Imaging evaluation of ovarian masses, *Radiographics* 20:1445, 2000.

Cross-Reference

Zagoria RJ, *Genitourinary Radiology: THE REQUISITES,* 2nd ed, pp 267–270.

Comment

MRIs show a T1-bright, T2-dark lesion in the left adnexa that shows no change with fat suppression. There is a low signal rim. This indicates a hemorrhage-filled cyst. Endometriomas ("chocolate cysts") of the ovary are a manifestation of endometriosis. Patients usually present with one or all of a classic triad of symptoms, including dysmenorrhea, dyspareunia, and infertility. Endometriomas are frequently multiple and bilateral and can be differentiated from other adnexal masses based on their MRI characteristics. Endometriomas are usually multiloculated lesions that are hyperintense on T1-weighted sequences with relatively low signal intensity on T2-weighted sequences, sometimes called shading. The typical appearance on T2-weighted imaging is due to high concentrations of proteins such as intracytoplasmic methemoglobin as well as iron products. Some endometriomas demonstrate heterogeneous signal intensity due to blood products. Identification of iron (hemosiderin) helps differentiate an endometrioma from a cystadenocarcinoma. Endometriomas may demonstrate a peripheral rim of low signal intensity on both T1- and T2-weighted images corresponding to a hemosiderin or a fibrous capsule. Large endometriomas may show hematocrit levels or contain thin septations.

Ovarian torsion is less often seen with endometriomas compared with other ovarian masses. This may be secondary to surrounding adhesions resulting in less mobility of the endometrioma. Malignant transformation is a rare complication of endometriosis. Solid components of intermediate to high signal on T2-weighted images, or enhancing papillary projections on T1-weighted images are suggestive of malignancy.

Notes

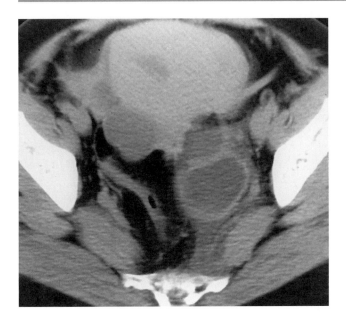 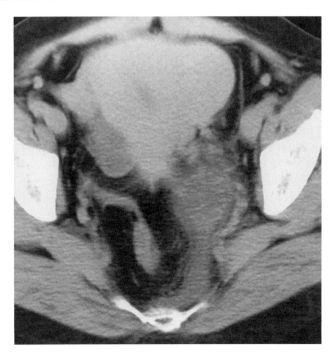

1. What are the most likely diagnoses for these imaging findings?

2. What should be done next?

3. It has been determined that an infection is most likely. True or false: Percutaneous drainage is the treatment of choice.

4. What are the complications of this disease?

Ob/Gyn: Tuboovarian Abscess

1. Pelvic inflammatory disease, abscess, ovarian torsion or less likely neoplasm.

2. Determine clinical history and physical examination findings.

3. False. Antimicrobial therapy is the first line of therapy. Percutaneous aspiration is useful to decrease the volume of the ovarian abscess and to determine the causative organisms in patients who do not respond to antibiotic therapy.

4. Fallopian tube scarring and paratubal adhesions, recurrent pelvic inflammatory disease, infertility, and chronic pelvic pain.

References

Caspi B, Zalel Y, Or Y, et al: Sonographically guided aspiration: an alternative therapy for tubo-ovarian abscess (see comments), *Ultrasound Obstet Gynecol* 7:439–442, 1996.

Sam JW, Jacobs JE, Birnbaum BA: Spectrum of CT findings in acute pyogenic pelvic inflammatory disease, *Radiographics* 22:1327–1334, 2002.

Cross-Reference

Zagoria RJ, *Genitourinary Radiology: THE REQUISITES*, 2nd ed, pp 270–274.

Comment

Pelvic inflammatory disease (PID) is a term used to describe ascending infection and inflammation of the endometrium, fallopian tubes, and ovaries. PID refers to a disease continuum that may progress from cervicitis, to endometritis, to salpingitis, to pelvic peritonitis. Tuboovarian abscess (TOA) refers to a more advanced form of the disease in which there are microabscesses involving the tubes and ovaries. Approximately 1% of patients treated for acute PID progress to development of a TOA, as in this case.

Imaging plays a role in cases in which the clinical diagnosis is unclear. Ultrasonography is the first-line imaging modality for evaluation of pelvic pain in young women. Ultrasonography of TOAs typically demonstrates an enlarged ovary in or adjacent to a heterogeneous mass. A heterogeneous mass is detected in more than 90% of patients with proven TOAs. On CT a TOA may appear as a complex mass with heterogeneous enhancement and thickened internal septations. The inflammation causes stranding of the adnexal fat. TOAs have a similar imaging appearance to ovarian carcinoma, but the clinical presentation is quite different. Patients who have a TOA are acutely ill, with fever and marked tenderness on examination, whereas patients with ovarian carcinoma have fewer clinical symptoms.

Notes

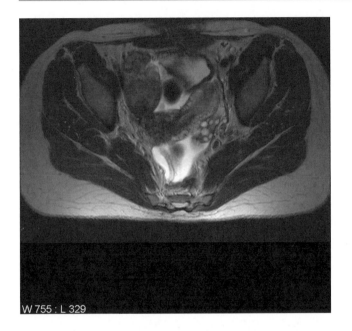

W 755 : L 329

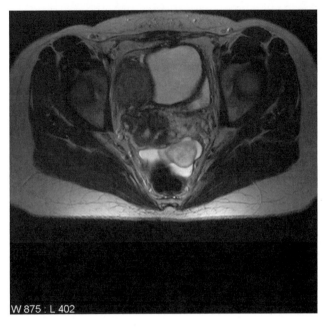

W 875 : L 402

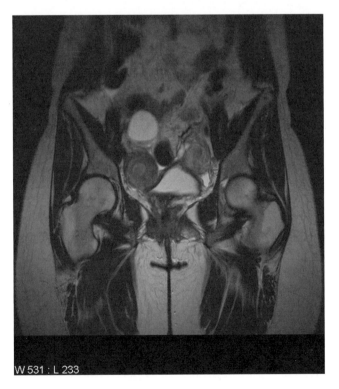

W 531 : L 233

1. What is this anomaly?

2. What is the most commonly associated renal anomaly?

3. Why is the right uterine horn dilated?

4. What is the embryologic origin of this anomaly?

Ob/Gyn: Uterus Didelphys with Obstructed Right Horn

1. Uterus didelphys with cervical stenosis of the right horn.

2. Unilateral renal agenesis.

3. Transverse vaginal septum or cervical stenosis.

4. Complete failure of fusion of the müllerian ducts.

References

Reinhold C, Hricak H, Forstner R, et al: Primary amenorrhea: evaluation with MR imaging, *Radiology* 203:383–390, 1997.

Troiano RN, McCarthy SM: Müllerian duct anomalies: imaging and clinical issues, *Radiology* 233:19–34, 2004.

Cross-Reference

Zagoria RJ, *Genitourinary Radiology: THE REQUISITES*, 2nd ed, p 264.

Comment

Uterus didelphys is the culmination of complete failure of fusion of the müllerian ducts. The result is two hemi-uteri each with its own myometrium, junctional zone, and endometrium visible on T2-weighted imaging. There are also two low signal cervices and two cephalad vaginas. As with all müllerian anomalies, associated renal anomalies, and particularly renal agenesis, may be present. On physical examination, often for infertility, the two vaginas and cervices are identified; however, a complete septate uterus remains in the differential until the external contour of the uterus is examined. Uterus didelphys has widely separated horns, completely unlike the flat or convex surface of the septate uterus. Occasionally, a transverse septum obstructs one of the horns, usually at the level of the vagina. This leads to hematometra and sometimes endometriomas from retrograde extension of endometrial tissue beyond the fimbria. In this case cervical stenosis was present on the right, leading to the presence of dark T2 signal blood products in the dilated horn as well as an endometrioma along the right fallopian tube. Treatment to resolve the obstruction is simple excision of the septum, or dilation of the stenotic cervix. There is no treatment for the associated infertility; however, many women with uterus didelphys or unicornuate uterus can carry a fetus to term.

Notes

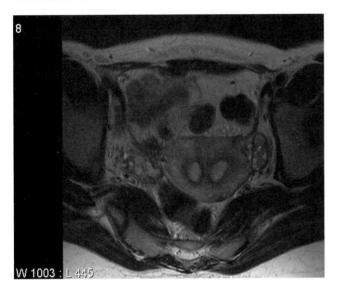 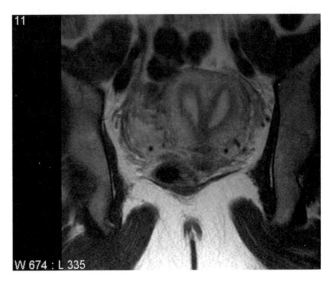

1. What is the müllerian anomaly?

2. What is the most important feature in distinguishing a bicornuate from a septate uterus?

3. Why is it important to do so?

4. What is the most commonly associated renal anomaly?

Ob/Gyn: Septate Uterus

1. Subseptate uterus; there has been resorption of the caudal portion of the septum.

2. External fundal contour.

3. Determination of therapy; septate uterus may be repaired using a hysteroscopy metroplasty.

4. Unilateral renal agenesis.

Reference

Troiano RN, McCarthy SM: Müllerian duct anomalies: imaging and clinical issues, *Radiology* 233:19–34, 2004.

Cross-Reference

Zagoria RJ, *Genitourinary Radiology: THE REQUISITES,* 2nd ed, pp 262–263.

Comment

MRI is used to definitively identify müllerian duct anomalies. In the general population, müllerian anomalies occur in less than 1% of women. For women with infertility issues, and specifically those who have suffered two or more spontaneous abortions, the incidence is approximately 15%. Usually an hysterosalpingogram or sonohysterogram is performed to confirm tubal patency. When a duplication anomaly is suspected by the demonstration of an abnormal internal uterine contour, and surgery is considered a therapeutic option, the radiologist must clearly demonstrate the presence of a septate or bicornuate uterus. This is because the septate uterus is treated using a hysteroscopic metroplasty instead of open surgery. Conception can be attempted within 6 weeks.

On MRI or ultrasonography, separation of the bicornuate from the septate uterus rests entirely on the external uterine contour. Because the bicornuate uterus is a failure of fusion, there is incomplete joining of the uterine horns, leaving an external fundal contour with a sharply defined concavity. The septate uterus is a failure of septal resorption following complete fusion. The external contour of the uterus is flat or convex. The septum of both the bicornuate and septate uterus contains myometrial tissue at the cephalad portion.

In the case of a complete septate uterus, the more caudal portion of the septum usually consists of low T2 signal, presumed fibrous tissue.

Notes

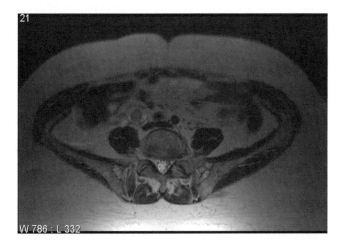

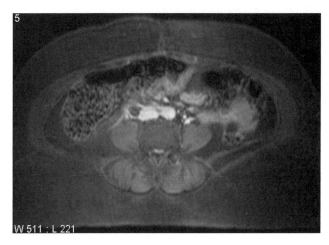

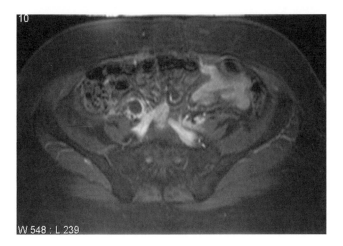

1. In this patient who underwent pelvic laparoscopy, what is the round-appearing structure in the posterior aspect of the pelvis to the right of midline?

2. Explain the change in signal intensity from T2 to contrast-enhanced T1-weighted images?

3. What is the most common cause of this disorder?

4. What are the best tests to diagnose this condition?

Ob/Gyn: Ovarian Vein Thrombosis

1. Right ovarian vein.

2. Thrombosed blood is bright on the T2-weighted spin-echo image and dark on the contrast-enhanced T1-weighted gradient-echo image.

3. Pelvic surgery, usually oncologic.

4. Contrast-enhanced CT or MRI.

Reference

Yassa NA, Ryst E: Ovarian vein thrombosis: a common incidental finding in patients who have undergone total abdominal hysterectomy and bilateral salpingo-oophorectomy with retroperitoneal lymph node dissection, *Am J Roentgenol* 172:45–47, 1999.

Cross-Reference

Zagoria RJ, *Genitourinary Imaging: THE REQUISITES,* 2nd ed, pp 36–37.

Comment

Ovarian vein thrombosis is a common sequela of gynecologic oncologic surgical procedures, occurring in as many as 80% of cases. These surgeries include total abdominal hysterectomy, oophorectomy, and pelvic sidewall and retroperitoneal lymph node dissection. Thrombosis may also follow abortion or an infection of the ovary such as occurs with tuboovarian complex. In asymptomatic patients, the finding is likely of no clinical significance. In this case of a patient with pelvic pain following laparoscopy for benign disease, the thrombus is seen to fill and expand the right ovarian vein, appearing bright on the T2-weighted image and dark on contrast-enhanced fat-saturated T1-weighted images. Other images showed that the thrombus extended from the ovary to the level of insertion into the inferior vena cava. The high signal fluid surrounding the vein was thought most likely due to the recent surgery, although infection can lead to adjacent edema. Ovarian vein thrombosis can also be diagnosed using contrast-enhanced CT scans. A completely thrombosed vein will appear as a target lesion on individual axial sections with a low signal center and high signal, enhancing the periphery. The ovarian vein is located too far posteriorly to be identified using ultrasonography. In asymptomatic patients, anticoagulation remains controversial. Over time, the thrombus will decrease in size and recanalization of the vein may occur. Alternatively, the ovarian vein may become permanently thrombosed.

Notes

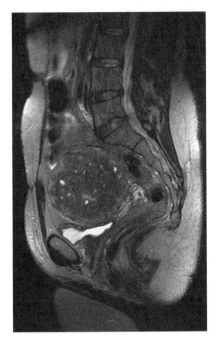

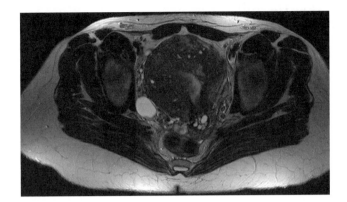

1. What is the normal thickness of the junctional zone?

2. What do the high signal areas in the abnormal myometrium contain?

3. What are the possible presenting symptoms associated with this diagnosis?

4. How does this condition differ in appearance from fibroids?

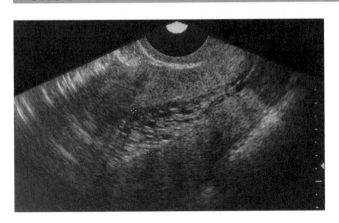

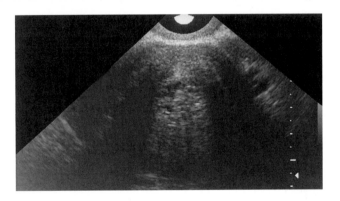

1. During which phase of the menstrual cycle is the endometrium normally thickest? What is the range of thickness (in millimeters) during this phase?

2. True or false: In women treated with tamoxifen, endometrial hyperplasia is the most common histopathologic abnormality resulting in abnormal endometrial thickening.

3. True or false: The relative risk of tamoxifen use leading to endometrial cancer is not dose dependent.

4. True or false: The prevalence of abnormal endometrial thickening depends on the duration of tamoxifen use.

Ob/Gyn: MR Adenomyosis

1. Less than 12 mm.

2. Islands of ectopic endometrium, cystically dilated endometrial glands, or hemorrhagic fluid.

3. Patients may be asymptomatic or present with pelvic pain, hypermenorrhea, and uterine enlargement.

4. Fibroids are round and well-defined on T2-weighted images. Adenomyosis is thickening of the junctional zone leading to an ovoid appearance with poorly defined peripheral margins.

Reference

Tamai K, Togashi K, Ito T, et al: MR imaging findings of adenomyosis: correlation with histopathologic features and diagnostic pitfalls, *Radiographics* 25:21–40, 2005.

Cross-Reference

Zagoria RJ, *Genitourinary Radiology: THE REQUISITES,* 2nd ed, pp 267–272.

Comment

Uterine adenomyosis is a common disease affecting women of menstrual age and is noted in up to 25% of hysterectomy specimens. Clinical symptoms include dysmenorrhea and menorrhagia and are similar to symptoms associated with uterine fibroids. Adenomyosis is defined as aberrant endometrial glands/stroma located in the myometrium. These aberrant glands/stroma may be diffuse, microscopic, or focal (adenomyoma represents a focal nodular form).

On MRI, diagnosis is based on T2-weighted images. Thickening of the hypointense junctional zone of 12 mm or greater is diagnostic. The myometrium may also contain hyperintense foci of T2 signal representing ectopic endometrial glands or hemorrhagic fluid.

T1-weighted imaging can show foci of hyperintensity in the myometrium representing areas of hemorrhage. When this hemorrhage becomes severe, cystic adenomyosis is present.

The diffuse form affects the entire uterus with subsequent uterine enlargement. Focal adenomyosis, adenomyoma, can affect any portion of the myometrium and presents as a focal region of junctional zone thickening. Associated findings include blurring of the myometrial border in this region or a low signal myometrial mass with ill-defined borders.

The main differential diagnosis for adenomyosis is leiomyoma. Factors favoring adenomyosis include a lesion with poorly defined borders, an oval-shaped lesion oriented along the endometrium, small high foci signal within the junctional zone, and a relative lack of mass effect.

Notes

Ob/Gyn: Endometrial Changes in Patients Treated with Tamoxifen

1. Secretory phase; between 8 and 12 mm.

2. False.

3. False.

4. True.

Reference

Hann LE, Giess CS, Bach AM, et al: Endometrial thickness in tamoxifen-treated patients: correlation with clinical and pathologic findings, *Am J Roentgenol* 168:657–661, 1997.

Cross-Reference

Zagoria RJ, *Genitourinary Radiology: THE REQUISITES,* 2nd ed, p 258.

Comment

Tamoxifen is a synthetic estrogen antagonist that has been used in the treatment of breast cancer. Paradoxically, tamoxifen has estrogenic effects on the endometrium. The association between tamoxifen treatment and endometrial cancer was first reported in 1985. When compared with historical controls, the relative risk ratio of endometrial cancer is 2.2 when tamoxifen is given at a dose of 20 mg/day, and the risk ratio increases to 6.4 with a dose of 40 mg/day.

In the study referenced above, Hann and her colleagues found that about half of 91 postmenopausal patients being treated with tamoxifen (20 mg/day) had an endometrial thickness of 8 mm or more on transvaginal sonography. Histologic abnormalities, including polyps (both endometrial and endocervical) and carcinoma, were found in about half of these patients; other studies have found subendometrial cysts and hyperplasia as well. Endometrial polyps were the most frequent abnormality. There was no association between abnormal endometrial thickness and postmenopausal bleeding, and more than half of the women with endometrial histologic abnormalities were asymptomatic. The authors found a correlation between duration of tamoxifen use and increased endometrial thickness; patients on tamoxifen for less than 5 years had a median endometrial thickness of 5 mm, whereas those receiving tamoxifen for 5 years or more had a median endometrial measurement of 14 mm.

Multiple studies suggest that the incidence of endometrial carcinoma is increased in patients treated with tamoxifen, but the incidence is less than 1%. It appears that the risk increases as the duration of tamoxifen use increases, particularly when use exceeds 5 years.

Notes

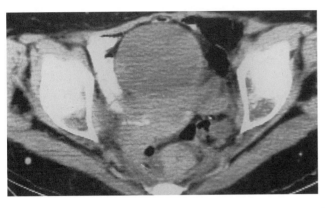 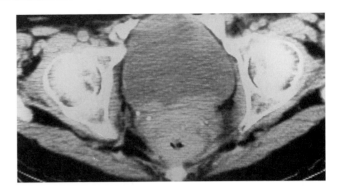

1. What are the treatment implications when bladder cancer invades through the bladder wall?

2. Which pelvic primary tumors may secondarily invade the urinary bladder?

3. What is a "herald" lesion?

4. True or false: All forms of bladder invasion by extravesical inflammation or tumor can be detected by cystoscopy.

Ob/Gyn: Invasion of the Urinary Bladder by Uterine Cervical Carcinoma

1. Complete resection of the tumor may not be possible; radiation therapy may be necessary.

2. Neoplasms of the uterine cervix, prostate, urethra, and rectum.

3. A bladder mucosal lesion with inflammatory features that results from extravesical tumor or inflammation.

4. False.

Reference

Kim SH, Han MC: Invasion of the urinary bladder by uterine cervical carcinoma: evaluation with MR imaging, *Am J Roentgenol* 168:393–397, 1997.

Cross-Reference

Zagoria RJ, *Genitourinary Radiology: THE REQUISITES,* 2nd ed, p 309.

Comment

Mucosal invasion of the urinary bladder or rectum by uterine cervical cancer is designated stage IVa disease and is treated with chemotherapy and radiation therapy. Chemotherapy that reduces a locally advanced tumor can improve the effectiveness of radiation therapy or reduce the size of a tumor sufficiently to make surgery feasible. In studies of cisplatin-based regimens administered to patients with locally advanced cervical carcinoma, response rates of 90% have been reported.

"Herald" lesions are vesical mucosal lesions caused by extravesical tumor or inflammation. On cystoscopy a sessile and shaggy mucosal lesion surrounded by telangiectasia, bullous edema, or hemorrhage may be visible. However, endoscopy may not identify all forms of bladder wall invasion by perivesical lesions; local invasion of the bladder that is confined to the serosa or muscular wall may go undetected and has treatment implications similar to mucosal disease.

Cross-sectional imaging is useful in staging locally advanced cervical carcinoma. Discrete masses protruding into the lumen of the bladder or sessile nodularity of the posterior bladder wall contiguous with a uterine cervical mass should suggest the diagnosis on CT or MRI. In addition, on MRI, abnormally high signal within the posterior bladder wall (which is normally hypointense on T2W images) and strands of abnormal soft tissue signal in the uterovesical space are other clues to stage IVa disease. However, abnormal signal or contrast enhancement of the uterovesical space may not indicate serosal invasion by tumor but a desmoplastic or inflammatory response to the cervical tumor.

Notes

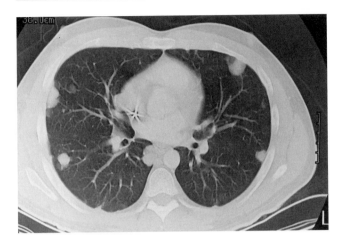

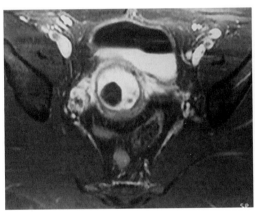
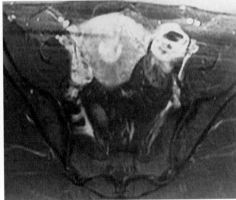

1. What is the differential diagnosis based on the chest CT?

2. What is most likely cause of the endocervical mass?

3. True or false: Endometrial carcinoma metastasis to the lungs is uncommon in the absence of metastatic lymphadenopathy.

4. True or false: After the administration of gadopentetate dimeglumine, most endometrial carcinomas enhance.

Ob/Gyn: Benign Metastasizing Leiomyoma

1. Lung metastases, fungal disease, septic pulmonary emboli, and vasculitis.

2. Endometrial carcinoma.

3. True.

4. True.

References

Maredia R, Snyder BJ, Harvey LA, Schwartz AM: Benign metastasizing leiomyoma in the lung, *Radiographics* 18:779–782, 1998.

Martin E: Leiomyomatous lung lesions: a proposed classification, *Am J Roentgenol* 141:269–272, 1983.

Cross-Reference

Zagoria RJ, *Genitourinary Radiology: THE REQUISITES*, 2nd ed, pp 276–281.

Comment

Martin classifies smooth muscle-containing pulmonary lesions into three general groups. The first group is primary leiomyoma of the lung, which is a benign fibroleiomyomatous hamartoma. The second group is metastatic leiomyoma that arises from extrauterine sites; growth of these tumors is not responsive to hormones, and they may represent low-grade sarcomas. The third group of lesions is exemplified by this case of benign metastasizing leiomyoma (BML).

In this case the uterine mass was an endocervical leiomyoma. Women with uterine leiomyoma have a higher prevalence of endometrial carcinoma. Malignant dedifferentiation of a leiomyoma rarely occurs. An even rarer occurrence is metastasis of histologically benign myomas to pelvic lymph nodes, the abdominopelvic peritoneum, the heart, and the lungs. Approximately 50 cases of BML have been reported in the medical literature, and multiple pulmonary nodules are the most common radiologic presentation. Other reported radiologic patterns include miliary nodules and a giant cystic mass obstructing the mainstem bronchus. The pulmonary lesions of BML are fibroleiomyomatous tumors containing variable mucinous glands. The tumors lack histologic features of malignancy (i.e., nuclear atypia, mitoses, or vascular invasion), and most have both estrogen and progesterone receptors. The clinical course of the disease parallels the estrogen status of the patient. In premenopausal women the disease progression may be difficult to control, but in postmenopausal women the course tends to be more indolent.

Notes

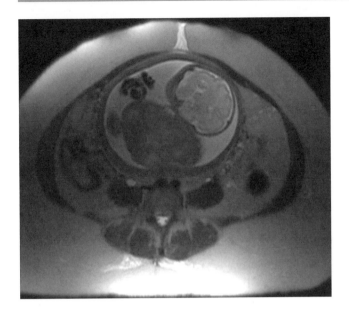

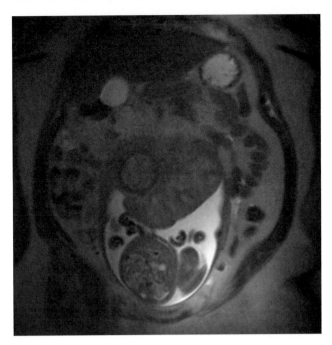

1. What is the diagnosis?

2. What specific type of degeneration of this lesion is associated with pregnancy?

3. What appearance is associated with this type of lesion?

4. What other lesions should be considered in the differential diagnosis of a pregnant patient with pelvic pain?

Ob/Gyn: Degenerating Fibroid in Pregnancy

1. Degenerating fibroid in pregnancy.

2. Red or hemorrhagic degeneration.

3. Peripheral or diffuse high signal on T1-weighted images with variable signal on T2-weighted images. A low signal hemosiderin rim may be present.

4. Adenomyosis, solid adnexal masses, focal myometrial contractions, and subchorionic hematoma.

Reference

Leyendecker JR, Gorengaut V, Brown JJ: MR imaging of maternal diseases of the abdomen and pelvis during pregnancy and the immediate postpartum period, *Radiographics* 24:1301–1316, 2004.

Cross-Reference

Zagoria RJ, *Genitourinary Radiology: THE REQUISITES,* 2nd ed, pp 276–281.

Comment

These single-shot, long echo train, spin-echo, T2-weighted sequences demonstrate a patient with a single intrauterine gestation. The placenta is implanted near the fundus. This case also demonstrates a well-demarcated mass in the intramural portion of the right aspect of the uterine fundus. This has a heterogeneous T2 intensity with a low-signal-intensity rim. No associated adnexal lesions are seen. The findings are typical of a degenerating leiomyoma in pregnancy.

Ultrasonography is the initial imaging modality of choice to evaluate various symptoms that may arise during the course of pregnancy. The lack of ionizing radiation in MRI make it an excellent choice when further imaging is required. MRI may be helpful in the setting of acute abdomen in pregnancy and for evaluation of extent and origin of abdominopelvic tumors.

Leiomyomas are the most common tumor of the uterus. They increase the likelihood of complications in pregnancy, including pain, bleeding, spontaneous abortion, placental abruption, fetal malposition, and mechanical obstruction of the uterus. Leiomyomas may outgrow their blood supply, which results in degeneration, and this may manifest clinically with pain, fever, and leukocytosis. A subtype of hemorrhagic infarction that often occurs in pregnancy is red degeneration, a description referring to the hemorrhagic appearance at gross examination. This occurs secondary to venous thrombosis of the peripheral tumor with rupture of the arteries within the tumor.

The majority of leiomyomas appear as masses that are isointense on T1 with low signal intensity on T2-weighted images. However, the appearance is variable, related to the histologic composition. Their location should be classified as submucosal, intramural, or subserosal. Red degeneration has an unusual appearance of peripheral or diffuse high T1 signal that is variable on T2 with or without a low signal rim. The T1 high signal is likely secondary to methemoglobin, and when the finding is localized to the periphery it may be secondary to blood products within thrombosed peripheral vessels. One sign that has been utilized to help to distinguish pedunculated leiomyomas from adnexal masses is the "bridging vascular sign," in which the vascular supply is seen as signal voids extending from the uterus to the mass.

Notes

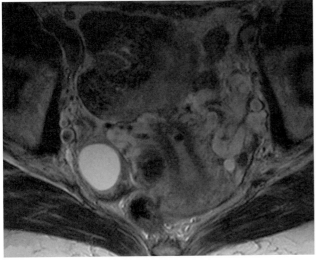

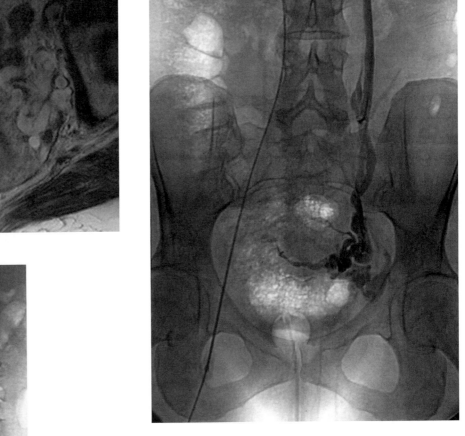

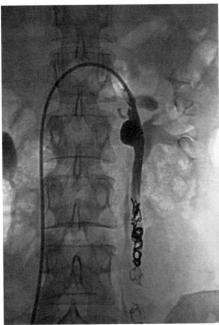

1. What is the abnormal finding on the T2W pelvic MRI (first image)?

2. Which vessel is cannulated in the second image and what is the access route?

3. What are the indications for pelvic/ovarian vein embolization in pelvic congestion syndrome?

4. What effect does this treatment have on menstrual cycle or fertility?

Ob/Gyn: Pelvic Congestion Syndrome

1. Pelvic varices.

2. Left ovarian vein. Access via right femoral vein, iliac vein, interior vena cava, left renal vein, to left ovarian vein.

3. Pelvic pain and fullness, and dyspareunia not relieved by hormonal therapy.

4. None.

References

Maleux G, Stockx L, Wilms G, Marchal G: Ovarian vein embolization for the treatment of pelvic congestion syndrome: long term technical and clinical results, *J Vasc Interv Radiol* 11:859–864, 2000.

Venbrux AC, Chang AH, Kim HS, et al: Pelvic congestion syndrome (pelvic venous incompetence): impact of ovarian and internal iliac vein embolotherapy on menstrual cycle and chronic pelvic pain, *J Vasc Interv Radiol* 13:171–178, 2002.

Cross-Reference

Zagoria RJ, *Genitourinary Radiology: THE REQUISITES*, 2nd ed, pp 266–281.

Comment

Pelvic congestion syndrome is a rare cause of chronic (greater than 6 months) pelvic pain due to reflux in the gonadal vein which results in varicosities of the ovarian or internal iliac veins (pelvic varices). The classic presentation is pelvic fullness, heaviness, or pain that is worst at the end of the day after standing and often resolves by the morning. Dyspareunia is another frequent complaint. Vulvar and/or lower extremity varicosities may also be present. The etiology of the reflux is not known. Possible causes include absence of venous valves, valvular incompetence of the ovarian and pelvic veins in multiparous women, and "nut cracker" phenomenon (extrinsic compression of the left renal vein by the aorta and superior mesenteric artery resulting in increased pressure in the left ovarian vein). The diagnosis is suggested by clinical history and supported by the findings of varicosities on pelvic MRI, CT, or ultrasonography. Treatment options include hormonal manipulation, laparoscopic ligation, and transcatheter embolotherapy. Embolotherapy of the ovarian veins via the inferior vena cava and renal veins can be performed with coils or sclerosing agents. Technical and clinical success is high and durable—some authors recommend embolization of both the ovarian and internal iliac veins to reduce the risk for recurrence. There is no clinically significant postprocedural effect on menstrual pattern or fertility.

This patient had persistent pelvic pain and the MRI (first image) demonstrates enlarged tubular structures in the pelvis. The second image is a selective left ovarian vein injection documenting reflux through the vein to the level of the uterus. After transcatheter embolization with metallic coils, the left gonadal vein injection confirms successful embolization and cessation of reflux (third image).

Notes

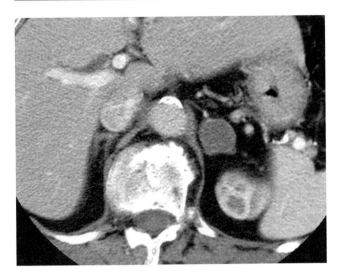

1. What is the differential diagnosis for this lesion?

2. On unenhanced CT, what is the density value that helps to distinguish a benign adenoma from a malignant mass?

3. If this lesion is seen at the time of unenhanced CT, what can be done to further characterize this mass?

4. What are the essential clinical questions that should guide management of this lesion?

Adrenal: Evaluation of an Incidental Adrenal Mass on CT

1. Adenoma, metastasis, and pheochromocytoma.

2. 10 Hounsfield units.

3. Calculate percentage washout on 10- or 15-minute delayed enhanced CT.

4. Is there biochemical evidence of adrenal hyperfunction? Is there a clinical history of primary tumor metastasizing to the adrenal gland?

References

Caoili EM, Korobkin M, Francis IR, et al: Adrenal masses: characterization with combined unenhanced and delayed enhanced CT, *Radiology* 222:629–633, 2002.

Mayo-Smith WW, Boland GW, Noto RB, Lee MJ: State of the art adrenal imaging, *Radiographics* 21:995–1012, 2001.

Cross-Reference

Zagoria RJ, *Genitourinary Radiology: THE REQUISITES,* 2nd ed, pp 369–379.

Comment

Adrenal masses have been found in up to 1% of abdominal CT examinations, and adrenal adenomas are very common tumors in the adrenal gland (1.5% in one autopsy series). In addition, the adrenal gland is a common site of metastases, particularly from patients with lung carcinoma. However, given the high incidence of adrenal adenomas, an isolated adrenal mass in a patient with known lung carcinoma is still most likely an adrenal adenoma. In addition to adenomas and metastases, hyperfunctioning adrenal neoplasms also occur. Finally, adrenocortical carcinoma is a rare neoplasm of the adrenal gland.

The role of the radiologist is to work with the referring physician to differentiate these entities. The first steps to be taken are to determine the patient's history and symptoms. Does the patient have a known malignancy? Does the patient have symptoms of a hyperfunctioning adrenal neoplasm (Cushing's syndrome, pheochromocytomas, aldosteronoma, virilizing tumor)? The clinical history should direct the imaging strategy, as will be defined in other cases in this book. If the patient has no history of neoplasm and does not have symptoms related to increased biochemically active mass, an incidental nonfunctioning adenoma should be strongly considered. Adenomas tend to be round or oval, have a well-defined margin, and are usually less than 3 cm in diameter. Because of the large amount of intracytoplasmic lipid, measured attenuation values are useful for characterizing adenomas. A Hounsfield unit (HU) measurement of less than 10 on unenhanced CT is diagnostic for an adenoma; however, there is no reliable HU to differentiate adenomas from metastases on dynamic enhanced CT as in this case. This 65-year-old patient with abdominal pain had no history of malignancy and had this mass discovered incidentally on dynamic outpatient contrast-enhanced CT. The density of the left adrenal measured 35 HU, which is not specific. She returned for an unenhanced CT, and the adrenal mass density measured −20 HU, which is diagnostic for a benign adenoma.

Notes

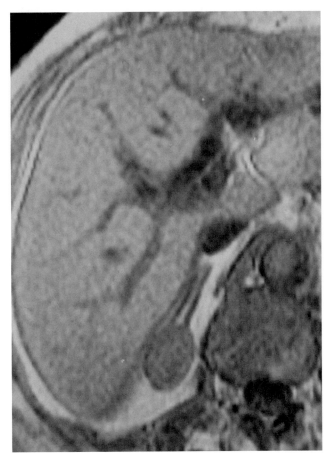
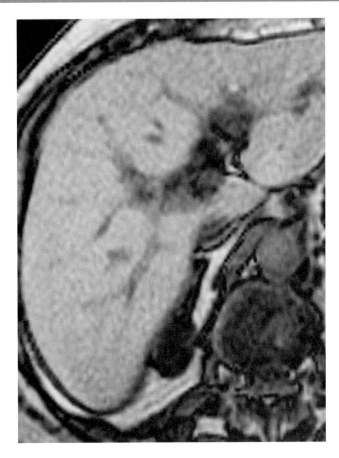

1. Name the imaging sequences in these two images performed at the same level.

2. What parameter is varied in the imaging sequence?

3. What is the cause of loss of signal in the second image?

4. What is the diagnosis?

Adrenal: Characterization of the Adrenal Mass with Chemical Shift MRI

1. In phase (left image) and out of phase T1W sequences.

2. Echo time.

3. Phase cancellation caused by the presence of both fat and water protons within the same voxel.

4. Adrenal adenoma.

References

Haider MA, Ghai S, Jhaveri K, Lockwood G: Chemical shift MR imaging of hyperattenuating (>10 HU) adrenal masses: does it still have a role? *Radiology* 231:711–716, 2004.

Israel GM, Korobkin M, Wang C, et al: Comparison of unenhanced CT and chemical shift MRI in evaluating lipid-rich adrenal adenomas, *Am J Roentgenol* 183: 215–219, 2004.

Cross-Reference

Zagoria RJ, *Genitourinary Radiology: THE REQUISITES,* 2nd ed, pp 354–356.

Comment

Adrenal cortical cells and benign tumors derived from these cells (adenomas) contain a large amount of cytoplasmic cholesterol, fatty acids, and neutral fat. Adrenal adenomas can be characterized on both CT and chemical shift MRI because they contain large numbers of "clear" cells (cortical cells with abundant lipids).

On MRI, the local chemical environment of a proton (specifically magnetic shielding by nearby electrons) may result in a change or shift in the resonance frequency of that proton. When a slice of tissue is first excited, all of the protons resonate synchronously (in phase) with one another, but very soon thereafter, water and fat protons resonate asynchronously (out of phase) with one another because of this chemical shift. The temporal periodicity of this cyclic phase synchrony-asynchrony can be approximated by the quotient of 3.4 ms/T divided by the magnet field strength (in units of Tesla). The signal intensity of a voxel is determined by a vectorial average of the amplitude and phase of its constituent protons. If the echo time of a gradient-echo pulse sequence corresponds with one of the out-of-phase times, then the signal intensity of a voxel containing equal populations of both fat and water decreases because of intravoxel phase cancellation. However, a voxel containing either mostly fat or mostly water protons will not have significant phase dispersion and therefore will not lose signal on the opposed-phase image. In most cases visual assessment of signal loss is as accurate as quantitative measurements (e.g., lesion-to-spleen signal intensity ratios). The role of MRI to characterize adrenal lesions has decreased in the past decade in the United States with development of washout calculations using CT and the expanding role of PET in oncologic patients.

Notes

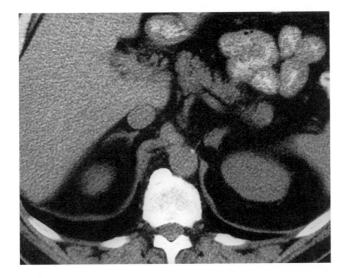

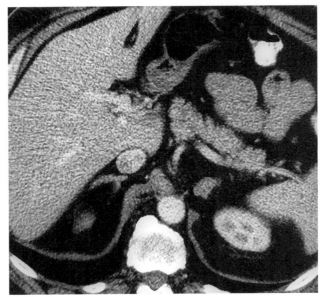

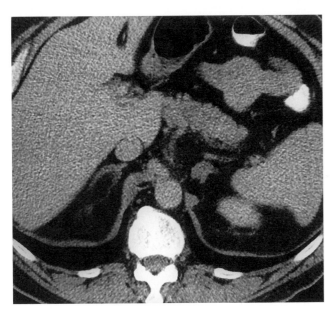

1. On a noncontrast CT of the abdomen (the first image), the left adrenal mass has an attenuation measurement of 23 Hounsfield units (HU). On noncontrast CT, what attenuation measurement HU value is used to characterize an incidental adrenal mass as an adenoma?

2. On CT performed after dynamic administration of intravenous contrast material (the second image), the measured attenuation of the left adrenal mass is 81 HU. What attenuation measurement value is used to diagnose an adrenal adenoma on early dynamic postcontrast CT?

3. The third image was performed 15 minutes after the administration of contrast medium and was used to calculate the value for the adrenal "washout" of contrast; the attenuation measurement of the left adrenal mass was 31 HU. What is the meaning of the term *adrenal washout?*

4. What is meant by relative and absolute washout?

Adrenal: Evaluation of an Adrenal Mass with Dynamic CT

1. A measurement of less than 10 HU.

2. A specific HU has not been found to be useful to discriminate between adenomas and metastases due to the overlap in enhancement patterns on dynamic CT. Fifteen-minute delayed imaging and washout calculations are required to differentiate these entities.

3. It refers to the relative decrease in attenuation or signal intensity in an adrenal mass on delayed imaging when compared with immediate postcontrast imaging.

4. Absolute washout is calculated from non-contrast-enhanced images, dynamic contrast-enhanced images, and 15-minute delayed contrast-enhanced images. An absolute washout value of greater than or equal to 60% is diagnostic of an adenoma. Relative washout is calculated from dynamic contrast-enhanced CT and 15-minute delayed contrast-enhanced CT. A non-contrast-enhanced CT in not required. A relative washout value of greater than or equal to 40% is diagnostic for an adrenal adenoma.

References

Caoili EM, Korobkin M, Francis IR, et al: Adrenal masses: characterization with combined unenhanced and delayed enhanced CT, *Radiology* 222:629–633, 2002.

Mayo-Smith WW: CT characterization of adrenal masses [Letter], *Radiology* 226:289–290, 2003.

Cross-Reference

Zagoria RJ, *Genitourinary Radiology: THE REQUISITES,* 2nd ed, pp 369–374.

Comment

Adrenal adenomas are the most common benign tumors of the adrenal gland. They are found in up to 1.5% of autopsy cases and 1% of CT examinations. The adrenal glands also are common sites of metastases, particularly from bronchogenic carcinoma. A common clinical problem encountered by the radiologist is the evaluation of an enlarged adrenal gland on CT in a patient who has a known malignancy. Much clinical research in the past decade has been dedicated to differentiating between adrenal adenomas and adrenal metastases on CT, MRI, and PET. Differentiation of these entities is based on two different parameters, histology and physiology. The histopathologic basis for differentiation is based on the increased cytoplasmic lipid content of adenomas. This finding accounts for the low density of an adenoma on noncontrast CT and the signal loss on chemical shift MRI. The physiologic differences between adenomas and metastases relates to differences in perfusion and washout of intravenous contrast. In dynamic post-contrast-enhanced images (performed approximately 90 seconds after administration of contrast), there is rapid enhancement of both adenomas and metastases with overlapping density values within the adrenal gland. However, the contrast "washes out" of adenomas more rapidly, so adenomas have a lower density on 15-minute delayed images when compared with metastases. Metastases do not "wash out" contrast as rapidly and thus have higher densities on delayed imaging. Different types, concentrations, and volumes of contrast agents are used at different institutions, so an absolute density in Hounsfield units cannot be applied on delayed imaging. However, washout values comparing early dynamic densities to delayed densities are useful. By comparing the density of an adrenal mass on delayed images to its density on early, enhanced images, the variation in attenuation caused by the type, concentration, and amount of contrast administered can be minimized.

Caoili and colleagues performed a study to differentiate adrenal adenomas from metastases using unenhanced and delayed enhanced CT and found they were able to correctly characterize 160 (96%) of 166 adrenal masses. Absolute washout is calculated as ([HU at dynamic CT − HU at 15-minute delayed CT] / [HU at dynamic CT − HU noncontrast CT]) × 100. Relative washout is used when no precontrast imaging is available. Relative washout is calculated as ([HU at dynamic CT − HU at 15-minute delayed CT] / [HU at dynamic CT]) × 100.

In this patient, the unenhanced CT value of 23 HU is not diagnostic for an adenoma. However, the absolute washout was 86%, which is diagnostic of an adenoma. This is an example of a "lipid-poor" adrenal adenoma.

Notes

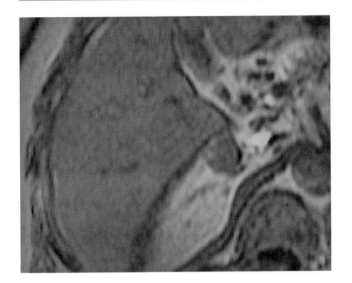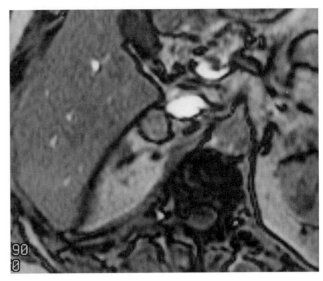

1. Identify the type (pulse sequence and weighting) of the MRIs shown.

2. What is the typical appearance of an adrenal metastasis on chemical shift images?

3. With regard to chemical shift MRI of adrenal adenomas, what is the explanation for false-negative cases?

4. Besides intracellular lipid content, what other parameter of adrenal physiology can be used to differentiate adenomas from metastases?

Adrenal: Adrenal Chemical Shift Imaging: False Negatives and False Positives

1. In-phase and out-of-phase T1W gradient-echo MRIs of a right adrenal mass.

2. On in-phase imaging, isointense with spleen or muscle. On out-of-phase imaging, metastases maintain signal compatible to spleen or muscle (do not lose signal intensity).

3. Histologic variability. Approximately 80% of adrenal adenomas have intracellular lipid. Thus, approximately 20% of adenomas are "lipid poor" and would not demonstrate signal drop-off on out-of-phase imaging (or measure less than 10 Hounsfield units on noncontrast CT).

4. Washout of intravenous contrast.

References

Haider MA, Ghai S, Jhaveri K, Lockwood G: Chemical shift MR imaging of hyperattenuating (>10 HU) adrenal masses: does it still have a role? *Radiology* 231:711–716, 2004.

Israel GM, Korobkin M, Wang C, et al: Comparison of unenhanced CT and chemical shift MRI in evaluating lipid-rich adrenal adenomas, *Am J Roentgenol* 183: 215–219, 2004.

Mayo-Smith WW, Boland GW, Noto RB, Lee MJ: State of the art adrenal imaging, *Radiographics* 21:995–1012, 2001.

Cross-Reference

Zagoria RJ, *Genitourinary Radiology: THE REQUISITES,* 2nd ed, pp 355–358, 369–374.

Comment

Chemical shift imaging is the method of choice for characterizing adrenal masses using MRI. However, like many noninvasive imaging tests, chemical shift imaging is imperfect. The chemical shift MRIs presented show a false-negative case of a biopsy-proven right adrenal adenoma.

For the diagnosis of adrenal adenoma, the sensitivity of chemical shift imaging is lower than its specificity. The rate of false negatives (i.e., no loss of signal in the mass on an opposed-phase T1W gradient-echo image compared with an in-phase image) may be as high as 20%. The explanation is that adenomas contain variable amounts of cytoplasmic fat. Approximately 80% of non-hyperfunctional adenomas consist of "clear" cells with abundant intracytoplasmic cholesterol, fatty acids, and neutral fat. The remaining 20% of adenomas are composed of relatively lipid-poor "compact" cells.

Conversely, in most reported series the specificity of chemical shift imaging for characterizing an adrenal adenoma is close to 100%. False-positive cases from metastases containing lipid (renal cell carcinoma and liposarcoma metastases to the adrenal) are largely theoretical. The take-home point is that signal drop-off in an adrenal mass on out-of-phase imaging is diagnostic of an adenoma; however, no signal drop-off is not diagnostic of a metastasis. If there is no signal drop-off in an adrenal mass and a metastasis is suspected, then further imaging characterization or a biopsy should be considered.

The expanding role of CT in diagnosing and staging oncologic patients, and the more recent literature applying washout of intravenous contrast, has limited the role of MRI in characterizing adrenal masses in the United States. In addition, PET has been shown to be quite useful in differentiating benign adenomas from metastases in patients with a known primary malignancy. The most efficacious noninvasive imaging examination to differentiate adenomas from metastases is evolving and depends on the patient's clinical presentation.

Notes

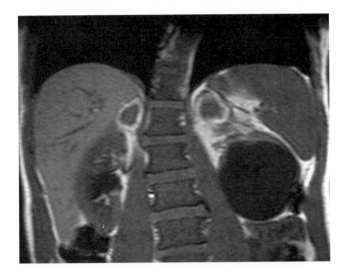

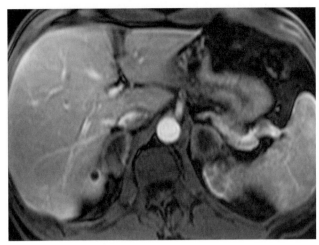

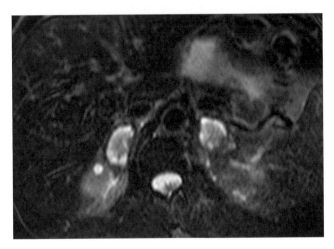

1. A coronal T1W gradient-echo image, an axial T1W image with fat saturation after administration of intravenous gadolinium contrast, and a fat-saturated turbo T2W spin-echo image are shown. What is the diagnosis?

2. Name three etiologies for this lesion.

3. What causes the dark region around the adrenal glands on the T2W image?

4. What is Waterhouse-Friderichsen syndrome?

Adrenal: Adrenal Hemorrhage on MRI

1. Adrenal hemorrhage.

2. Anticoagulation, trauma, surgery.

3. Signal loss from magnetic susceptibility of hemosiderin (most likely in macrophages).

4. Hemorrhagic destruction of both adrenal glands caused by overwhelming meningococcemia that results in acute adrenocortical insufficiency.

References

Kawashima A, Sandler CM, Ernst RD, et al: Imaging of nontraumatic hemorrhage of the adrenal gland [Review], *Radiographics* 19:949–963, 1999.

Mayo-Smith WW, Boland GW, Noto RB, Lee MJ: State of the art adrenal imaging, *Radiographics* 21:995–1012, 2001.

Cross-Reference

Zagoria RJ, *Genitourinary Radiology: THE REQUISITES,* 2nd ed, p 366.

Comment

There are multiple causes of adrenal hemorrhage. In neonates, hemorrhage may be the result of birth trauma, anoxia, dehydration, renal vein thrombosis, or systemic coagulopathy; the major differential diagnosis is neuroblastoma. Spontaneous adrenal hemorrhage in adults may be caused by the systemic "stress" of surgery, extensive body burns, sepsis, or hypotension. Anticoagulants, disseminated intravascular coagulation, and antiphospholipid antibody syndrome may result in a bleeding diathesis that predisposes to adrenal hemorrhage. The majority of cases caused by anticoagulant administration occur within the first 3 weeks after use of the anticoagulant; patients are not necessarily over-anticoagulated when bleeding complications occur.

Iatrogenic causes of adrenal hemorrhage include open and percutaneous biopsy, adrenal venous sampling, exogenous adrenocorticotropic hormone or other corticosteroid administration, and orthotopic liver transplantation. After liver transplantation, hemorrhagic infarction or hematoma of the right adrenal gland is thought to result from the ligation and division of the right adrenal vein during hepatectomy. Blunt traumatic hematoma is also more common in the right adrenal gland.

Adrenal hemorrhage can very rarely cause acute adrenal insufficiency when it is bilateral. MRI is the most sensitive and specific imaging technique for detecting and characterizing adrenal hemorrhage. Adrenal hemorrhage does not enhance with either iodinated intravenous contrast on CT or with gadolinium contrast on MRI.

Notes

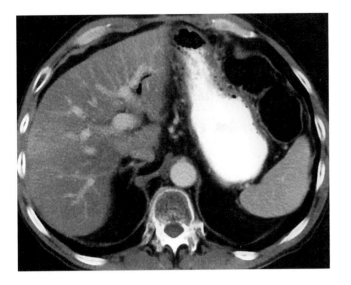
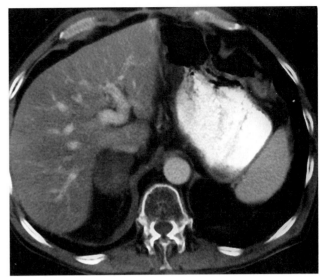
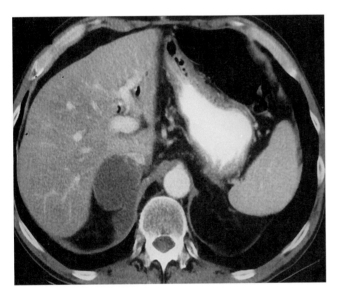

1. Three abdominal CT scans, each performed 2 months apart, are shown. What is the diagnosis? What is the cause of this abnormality?

2. Which primary adrenal tumors may present as a predominantly cystic mass?

3. What are some indications for surgical removal of an adrenal cyst?

4. What is the expected natural history of this lesion?

Adrenal: Adrenal Pseudocyst

1. Adrenal pseudocyst secondary to hemorrhage.

2. Adenoma, necrotic metastases, and very rarely pheochromocytoma.

3. Symptoms that can be attributed to the size of the cyst, endocrinologic hyperfunction, infection, or possibility of malignancy.

4. Involution with time.

References

Castillo OA, Litvak JP, Kerkebe M, Urena RD: Laparoscopic management of symptomatic and large adrenal cysts, *J Urol* 173:915–917, 2005.

Rozenblit A, Morehouse HT, Amis ES Jr: Cystic adrenal lesions: CT features, *Radiology* 201:541–548, 1996.

Cross-Reference

Zagoria RJ, *Genitourinary Radiology: THE REQUISITES,* 2nd ed, pp 366–367.

Comment

Adrenal cysts can be divided into several pathologic subtypes: true cysts, pseudocysts, and infectious cysts. Some true adrenal cysts arise from endothelium; of this type, lymphangiomatous cysts are much more common than adrenal hemangiomas. Epithelial cysts are the other type of true adrenal cyst and are divided into retention, embryonal, and adenomatous types. Infectious cysts are the least common, and the majority of infectious adrenal cysts are echinococcal in origin.

Adrenal pseudocysts are so named because the wall in these types of cysts does not have a benign endothelial or epithelial lining. Instead, the pseudocyst wall has variable composition depending on its etiology; pseudocysts can be the sequela of chronic adrenal hemorrhage (as in this case), a hemorrhagic complication of benign vascular neoplasm or malformation, or cystic degeneration of a primary or metastatic tumor. Benign primary adrenal tumors that can rarely present as pseudocysts include cystic adenomas, pheochromocytomas, adenomatoid tumors, and schwannomas. Many cysts with attenuation values in excess of 30 Hounsfield units have evidence of organizing hemorrhage pathologically; intracystic proteinaceous debris or calcification also may account for an attenuation higher than that of water.

Notes

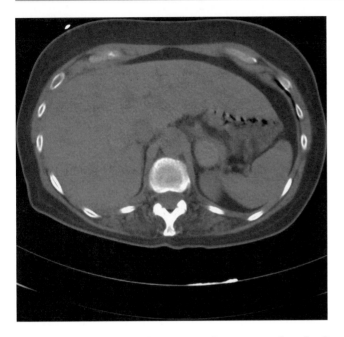 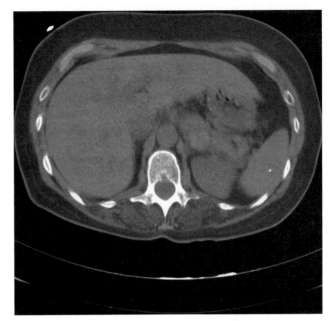

1. What clinical conditions predispose to this finding?

2. What is Waterhouse-Friderichsen syndrome?

3. What is the term for a chronic cystic adrenal mass that has evolved from prior adrenal hematoma?

4. In the setting of trauma, which side of the body is more commonly affected?

Adrenal: Adrenal Hemorrhage

1. Trauma, severe systemic stress, coagulopathy, neonatal stress, and adrenal mass.

2. Adrenal hemorrhage associated with fulminant meningococcemia.

3. Adrenal pseudocyst.

4. The right adrenal gland is more prone to traumatic hemorrhage, likely due to compression by the adjacent liver.

References

Elsayes KM, Mukundan G, Narra VR, et al: Adrenal masses: MR imaging features with pathologic correlation, *Radiographics* 24:573–586, 2004.

Kawashima A, Sandler CM, Ernst RD, et al: Imaging of nontraumatic hemorrhage of the adrenal gland, *Radiographics* 19:949–963, 1999.

Cross-Reference

Zagoria RJ, *Genitourinary Radiology: THE REQUISITES,* 2nd ed, p 366.

Comment

The unenhanced CT images show a slightly hyperdense lesion in the left adrenal gland with periadrenal soft tissue stranding. This indicates an adrenal hematoma. Adrenal hemorrhage generally occurs in one or more of the following situations: trauma, states of severe systemic stress such as sepsis, coagulopathy, neonatal stress, or underlying adrenal mass. The spectrum of clinical manifestations is variable and the condition may be clinically occult. Alternatively, cases of massive bilateral adrenal hemorrhage, as can be seen with systemic stress or coagulopathy, may damage enough adrenal tissue to cause life-threatening adrenal insufficiency.

In general, adrenal hemorrhage demonstrates imaging characteristics and evolution similar to hematomas elsewhere in the body. In the acute to subacute phase as seen here, CT typically reveals a fairly homogeneous round or oval mass with attenuation values ranging from 50 to 90 Hounsfield units. This may be accompanied by stranding in the periadrenal fat and extension into the perinephric space. Over time, the mass will decrease in attenuation and may resolve completely, or may organize into a chronic low-density cystic collection with or without calcifications. This entity is termed an adrenal pseudocyst.

In neonates, adrenal hemorrhage may present as a flank mass and is typically diagnosed by ultrasonography. Acutely, adrenal hemorrhage presents as a solid mass with absent flow on Doppler imaging. Follow-up studies reveal reduction in size, and the lesion may progress to an anechoic, cyst-like appearance. Calcifications may develop as early as 1 to 2 weeks.

MRI may be useful to determine the age of the hematoma, or to evaluate for an underlying mass when no other predisposing factors are evident. The classic appearance of the subacute adrenal hematoma is hyperintensity on precontrast T1 imaging secondary to methemoglobin, which can be seen peripherally as early as 7 days posthemorrhage. The presence of marked heterogeneity, central stromal enhancement, or failure to decrease in size over time may indicate the presence of an underlying adrenal tumor. For example, a central fat component within an adrenal hematoma suggests an underlying myelolipoma.

Notes

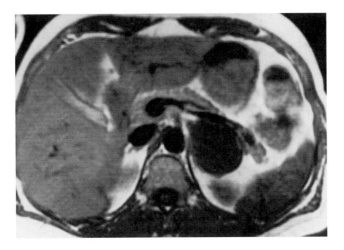 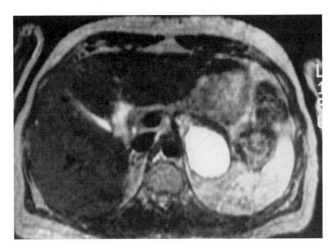

1. True or false: This adrenal lesion is diagnostic of a pheochromocytoma because it is T2 bright.

2. What is the most common type of true adrenal cyst?

3. Is mural calcification a common feature of adrenal cysts?

4. What is the most common cause of adrenal pseudocysts?

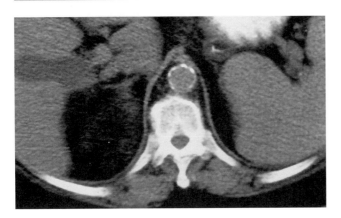 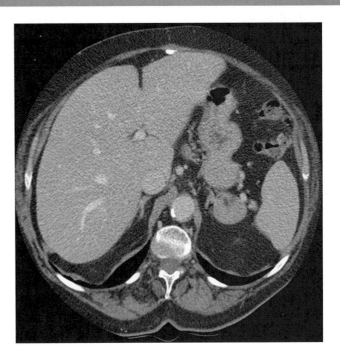

1. These are two different patients with the same diagnosis. What are the histologic constituents of this tumor?

2. What is the most common presentation of patients with this entity?

3. Can patients have endocrine disturbances with this tumor?

4. Is there malignant potential?

CASE 152

Adrenal: Adrenal Cyst

1. False. T2 hyperintensity is not sensitive or specific for the diagnosis of pheochromocytoma.

2. Endothelial cyst. Lymphangioma is much more common than hemangioma.

3. Yes. 15% to 54% of adrenal cysts showed calcification on CT scans.

4. Adrenal hemorrhage.

References

Otal P, Escourrou G, Mazerolles C, et al: Imaging features of uncommon adrenal masses with histopathologic correlation, *Radiographics* 19:569–581, 1999.

Rozenblit A, Morehouse HT, Amis ES Jr: Cystic adrenal lesions: CT features, *Radiology* 201:541–548, 1996.

Cross-Reference

Zagoria RJ, *Genitourinary Radiology: THE REQUISITES,* 2nd ed, pp 366–369.

Comment

True cysts of the adrenal gland are rare. Cysts are typically nonfunctional and can present as large masses up to 20 cm in diameter. Some patients complain of back or flank pain when very large cysts compress surrounding organs; symptoms also may develop when hemorrhage or infection complicates an adrenal cyst.

One study has reported that 60% of adrenal cysts are true cysts in that they have an epithelial lining and 40% are pseudocysts that are the sequela of chronic adrenal hemorrhage. Adrenal cysts can have a variable appearance and up to 54% of adrenal cysts may have peripheral calcification. Complicated cysts with thick walls and mural enhancement are difficult to differentiate from necrotic or cystic neoplasms and either cyst aspiration of surgical resection should be considered. Evaluation of cyst fluid, obtained by fine-needle aspiration, may confirm the benign nature and adrenal origin of these indeterminate cysts by revealing high concentrations of cortisol or weak adrenal androgens or visible cholesterol crystals. Pheochromocytomas can rarely present as cystic adrenal masses so appropriate biochemical workup should be performed in the correct clinical setting.

Notes

CASE 153

Adrenal: Adrenal Myelolipoma

1. Mature adipose and hematopoietic tissue.

2. None. Usually the mass is discovered incidentally, although larger lesions can hemorrhage, causing pain.

3. Yes, very rarely.

4. No.

References

Elsayes KM, Mukundan G, Narra VR, et al: Adrenal masses: MR imaging features with pathologic correlation, *Radiographics* 24(Suppl 1):73–86, 2004.

Mayo-Smith WW, Boland GW, Noto RB, Lee MJ: State of the art adrenal imaging, *Radiographics* 21:995–1012, 2001.

Cross-Reference

Zagoria RJ, *Genitourinary Radiology: THE REQUISITES,* 2nd ed, pp 368–369.

Comment

Adrenal myelolipomas are benign tumors of the adrenal cortex. The overall incidence is estimated to be between 0.08% and 0.20% of the population based on autopsy series. The tumor is composed of mature adipose tissue and hematopoietic elements similar to bone marrow. Approximately one third have calcification.

The tumor is usually asymptomatic and is discovered incidentally. However, larger lesions (greater than 10 cm) may hemorrhage, resulting in pain and or hypotension. These tumors are rarely associated with endocrine dysfunction (e.g., Cushing's syndrome or Conn's syndrome). The diagnosis can be established by CT if there is macroscopic fat within an adrenal mass, and follow-up is usually not required unless the patient becomes symptomatic or endocrine dysfunction is present.

The imaging hallmark of adrenal myelolipoma is macroscopic fat within an enlarged adrenal gland. On ultrasonography, these masses are typically hyperechoic with hypoechoic marrow elements within the lesion. On CT, they are well-defined heterogeneous lesions with layers of fat interspersed among higher-attenuation tissue as demonstrated in these two cases. The two patients presented here have variable amounts of fat within the adrenal myelolipoma. The patient imaged on the left has large amounts of macroscopic fat in the enlarged right adrenal. The patient imaged on the right has a smaller amount of macroscopic fat in the enlarged left adrenal.

Notes

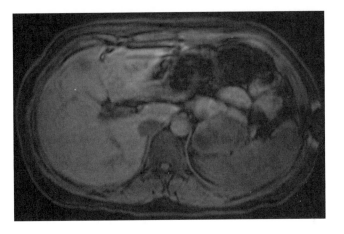 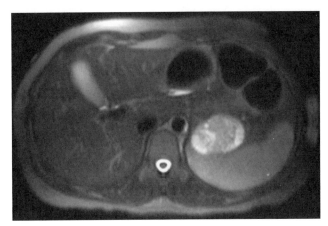

1. What is the differential diagnosis for the mass?

2. How is the final diagnosis made?

3. What percentages of these tumors are of high T2 signal on MRI?

4. What are three alternative imaging methods for the adrenal gland?

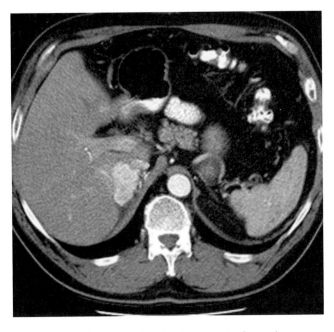 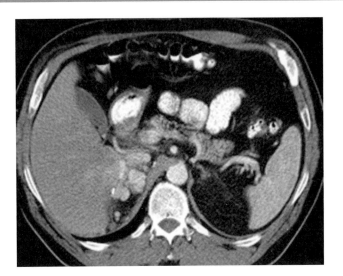

1. What is the most likely diagnosis for a hypervascular adrenal mass?

2. This is a 52-year-old man 5 years after laparoscopic resection of a right 5-cm pheochromocytoma. Where do these recur?

3. How is this diagnosis established?

4. What is the imaging modality of choice to assess for recurrent disease?

CASE 154

Adrenal: Pheochromocytoma

1. Pheochromocytoma and metastasis.

2. Clinical symptoms, and blood and urine chemistries.

3. 85%.

4. CT with washout technique is useful for diagnosing adenomas, octreotide and ^{131}I meta-iodobenzylguanidine (MIBG) studies can locate biochemically active tumors, and PET scanning is often appropriate for the diagnosis of metastatic disease.

Reference

Elsayes KM, Narra VR, Leyendecker JR, et al: MRI of adrenal and extraadrenal pheochromocytoma, *Am J Roentgenol* 184:860–867, 2005.

Cross-Reference

Zagoria RJ, *Genitourinary Imaging: THE REQUISITES,* 2nd ed, pp 358–365.

Comment

The usual differential diagnosis for a solid adrenal mass is adenoma, metastasis, pheochromocytoma, and primary adrenocortical carcinoma. In general, the diagnosis of pheochromocytoma is a clinical one based on symptomatology and laboratory values. In particular, elevation of vanillylmandelic acid levels in the urine is an important marker for an actively secreting pheochromocytoma. Once this tumor is suspected, imaging is often employed to identify the site of origin. The majority of pheochromocytomas arise from the adrenal gland, with the remainder arising from the retroperitoneum (especially adjacent to the original of the inferior mesenteric artery) and, less commonly, other organs such as the bladder or heart. In the adrenal, this tumor arises from the medullary portion of the gland; therefore, it is usually ovoid or round rather than adreniform in shape. The cells contain a significant amount of fluid and the majority of tumors (85%) are of bright signal on T2-weighted imaging. Because they do not contain intracytoplasmic lipid, there is no signal loss on out-of-phase imaging, unlike most adenomas. When the clinical findings are appropriate and imaging of the abdomen is negative, nuclear medicine tests using octreotide or ^{131}I MIBG are often helpful in locating multiple or ectopic tumors.

Notes

CASE 155

Adrenal: Recurrent Pheochromocytoma (Pheochromocytomatosis)

1. Metastasis or pheochromocytoma.

2. Recurrent pheochromocytomas can occur at the operative site as in this case or by local metastases to the ipsilateral retroperitoneum.

3. Biochemical assessment with serum plasma catecholamine levels, 24-hour urine vanillylmandelic acid, and metanephrine levels.

4. CT. If CT is not diagnostic in the setting of elevated catecholamines, MRI or nuclear medicine studies can be performed.

References

Blake MA, Kalra MK, Maher MM, et al: Pheochromocytoma: an imaging chameleon, *Radiographics* 24(Suppl):87–99, 2004.

Li ML, Fitzgerald PA, Price DC, Norton JA: Iatrogenic pheochromocytomatosis: a previously unreported result of laparoscopic adrenalectomy, *Surgery* 130: 1072–1077, 2001.

Cross-Reference

Zagoria RJ, *Genitourinary Radiology: THE REQUISITES,* 2nd ed, pp 358–365.

Comment

This patient had previous laparoscopic resection for an adrenal pheochromocytoma and presented with recurrence of symptoms 5 years later. Recurrence of tumor was thought to be iatrogenic from seeding. Pheochromocytomas are hyperfunctioning catecholamine-secreting neoplasms of the adrenal medulla. First-line tests for evaluating a patient with suspected pheochromocytoma are plasma catecholamine levels, 24-hour urine vanillylmandelic acid, and metanephrine levels.

This is an unusual case, but if the patient presents with recurrent symptoms, the diagnosis of recurrent pheochromocytoma should be entertained. In the study cited above, three patients who underwent laparoscopic adrenalectomy for pheochromocytoma had recurrences at the laparoscopic site. The original tumors were 5 to 6 cm in size, not malignant, and the average recurrence time was 3 to 4 years after the original resection. The presumed etiology was tumor fragmentation and seeding at the time of laparoscopic resection. The patient in this case had resolution of symptoms and restoration of normal catecholamine levels after repeat surgical resection.

Notes

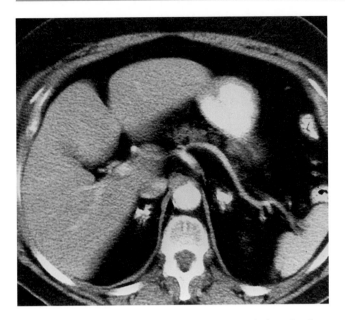

1. What is the differential diagnosis of this finding?

2. What is the expected biochemical abnormality?

3. What is the treatment for this disease?

4. Which U.S. president had this disease?

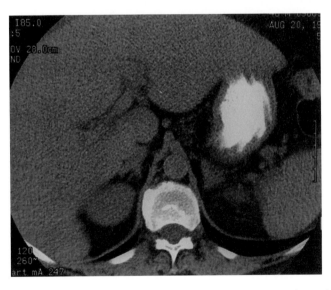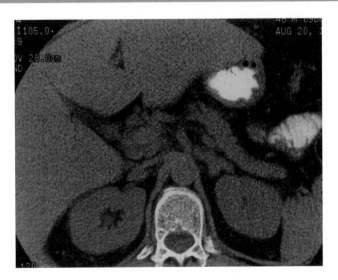

1. Given the clinical history of insulin-dependent diabetes, autoimmune thyroiditis, and Addison's disease, what is the most likely diagnosis?

2. What are some of the clinical manifestations of Addison's disease?

3. What is the differential diagnosis for adrenal enlargement and Addison's disease?

4. In idiopathic Addison's disease, what are the primary autoantigens?

CASE 156

Adrenal: Adrenal Calcifications Caused by Addison's Disease

1. Granulomatous disease (e.g., tuberculosis or histoplasmosis), prior adrenal hemorrhage, and treated metastases.

2. Reduced serum levels of aldosterone and cortisol.

3. Oral supplements of cortisol and mineralocorticoids.

4. John F. Kennedy.

References

Ammini AC, Gupta R, Mukopadhyay C, et al: Computed tomography morphology of the adrenal glands of patients with Addison's disease, *Australas Radiol* 40:38–42, 1996.

Morgan HE, Austin JH, Follet DA: Bilateral adrenal enlargement in Addison's disease caused by tuberculosis: nephrotomographic demonstration, *Radiology* 115:357–358, 1975.

Cross-Reference

Zagoria RJ, *Genitourinary Radiology: THE REQUISITES*, 2nd ed, pp 367–369.

Comment

Addison's disease is the result of decreased production of steroid hormones by the adrenal cortex. It may be primary, when there is insufficient adrenal tissue to produce steroid hormones, or secondary, when there is insufficient adrenocorticotropic hormone (ACTH) produced by the pituitary to stimulate the adrenal glands. Primary Addison's disease has an autoimmune etiology in more than half of all cases. In these patients the adrenal glands are small on CT or MRI. Addison's disease also may result from destruction of the adrenal gland caused by hemorrhage or infection with tuberculosis, histoplasmosis, coccidioidomycosis, or cryptococcosis. Bilateral metastases are a rare cause of Addison's disease. More than 90% of the adrenal gland must be destroyed for hypofunction to occur.

Typically, short-term involvement with an infectious process, such as tuberculosis, results in an enlargement of the adrenal glands, with or without calcification. Long-term involvement after treatment of the infection results in decreased gland size and dense calcification.

The diagnosis of Addison's disease is made by ACTH stimulation testing but can be suggested if small adrenal glands or enlarged and calcified adrenal glands are demonstrated on CT.

Notes

CASE 157

Adrenal: Schmidt's Syndrome

1. Polyglandular syndrome type 2 (Schmidt's syndrome).

2. Asthenia (weakness and fatigue), arterial hypotension, anorexia, weight loss, pain, nausea, vomiting, and diarrhea, and hyperpigmentation.

3. Granulomatous adrenalitis, adrenal hemorrhage, metastatic disease, lymphoma, sarcoidosis, and amyloidosis.

4. Enzymes involved with steroidogenesis (17-alpha hydroxylase, 21-alpha hydroxylase, and side-chain cleavage enzymes).

Reference

Baker JR Jr: Autoimmune endocrine disease, *JAMA* 278: 1931–1937, 1997.

Cross-Reference

Zagoria RJ, *Genitourinary Radiology: THE REQUISITES*, 2nd ed, pp 377–379.

Comment

In the United States, primary adrenal insufficiency presents most commonly in middle-aged women; idiopathic adrenal atrophy is the most common cause of Addison's disease. Immunohistochemical staining reveals the antibody and complement on the few remaining glandular cells. Primary ovarian failure caused by autoimmune oophoritis also may occur. Addison's disease also can be a part of an autoimmune endocrinopathy called polyglandular syndrome (PGS). This syndrome accounts for all of the cases of Addison's disease in juveniles and more than one third of all cases in adults. There are three types of PGS. Type 1 PGS usually begins in early childhood and is defined by mucocutaneous candidiasis and hypoparathyroidism. More than half of these patients develop Addison's disease; gonadal failure, chronic hepatitis, and alopecia also may occur. Addison's disease and either insulin-dependent diabetes or autoimmune thyroid disease defines PGS type 2 (Schmidt's syndrome). Addison's disease does not occur in type 3 PGS, which consists of autoimmune thyroid disease together with any two other autoimmune disorders, including insulin-dependent diabetes, pernicious anemia, or any nonendocrine autoimmune disorder (e.g., myasthenia gravis).

This case is unusual because the adrenal glands are slightly enlarged rather than atrophic; adrenal insufficiency was biochemical (as evidenced by abnormal results of a corticotropin stimulation test), and the adrenal enlargement was incidentally discovered.

Notes

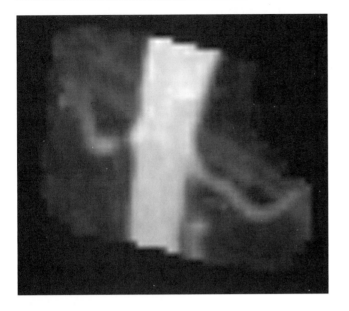

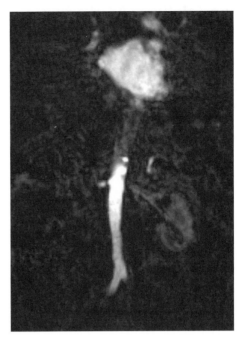

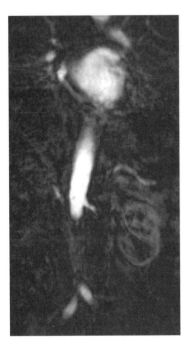

1. Given the images presented, what is the most likely cause of a small right kidney, and how does this lesion cause hypertension?

2. What is the difference between first image and the second and third images?

3. Name three imaging tests that can be used to screen for renovascular hypertension.

4. Given systemic hypertension, what is the success rate of angioplasty without stenting for ostial versus mid-renal artery stenosis?

Vascular and Interventional: Renal Artery Stenosis

1. Ostial renal artery stenosis, which causes glomerular hypoperfusion and primary hyperreninemic hypertension.

2. The first image is a maximum-intensity projection image and the other two are directly acquired T1W coronal images after administration of intravenous gadolinium chelate.

3. Captopril renal scan, MR-angiography, multidetector row CT-angiography, and digital subtraction angiography.

4. For ostial stenosis, angioplasty success rate is 30%; this rate is higher when intravascular stents are used. The angioplasty success rate is greater than 80% for stenoses in the mid-renal artery.

References

Vasbinder GB, Nelemans PJ, Kessels AG, et al: Renal Artery Diagnostic Imaging Study in Hypertension (RADISH) Study Group. Accuracy of computed tomographic angiography and magnetic resonance angiography for diagnosing renal artery stenosis, *Ann Intern Med* 141:674–682, 2004.

Volk M, Strotzer M, Lenhart M, et al: Time-resolved contrast-enhanced MR angiography of renal artery stenosis: diagnostic accuracy and interobserver variability, *Am J Roentgenol* 174:1583–1588, 2000.

Cross-Reference

Zagoria RJ, *Genitourinary Radiology: THE REQUISITES*, 2nd ed, pp 129–130, 406–407.

Comment

Arteriosclerosis is the most common cause of renal artery stenosis (RAS). The site of arterial narrowing is usually at the ostium or proximal 2 cm of the renal artery. RAS tends to occur in patients older than 50 years. Fibromuscular dysplasia accounts for up to 30% of renovascular hypertension cases, tends to occur in women between ages 20 and 50, and occurs in the middle to distal renal artery.

Screening for renovascular hypertension should be performed in a select group of patients because it accounts for only 1% to 5% of cases of systemic hypertension. Renal scintigraphy with an angiotensin-converting enzyme inhibitor (ACEI) has a reported sensitivity of 90% and specificity of greater than 95%. The ACEI blocks the production of angiotensin 2 and thus unmasks the compensating mechanism of the ischemic kidney. This effect results in a significant decrease in perfusion of the kidney with RAS. Thus, there is delayed function and tracer accumulation in the kidney with RAS. Catheter angiography is the gold standard for the evaluation of RAS, but it is invasive and costly and requires the use of iodinated contrast material. More recently, MR-angiography has proved useful as a screening test. The most effective technique is bolus chase, breath-hold, three-dimensional MR-angiography after administration of intravenous gadolinium chelate contrast agents. This technique offers excellent spatial resolution for detecting RAS and can be used to assess the symmetry of renal perfusion and contrast excretion. Gadolinium contrast agents are not nephrotoxic and can be used safely in patients with compromised renal function. Literature comparing imaging modalities is often difficult to evaluate due to the rapid evolution of imaging technologies. Multidetector row CT has improved spatial resolution over conventional CT, and careful timing of intravenous contrast administration (through use of bolus tracking techniques) has allowed lower volumes of contrast to be administered for diagnostic examinations evaluating renal artery stenosis. The use of ultrasonography to detect RAS has been advocated by some groups, but this technique is highly operator dependent and results are often difficult to reproduce.

Notes

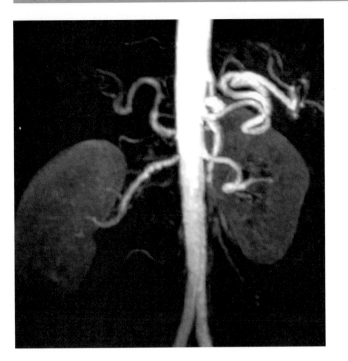 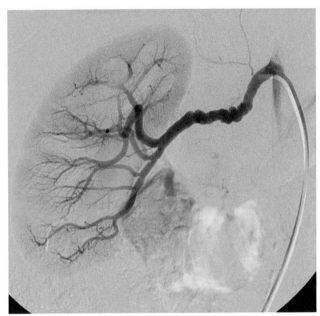

1. What is the diagnosis from these two studies?

2. Which two arterial systems are affected the most?

3. What is the gold standard for diagnosis?

4. What is the treatment of choice for the patient?

Vascular and Interventional: Fibromuscular Dysplasia

1. Fibromuscular dysplasia.

2. Renal and carotid arteries.

3. Conventional catheter angiography.

4. Percutaneous transluminal angioplasty.

References

Sharafuddin MJ, Stolpen AH, Dixon BS, et al: Value of MR angiography before percutaneous transluminal renal artery angioplasty and stent placement, *J Vasc Interv Radiol* 13(Pt 1):901–908, 2002.

Slovut DP, Olin JW: Fibromuscular dysplasia, *N Engl J Med* 350:1862–1871, 2004.

Uder M, Humke U: Endovascular therapy of renal artery stenosis: where do we stand today? *Cardiovasc Intervent Radiol* 28:139–147, 2005.

Cross-Reference

Zagoria RJ, *Genitourinary Radiology: THE REQUISITES*, 2nd ed, pp 406–407.

Comments

Fibromuscular dysplasia (FMD) is a nonatherosclerotic, noninflammatory narrowing of medium-sized arteries characterized by fibrodysplastic changes. It predominantly affects women of childbearing age. It most commonly affects the renal arteries (65%–75%) and can cause refractory renovascular hypertension. The carotid artery is the second most commonly affected vessel (25%–35%); however, FMD has been reported in virtually all vascular beds. The pathological classification of FMD for renal lesions is based on the vascular layer—intima, media, or adventitia—in which the lesion predominates. Medial fibroplasia is the most common subtype.

Angiography remains the gold standard for diagnosing FMD; however, MR- and CT-angiography are now being used successfully to establish the diagnosis (as in this case). The classic "string-of-beads" appearance with alternating areas of narrowing and mild dilation is considered pathognomonic for medial fibroplasia on catheter angiography. Aneurysms and dissections are considered complications of FMD, not part of its basic pathology. When the carotid arteries are involved, the cervical segment C1–C2 most often is affected.

Over the past 20 years, percutaneous transluminal angioplasty has emerged as the treatment method of choice for FMD involving the main renal artery or its primary branches. Angioplasty for FMD has a technical success rate of greater than 90% and a low morbidity rate. Stents are not generally used for FMD since the results with balloon angioplasty have been excellent, and the recurrence rate is far less than that for atherosclerotic renal artery stenosis. The patient in this example is a 38-year-old woman with recent onset of hypertension and FMD that was treated with angioplasty.

Notes

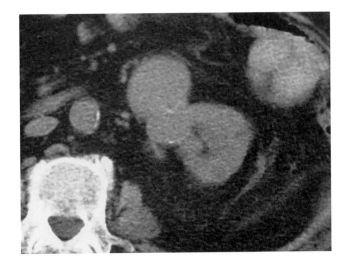
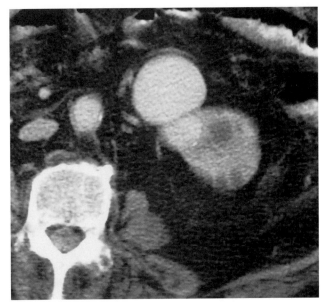
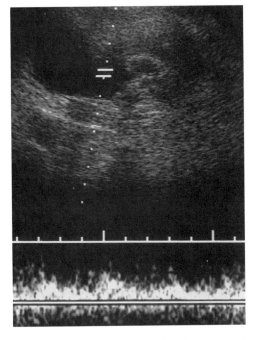

1. What is the most likely diagnosis for the mass adjacent to the lower pole of the left kidney?

2. Is this abnormality of clinical significance?

3. What CT features suggest that this is not a neoplasm?

4. How is this abnormality usually treated?

Vascular and Interventional: Renal Artery Aneurysm

1. Renal artery aneurysm.

2. Yes, because of the risk for rupture and renal embolization.

3. The degree of enhancement is identical to that of the aorta, and there is evidence of atherosclerotic calcification in the aorta and at the edges of the mass on the precontrast CT scan.

4. Renal artery aneurysms are usually treated surgically, although some lesions may be treated with selective endovascular obliteration.

References

Davidson AJ, Hartman DS, eds: *Radiology of the Kidney and Urinary Tract,* 2nd ed, Philadelphia, 1994, Saunders, pp 544–557.

Schiller VL, Sytner S, Sarti DA, Krisiloff M: Color Doppler sonography of renal artery aneurysm, *Am J Roentgenol* 169:1750, 1997.

Cross-Reference

Zagoria RJ, *Genitourinary Radiology: THE REQUISITES,* 2nd ed, p 385.

Comment

This patient has a 25-mm, bilobed mass with peripheral calcifications abutting the lower pole of the left kidney. This mass enhances to an identical degree as the aorta, and on sonography, turbulent flow is detected within the mass. These features suggest that this mass is an arterial structure. Adjacent scanning demonstrated continuity of this mass with the left renal artery. Most renal artery aneurysms are acquired and result from advanced atherosclerosis. Some develop as the result of fibromuscular disease of the renal artery, and others result from vasculitides. Even small renal artery aneurysms are significant because they may be the source of emboli to the kidney and may cause renal ischemia, oversecretion of renin, and renovascular hypertension. With increasing size, the risk for aneurysm rupture increases. When a mass in or near the kidney enhances to a degree equal to that of the arteries, an aneurysm or vascular malformation should be suspected. This diagnosis can be confirmed with conventional angiography, CT-angiography, or MR-angiography. Obviously, biopsy of this type of lesion should be avoided because of the risk of exsanguination. Most renal artery aneurysms are treated with renal artery bypass procedures. However, endovascular technology has been used to successfully treat some renal artery aneurysms with occlusion devices or stent-grafts.

Notes

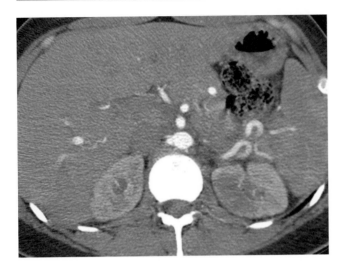
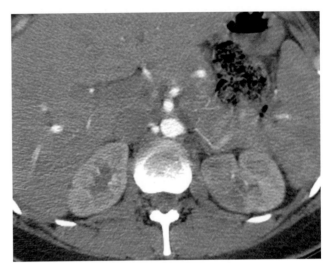
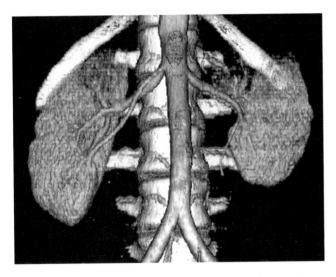

1. Identify this examination. What are the indications for this study?

2. What is the significance of the renal arterial anatomy in this renal donor?

3. What other noninvasive radiology examination offers comparable accuracy in evaluating renal vasculature?

4. What other information is required by the transplant surgeons?

Vascular and Interventional: CT-Angiography of Duplicated Renal Arteries

1. CT-angiography. To evaluate potential renal transplantation donors; performed less frequently to diagnose renal artery stenosis.

2. Duplicated right renal artery means that the left kidney will be chosen as the donor kidney.

3. MR-angiography.

4. Number, size, and location of renal arteries, veins, and ureters. The size and location of kidneys, presence of congenital or acquired renal disease.

References

Kawamoto S, Montgomery RA, Lawler LP, et al: Multi-detector row CT evaluation of living renal donors prior to laparoscopic nephrectomy, *Radiographics* 24:453–466, 2004.

Sahani DV, Rastogi N, Greenfield AC, et al: Multi-detector row CT in evaluation of 94 living renal donors by readers with varied experience, *Radiology* 235: 905–910, 2005.

Cross-Reference

Zagoria RJ, *Genitourinary Radiology: THE REQUISITES,* 2nd ed, pp 24–29.

Comment

Renal transplantation is the treatment of choice for end-stage renal disease. Donor kidneys can come from living related donors or from unrelated cadavers. HLA matching, better immunosuppression, and improvements in transplant surgical technique have resulted in a 75% to 90% 1-year graft survival rate.

The objectives of the pretransplant evaluation of the renal donor are to determine that there are (1) two viable kidneys without intrinsic disease, (2) no vascular abnormalities (arterial or venous) that might contraindicate transplantation or leave the donor with a single compromised kidney, and (3) no ureteral abnormalities that might contraindicate surgery. Duplication of the renal arteries or renal veins is estimated to occur in up to 35% of the healthy population. Duplication of renal arteries may be a contraindication to renal transplant, depending on the size and number of duplicated vessels. In general, small hypoplastic renal arteries can be sacrificed without a significant loss of renal function. The finding of multiple renal arteries of a similar size necessitates multiple anastomoses, which lengthens the transplant surgery and increases the likelihood of postoperative complications. The same caveat applies for duplicated renal veins. In general the left kidney is preferred for transplantation because the longer renal vein facilitates vascular anastomosis.

Multidetector row CT (MDCT)–angiography and MR-angiography have replaced conventional angiography for the evaluation of renal transplant donors. MDCT provides accurate information regarding the number, location, and size of renal arteries and veins. Experienced radiologists are more than 95% accurate in identifying accessory renal arteries and veins.

Notes

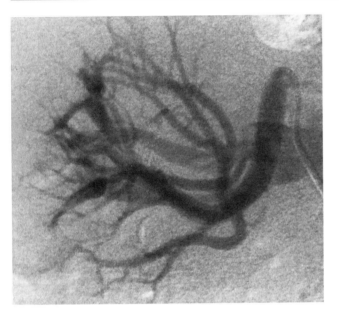 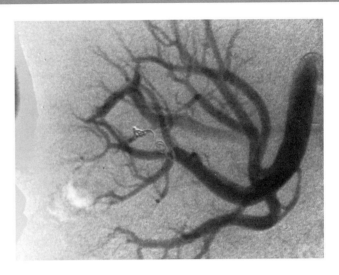

1. The image on the left is an arteriogram of a transplanted kidney after biopsy. What are the most common complications of renal biopsy?

2. What are the incidence and natural history of the lesion shown in the image on the left?

3. What are the Doppler sonographic characteristics of this lesion?

4. How is this lesion treated? (Hint: Refer to the image on the right.)

Vascular and Interventional: Arteriovenous Fistula after Biopsy in a Renal Transplant

1. Hematoma at the biopsy site, hematuria, perirenal hematoma, pseudoaneurysm, and arteriovenous (AV) fistula.

2. Incidence of AV fistula is approximately 9%; 70% to 95% spontaneously thrombose.

3. High-velocity and low-impedance arterial flow (with elevated end-diastolic flow); pulsatile, high-velocity flow through the draining vein.

4. Distal, superselective embolization is necessary to minimize the loss of renal parenchyma.

References

Benson DA, Stockinger ZT, McSwain NE Jr: Embolization of an acute renal arteriovenous fistula following a stab wound: case report and review of the literature, *Am Surg* 71:62–65, 2005.

Shlansky-Goldberg RD: Renal transplantation. In Baum S, ed: *Abrams' Angiography,* 4th ed, Boston, 1997, Little, Brown.

Cross-Reference

Zagoria RJ, Genitourinary Radiology: THE REQUISITES, 2nd ed, pp 400, 407–409.

Comment

Although many sonographic parameters have been suggested to differentiate acute tubular necrosis from cyclosporine toxicity, none are specific, and biopsy often is required. Ultrasonography is the imaging study of choice for guiding renal transplant biopsy. To avoid hilar vessels, biopsy should be performed in the renal poles. Arteriovenous (AV) fistulas occur in approximately 9% of patients undergoing biopsy. In this case the transplant biopsy was performed in the middle of the kidney, which may account for the formation of the fistula.

Renal transplant angiography is reserved for the investigation of either vascular complications of biopsy or hypertension resulting from suspected renal artery stenosis. The image on the left demonstrates a catheter in the transplant renal artery and early opacification of the renal vein. These findings are diagnostic of an AV fistula. Although most AV fistulas close spontaneously, there is the risk that thrombus may form. In a transplant kidney, thrombus may result in ischemia, acute tubular necrosis, or both, and early intervention is indicated. It is important for the radiologist to determine the type of vascular anastomosis before performing angiography. If an end-to-end anastomosis has been performed, arterial access should be attempted from the contralateral femoral artery. If an end-to-side anastomosis was performed, either an ipsilateral or a contralateral femoral approach is appropriate.

Notes

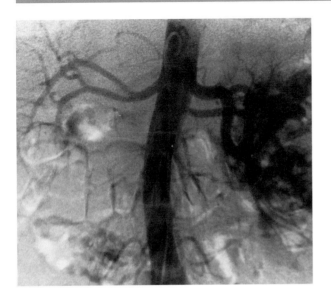 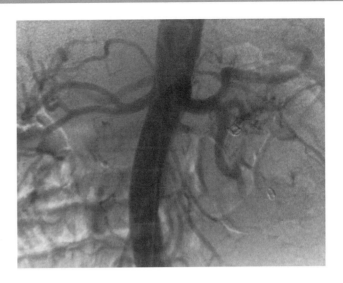

1. Two images from a renal embolization procedure are shown. In this case why was this procedure performed?

2. What is the time interval between this procedure and definitive surgery?

3. What are the other indications for this procedure?

4. What are the potential complications of this procedure?

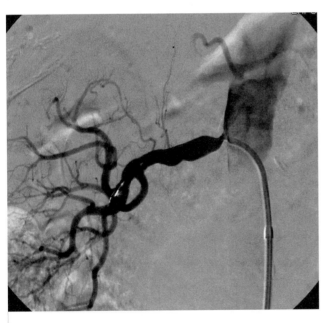 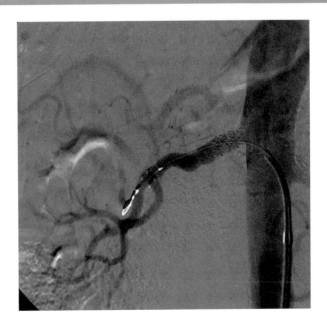

1. What are the secondary causes of hypertension?

2. What is the percentage of patients with hypertension who have renal artery stenosis as the etiology?

3. What are the complications of renal artery stenting?

4. What is the restenosis rate of atherosclerotic renal artery stenting?

Vascular and Interventional: Embolization of a Renal Cell Carcinoma

1. To reduce blood loss during nephrectomy performed to treat renal cell carcinoma.

2. Generally, nephrectomy is performed hours after the embolization.

3. Selective renal ablation before image-guided tumor ablation in nonoperative candidates, or to control bleeding after renal trauma.

4. Complications include renal abscess formation, transient elevation of blood pressure, temporary or irreversible renal failure, and embolization of nontarget tissues.

References

Bakal CW, Cynamon J, Lakritz PS, Sprayregan S: Value of preoperative renal artery embolization in reducing blood transfusion requirements during nephrectomy for renal cell carcinoma, *J Vasc Interv Radiol* 4: 727–731, 1993.

Hom D, Eiley D, Lumerman JH, et al: Complete renal embolization as an alternative to nephrectomy, *J Urol* 161:24–27, 1999.

Cross-Reference

Zagoria RJ, *Genitourinary Radiology: THE REQUISITES,* 2nd ed, pp 407–408.

Comment

The intent of renal artery embolization is to reduce blood loss in patients undergoing a nephrectomy to treat large hypervascular renal cell carcinomas. The technique of renal artery embolization and the embolic material used largely depend on the indications for the procedure. In most cases ablation with absolute (98%) ethanol is performed, and the entire arterial tree is embolized. Considerable controversy has surrounded this procedure, and although many urologists have abandoned preoperative renal ablation, citing the lack of proved efficacy, others still request it. Less commonly, renal artery embolization may be performed as a palliative treatment for inoperable and symptomatic cancer, cancer in patients with high surgical risk, cancer in the solitary kidney, or to reduce tumor volume in patients undergoing image-guided radiofrequency tumor ablation.

Embolization of the renal artery also is used to treat uncontrollable hematuria after incidental or iatrogenic trauma, which may result in arterial laceration or the formation of a pseudoaneurysm, arteriovenous fistula, or arteriocaliceal fistula. In these cases Gelfoam is used and is often supplemented with coils in larger vessels or in fast-flowing arteriovenous fistulas.

Vascular and Intraventional: Renal Artery Stenting for Renovascular Hypertension

1. Renal artery stenosis, pheochromocytoma, hyperaldosteronism, hyperthyroidism, kidney disease, Cushing's syndrome, and medications.

2. Approximately 1%.

3. Groin puncture site hematoma, pseudoaneurysm, renal artery rupture, dissection, thrombosis, peripheral emboli, infarction, and renal function compromise.

4. 10% to 25%.

References

American Heart Association. www.americanheart.org.

Leertouwer TC, Gussenhoven EJ, Bosch JL, et al: Stent placement for renal arterial stenosis: where do we stand? A meta-analysis, *Radiology* 216:78–85, 2000.

Cross-Reference

Zagoria RJ, *Genitourinary Radiology: THE REQUISITES,* 2nd ed, pp 406–407.

Comment

Sixty-five million Americans have high blood pressure. The cause in 90% to 95% of the cases is unknown. Five percent to 10% of patients have hypertension due to secondary causes, such as renal artery stenosis (RAS) and pheochromocytomas. RAS is mostly due to atherosclerosis, but also occurs with fibromuscular dysplasia. Narrowing in the renal artery acts as a barrier limiting blood flow through the kidneys, resulting in release of hormone renin that initiates a series of chemical events that result in hypertension.

RAS causes ischemic nephropathy in the kidneys. The other normal kidney can develop hypertensive nephrosclerosis. In this way both stenotic and nonstenotic kidneys can develop chronic renal failure. Nuclear medicine scintigraphy, CT, and MR-angiography are the primary screening tests for RAS.

RAS can be treated by medical therapy, renal artery stent placement, or surgical revascularization. Medications, particularly angiotensin-converting enzyme inhibitors, can control blood pressure, but they are not effective in all patients. Stent placement has lower morbidity and mortality than renal artery bypass surgery. Although stenting RAS has shown benefit, atheroembolism during stenting has been a concern, particularly wherever atherosclerotic lesions are treated. To protect the kidneys from emboli, the use of distal protection devices has become increasingly common. Restenosis of atherosclerotic renal narrowing ranges from 10% to 25%.

Notes

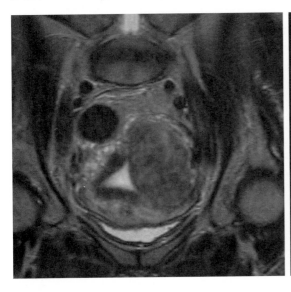
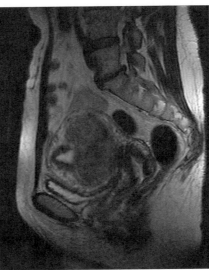

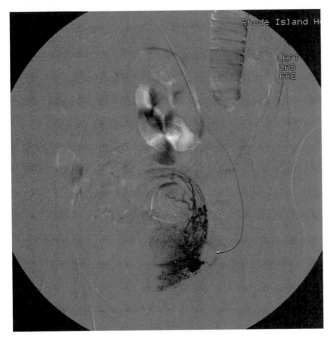
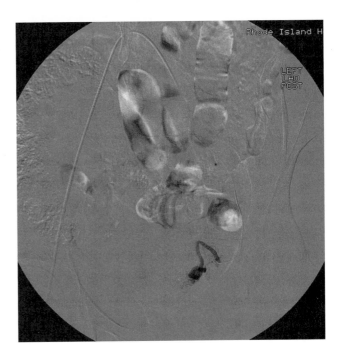

1. What significant finding does the MRI demonstrate?

2. What role does imaging play in the preprocedure evaluation of uterine artery embolization patients?

3. What are the indications for uterine artery embolization?

4. What is the clinical success of uterine artery embolization?

CASE 165

Vascular and Interventional: Uterine Artery Embolization

1. MRI documents an enlarged uterus with multiple fibroids with marked distortion of endometrial cavity and compression of bladder.

2. Imaging before uterine artery embolization is performed to evaluate the uterus and ovaries, confirm fibroids, and exclude other causes of pelvic pain.

3. Uterine leiomyomata causing pain and/or bleeding that are not responsive to medical (hormonal or analgesic) therapy. Other invasive options (myomectomy, hysterectomy, endometrial ablation) may also be considered.

4. 80% to 90%.

References

Spies JB, Spector A, Roth AR, et al: Complications after uterine artery embolization for leiomyomas, *Obstet Gynecol* 100:873–880, 2002.

Worthington-Kirsch R, Spies JB, Myers ER, et al, for the FIBROID Investigators: The Fibroid Registry for Outcomes Data (FIBROID) for uterine embolization: short-term outcomes, *Obstet Gynecol* 106:52–59, 2005.

Cross-Reference

Zagoria RJ, *Genitourinary Radiology: THE REQUISITES*, 2nd ed, pp 408–410.

Comment

Uterine artery embolization (UAE), or uterine fibroid embolization, is performed for the relief of symptomatic uterine leiomyomata. Leiomyomata are present in 20% to 40% of women over 35. Women may present with menorrhagia, menometrorrhagia, or pelvic "bulk" symptoms, which may include pain, pressure, fullness, urinary frequency, or dyspareunia. Preintervention evaluation includes gynecologic evaluation including Papanicolaou smear, consultation with an interventional radiologist, and a pelvic imaging study (ultrasonography and/or MRI) to confirm the diagnosis of fibroids, their location and size, and to exclude other etiologies including ovarian masses, pelvic inflammatory disease, endometriosis, and adenomyosis.

UAE involves selective catheterization of the uterine arteries followed by embolization using either polyvinyl alcohol or calibrated microspheres. The first angiographic image depicts the selective injection of the left uterine artery with a microcatheter, showing hyperemia of the uterus and uterine artery enlargement typical of fibroids. To prevent spasm, selection of the tortuous uterine artery is most safely performed with a microcatheter. The embolic agent is targeted to reach the perifibroid capillary plexus, and the second angiographic image depicts the selective injection of the left uterine artery after embolization, which documents minimal antegrade flow in main uterine artery with no filling of myometrial branches. Using 500- to 700-μm particles, most patients can be discharged to home the day following the procedure on oral nonsteroidal antiinflammatory drugs with antiemetic and narcotic prescriptions only as needed. Clinical success with significant improvement/resolution of symptoms can be expected in 80% to 90% of patients. Minor complications occur in less than 5% (severe pain/nausea, access site hematoma, amenorrhea) with significant complications in less than 0.5% (infection, deep venous thrombosis, and pulmonary emboli). Postprocedure imaging with MRI may be used to document the reduced size of fibroids or to evaluate inadequate clinical response and/or complications.

Notes

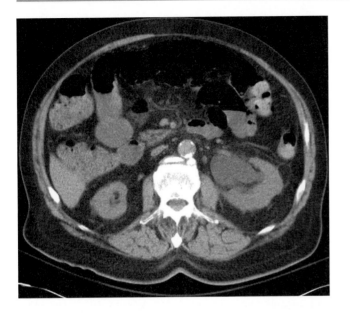

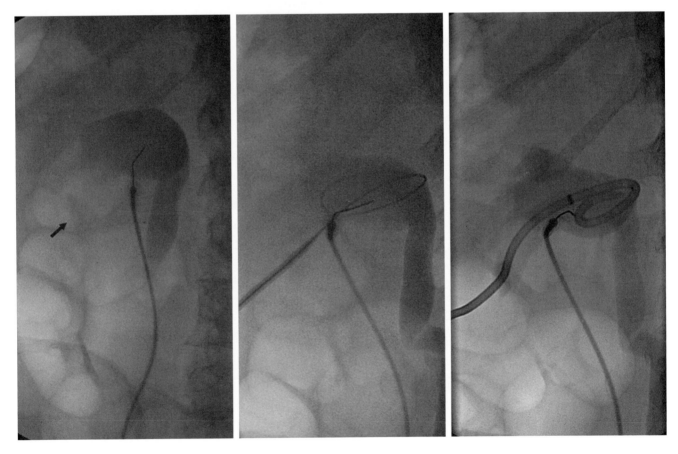

1. What significant findings does the CT demonstrate?

2. What are the common and uncommon causes of urinary tract obstruction?

3. What are the indications for percutaneous nephrostomy placement?

4. What are the potential complications of percutaneous nephrostomy placement?

Vascular and Interventional: Percutaneous Nephrostomy

1. Urinary tract obstruction with hydronephrosis, perinephric stranding, and renal enlargement.

2. Common: nephrolithiasis, ureteropelvic junction obstruction, and stricture. Less common: tumor (transitional cell carcinoma, pelvic tumor such as metastatic gynecologic or colon malignancy), hematoma, and fungus ball.

3. Relief of urinary tract obstruction, access to the renal collecting system/ureter for percutaneous nephrolithotomy, Whitaker test, ureteric dilation, urothelial biopsy, or ablation of urothelial tumor.

4. Septicemia and minor bleeding are most common but generally self-limited (stops in less than 48 hours). Renal artery laceration, pseudoaneurysm, or arteriovenous fistula occur in less than 2%.

References

Dyer RB, Regan JD, Kavanagh PV, et al: Percutaneous nephrostomy with extensions of the technique: step by step, *Radiographics* 22:503–525, 2002.

Wah TM, Weston MJ, Irving HC: Percutaneous nephrostomy insertion: outcome data from a prospective multi-operator study at a UK training centre, *Clin Radiol* 59:255–261, 2004.

Cross-Reference

Zagoria RJ, *Genitourinary Radiology: THE REQUISITES*, 2nd ed, pp 384–388.

Comment

Percutaneous nephrostomy (PCN) represents the mainstay uroradiologic approach to the upper urinary tract. The procedure is generally performed to relieve urinary tract obstruction. The most common cause of obstruction is nephrolithiasis, but PCN may be used effectively for other causes of obstruction, including congenital ureteropelvic junction obstruction, urothelial tumor, or ureteric obstruction from metastatic tumor (i.e., gynecologic or bowel malignancy). PCN may also be used to evaluate patients with partial obstruction using a Whitaker test or to allow access for other genitourinary interventions such as percutaneous nephrolithotomy, percutaneous nephroureterostomy, or ureteric dilation or biopsy.

PCN placement is most often performed in the setting of infection and/or compromised renal function and provides rapid relief. Preliminary CT or ultrasonography confirms renal obstruction and potentially its cause and level. For a PCN, patients are placed in the prone position and receive intravenous sedation and prophylactic antibiotics to minimize septicemia during the intervention. Fluoroscopy or ultrasonography may be used to assist initial access to the collecting system using a 22-gauge needle (first fluoroscopic image). This needle is used to opacify the collecting system with a small amount of contrast and air, which facilitates direct access to a posterior calyx. The posterior calyx is preferred to avoid major vascular structures and minimize the risk for vascular injury. A wire is placed through this needle (second fluoroscopic image) and the tract is dilated sequentially allowing placement of the 8- to 12-French PCN tube (third fluoroscopic image). Major complications occur in less than 4% of patients. Transient septicemia is common and requires close postprocedure monitoring. Minor bleeding generally stops in less than 48 hours. Bleeding persisting longer suggests arterial injury (laceration, pseudoaneurysm, arteriovenous fistula) and may require renal arteriography with embolization.

Notes

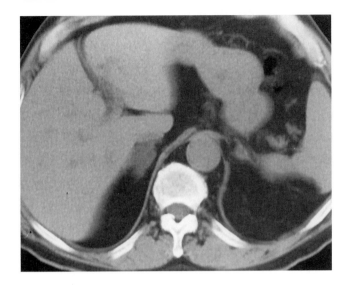

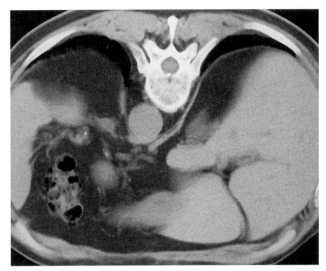

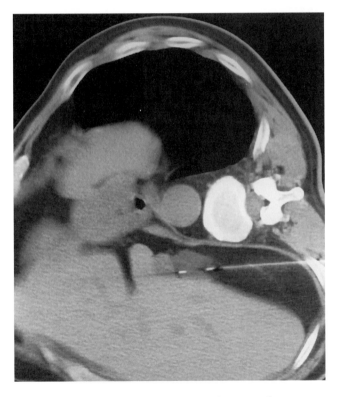

1. What is the most common indication for percutaneous adrenal biopsy?

2. Which occurs more often, a false-positive or false-negative percutaneous adrenal biopsy?

3. What are some of the complications of percutaneous adrenal biopsy?

4. What CT biopsy position is most useful to avoid a pneumothorax when performing an adrenal biopsy?

Vascular and Interventional: Percutaneous Adrenal Biopsy

1. Presence of an adrenal mass in a patient with a history of bronchogenic carcinoma.

2. False-negative.

3. Flank pain, hematoma, and pneumothorax.

4. Ipsilateral decubitus as in the third image.

References

Paulsen SD, Nghiem HV, Korobkin M, et al: Changing role of imaging-guided percutaneous biopsy of adrenal masses: evaluation of 50 adrenal biopsies, *Am J Roentgenol* 182:1033–1037, 2004.

Welch TJ, Sheedy PF, Stephens DH, et al: Percutaneous adrenal biopsy: review of a ten-year experience, *Radiology* 193:341–344, 1994.

Cross-Reference

Zagoria RJ, *Genitourinary Radiology: THE REQUISITES,* 2nd ed, p 373.

Comment

The number of percutaneous adrenal biopsies (PABs) performed has decreased in recent years in part because of the excellent performance characteristics of CT, chemical shift MRI, and more recently PET for adrenal mass characterization. Yet PAB still has an important role (1) when a specific tissue diagnosis of metastatic disease is necessary for management decisions or (2) there are equivocal or discordant results from imaging examinations.

In the authors' experience, CT is the imaging modality of choice for performing adrenal biopsies. Twenty- or 18-gauge cutting needles usually provide diagnostic samples. The right adrenal mass can be sampled via biopsy from a right-side-down decubitus position, posterior approach, or transhepatic approach. Left adrenal mass biopsies can be performed with a direct posterior approach or a left-side-down decubitus position. The authors use a coaxial technique to obtain a core biopsy and prefer to have the patient lie in the decubitus position with the enlarged adrenal in the dependent position. The dependent lung does not expand as much as the nondependent lung, and thus the lung rarely has to be transgressed to obtain an adequate specimen. This point is illustrated in the images accompanying this case. With the patient in the prone position, the position of the lungs is such that access to the adrenals is difficult. With the patient in the decubitus position, the dependent lung is hypoinflated, which creates a good window for a biopsy. Complications have been reported in 3% to 9% of biopsies and do not appear to be related to needle size.

A patient with an isolated adrenal mass who has no known primary tumor should undergo an endocrinologic workup to exclude a pheochromocytoma before undergoing an image-guided biopsy. Patients with biochemical evidence of a pheochromocytoma should have the lesion resected without a biopsy because there is a risk for malignant hypertension during biopsy of a pheochromocytoma without alpha- and beta-blockade.

Notes

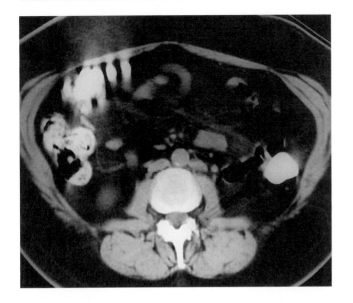

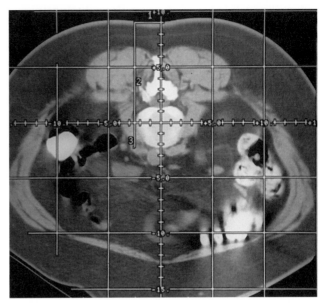

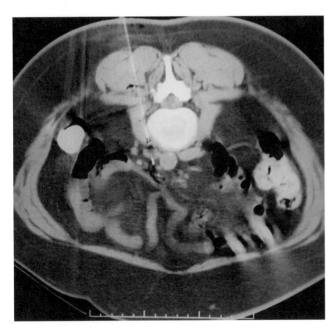

1. What is the abnormal finding in the first image?

2. What is the differential diagnosis for this finding?

3. What is the grid shown in the middle of the second image?

4. Name two percutaneous techniques for performing biopsy of a retroperitoneal mass.

Vascular and Interventional: Percutaneous Biopsy of Retroperitoneal Lymphadenopathy

1. Left paraaortic lymph node.

2. Based on this image alone, a lymph node or duplicated inferior vena cava. Other images showed a single inferior vena cava.

3. An electronic grid used for localization of a biopsy site. Paper grids can also perform this function, although they can be lost or contaminated and are more expensive.

4. Tandem and coaxial.

References

Gupta S: New techniques in image-guided percutaneous biopsy, *Cardiovasc Intervent Radiol* 27:91–104, 2004.

Silverman SG, Deuson TE, Kane N, et al: Percutaneous abdominal biopsy: cost-identification analysis, *Radiology* 206:429–435, 1998.

Cross-Reference

Zagoria RJ, *Genitourinary Radiology: THE REQUISITES,* 2nd ed, pp 400–401.

Comment

Staging CT was performed for this patient with carcinoma of the cervix. The only abnormal finding was a small paraaortic lymph node. Accurate staging of cervical carcinoma is critical because treatment may be altered significantly. If this retroperitoneal lymph node contains tumor, the patient has stage IV disease and is not a candidate for surgery. Instead, she must undergo pelvic and paraaortic radiation therapy and possibly chemotherapy. If this node does not contain malignant cells, the patient should undergo radical hysterectomy and pelvic lymph node dissection. The biopsy in this case was positive for carcinoma.

Image-guided biopsy is a routine procedure at most institutions and has achieved general acceptance in the medical community. The study referenced above by Silverman and colleagues compared the cost of percutaneous biopsy with surgical biopsy in 400 patients with a newly discovered abdominal mass. The study reported a cost savings of more than $3000 per patient when percutaneous biopsy was performed as the initial procedure to establish the diagnosis.

The techniques used to perform a biopsy vary depending on the institution, radiologist, and pathology department. A variety of needle types and sizes can be used, and the choice depends on radiologist preference, type of tumor being examined via biopsy, and preferences of the pathologists. As with radiology, provision of an accurate history to the pathologist is critical to establish a definitive and accurate diagnosis. Two techniques are used most commonly when performing an image-guided abdominal biopsy. The coaxial technique involves placement of a larger gauge needle at the edge of a lesion and sampling tissue through a smaller needle placed coaxially through the outer needle. This technique is used frequently for the biopsy of lung masses. In addition, this technique is preferable for difficult-to-access lesions because the outer guiding needle needs to be placed only once. Once the outer needle is in place, no further imaging is required to obtain multiple biopsy samples. For larger lesions, either a coaxial or tandem technique can be used. The tandem technique uses two needles adjacent to each other (in tandem). The first needle is used for localization and the second for performing the biopsy. Using imaging guidance, the first needle is placed in the lesion. Multiple biopsy samples can then be obtained from the second needle without additional imaging, with the first needle serving as a guide. The tandem technique can be used for larger masses that are easier to access.

Notes

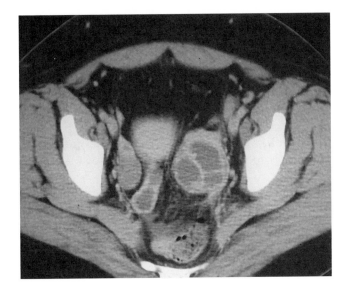

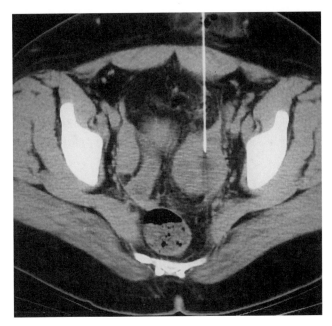

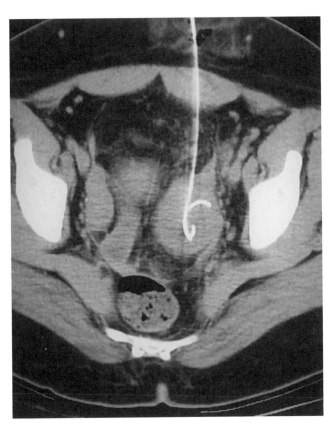

1. What is the differential diagnosis for the finding or findings in the first image?

2. True or false: The patient history and physical examination are not helpful in narrowing the differential diagnosis.

3. True or false: The treatment shown in the second and third images is the first-line treatment for this disease.

4. What alternative technique might be used to perform this procedure?

Vascular and Interventional: Percutaneous Drainage of a Tuboovarian Abscess

1. Tuboovarian or other pelvic abscess and ovarian neoplasm.

2. False. Patients with a tuboovarian abscess often have pain, fever, and tenderness associated with cervical motion. These symptoms are not common in patients with ovarian carcinoma.

3. False.

4. Needle aspiration using transvaginal ultrasonography.

References

Caspi B, Zalel Y, Or Y, et al: Sonographically guided aspiration: an alternative therapy for tubo-ovarian abscess (see comments), *Ultrasound Obstet Gynecol* 7:439–442, 1996.

Fabiszewski NL, Sumkin JH, Johns CM: Contemporary radiologic percutaneous abscess drainage in the pelvis, *Clin Obstet Gynecol* 36:445–456, 1993.

Cross-Reference

Zagoria RJ, *Genitourinary Radiology: THE REQUISITES*, 2nd ed, pp 273–275.

Comment

A tuboovarian abscess (TOA) typically presents as a complex adnexal mass on imaging studies. Because the adnexa are well visualized and no ionizing radiation is involved, ultrasonography is the initial imaging modality of choice when the diagnosis is suspected clinically. Using ultrasonography, a TOA typically appears as an enlarged complex adnexal mass with adjacent free pelvic fluid; the specificity of the diagnosis increases if a dilated tubular structure (the distended fallopian tube) is visible within or adjacent to the mass. For the woman with nonspecific pelvic pain, tenderness, and fever, renal calculus disease and appendicitis should be considered and evaluated by ultrasonography, CT, or both.

The first line of treatment for patients with a TOA is antibiotic therapy, hydration, and analgesics, and the majority of patients respond to this medical treatment. Percutaneous aspiration can be performed in patients who do not respond to antibiotics in 72 hours. If a percutaneous procedure is performed, aspiration of the infected material is usually sufficient treatment; placement of a drainage catheter is seldom necessary. One study has shown a reduction in hospital stays and a reduction in overall cost when patients undergo percutaneous aspiration for TOA.

Although this case demonstrates CT-guided drainage, some prefer transvaginal ultrasound-guided drainage and find it technically easier and more rapid to perform.

When using either technique, the clinician should perform the procedure during or after administration of intravenous antibiotics because transient bacteremia is common. Pelvic abscesses that result from perforated diverticulitis or surgery are most often drained percutaneously. Image-guided abscess drainage has a low morbidity and often results in rapid clinical improvement.

Notes

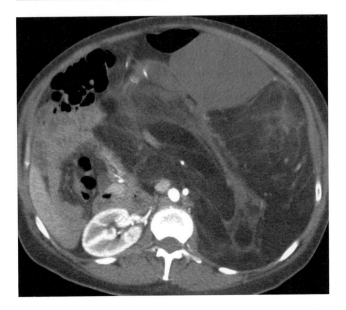 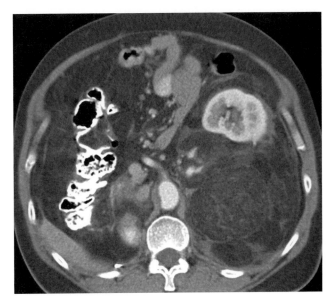

1. What type of tissue makes up the majority of the mass shown?

2. Is this mass more likely benign or malignant?

3. From what organ does this originate?

4. Is this more likely to be classified histologically as well differentiated or poorly differentiated?

Retroperitoneum: Liposarcoma

1. Fat.

2. The mass is large, contains tissue other than fat, and it does not originate from the kidney, making it likely to be malignant.

3. None identifiable, this is probably a primary retroperitoneal neoplasm.

4. Based on the presence of a large amount of fat, it is more likely well differentiated.

Reference

Nishino M, Hayakawa K, Minami M, et al: Primary retroperitoneal neoplasms: CT and MR imaging findings with anatomic and pathologic diagnostic clues, *Radiographics* 23:45–57, 2003.

Cross-Reference

Zagoria RJ, *Genitourinary Radiology: THE REQUISITES,* 2nd ed, pp 74–79.

Comment

The CT images show marked mass effect on the kidney and intraperitoneal structures. The mass effect is caused by a lesion composed predominantly of fat, but also containing soft tissue components. The mass is ill defined, and large. This has a typical appearance of a liposarcoma.

When evaluating retroperitoneal masses, it is helpful to determine the organ of origin. With some masses this can be difficult. Organs that are pushed or compressed without invasion are unlikely to be the organs of origin. If a "beak" of tissue in an organ can be identified surrounding a part of the tumor, then this supports the diagnosis of that organ as the site of tumor origination. If no originating organ is identified for a retroperitoneal mass, then it should be assumed to be a primary retroperitoneal neoplasm.

Liposarcomas are the most common type of retroperitoneal sarcoma. They usually occur in people in their fifth and sixth decades of life. Tumor grade, a key prognostic feature for sarcomas, is determined histologically and ranges from well differentiated to dedifferentiated, or poorly differentiated. Liposarcomas typically contain fat mixed with soft tissue components and are ill defined. Poorly differentiated liposarcomas may not contain any detectable fat. Treatment for liposarcomas is surgical excision. Masses that are well defined and contain only fat are lipomas.

Notes

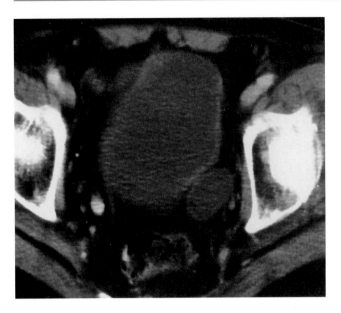
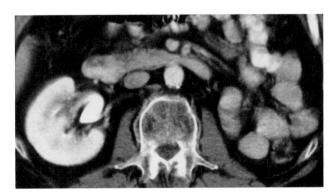

1. What is the differential diagnosis for a paraprostatic cyst?

2. What prostatic cysts are associated with renal agenesis?

3. What renal and ureteral anomalies are associated with seminal vesicle cysts?

4. Are seminal vesicle cysts congenital or acquired?

Prostate: Zinner Syndrome (Seminal Vesicle Cyst with Renal Agenesis)

1. Lateral paraprostatic cysts include seminal vesicle and vas deferens cysts; müllerian duct cysts tend to be midline. Bladder diverticula may be either lateral or midline.

2. Cysts of wolffian duct derivation; rarely renal agenesis is associated with utricular and müllerian duct cysts.

3. Ipsilateral renal agenesis, renal ectopia, adult polycystic kidney disease, collecting system duplication, and ectopic ureteral insertion.

4. Either.

Reference

King BF, Hattery RR, Lieber MM, et al: Congenital cystic disease of the seminal vesicle, *Radiology* 178:207–211, 1991.

Cross-Reference

Zagoria RJ, *Genitourinary Radiology: THE REQUISITES,* 2nd ed, p 314.

Comment

The duct of the seminal vesicle joins the ampulla of the vas deferens to form the ejaculatory duct. Cysts of the seminal vesicle may form after either congenital (atresia) or acquired obstruction of the ejaculatory duct. Some examples of acquired causes include chronic prostatitis and benign prostatic hyperplasia. Patients with seminal vesicle cysts may have an asymptomatic pelvic mass, infertility, hematuria, hemospermia, postejaculatory perineal pain, or epididymitis. Fluid aspirated from a seminal vesicle cyst is often hemorrhagic and contains inactive sperm.

Zinner syndrome, or the coexistence of renal dysgenesis or agenesis and ipsilateral seminal vesicle cysts, was first described in 1914. Approximately two thirds of patients with seminal vesicle cysts have ipsilateral renal agenesis. The association is explained by the common embryologic origin of the male internal genital system and the ureters. At about the fifth fetal week, the ureteric buds (metanephric ducts) branch from the mesonephric (wolffian) ducts and extend to the metanephric blastema; the ureteric bud eventually induces the formation of the permanent kidney. Later in normal development, the wolffian duct separates from the metanephric duct and persists in the male as the appendix of the epididymis, paradidymis, epididymis, vas deferens, ejaculatory duct, seminal vesicle, and hemitrigone of the bladder. Early dysgenesis of the mesonephric duct may explain the association of unilateral renal agenesis (which affects about 0.1% of the population) and ipsilateral genital tract anomalies.

Seminal vesicle cysts also are associated with cystic renal disease. Even in the absence of a family history, an evaluation of the kidneys for adult-type polycystic renal disease is warranted in patients with seminal vesicle cysts, particularly when bilateral.

Notes

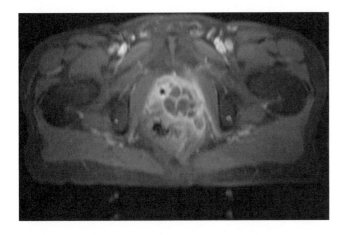

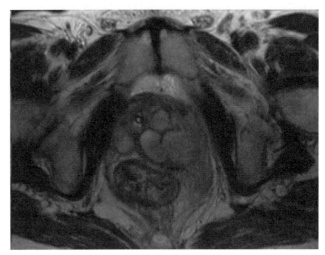

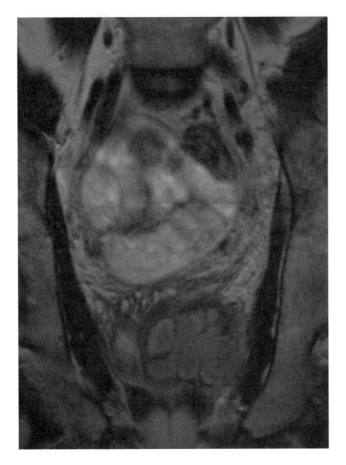

1. What is the diagnosis?

2. What is the usual organism responsible?

3. What are the ovoid high T2 signal structures posterior and superior to the prostate?

4. What other test may be helpful in initial evaluation?

Prostate and Seminal Vesicles: Prostatic Abscess

1. Prostatic abscess.

2. *Escherichia coli.*

3. Seminal vesicles.

4. Transrectal ultrasonography of the prostate.

Reference

Barozzi L, Pavlica P, Menchi I, et al: Prostatic abscess: diagnosis and treatment, *Am J Roentgenol* 170: 753–757, 1998.

Cross-Reference

Zagoria RJ, *Genitourinary Radiology: THE REQUISITES,* 2nd ed, p 345.

Comment

On MRI, enhancing and septated irregular fluid collections arise from the enlarged prostate. The anatomy of the gland is distorted. These findings are consistent with a prostatic abscess, in this case extending into the seminal vesicle.

Symptoms referable to the prostate along with signs such as leukocytosis, pyuria, and fluctuance on digital rectal examination may lead to the clinical diagnosis of prostatitis. It has been proposed that prostatic abscess represents a complication of bacterial prostatitis, either acute or chronic. However, hematogenous spread has also been described. Initial diagnosis may be confirmed with transrectal ultrasonography and aspiration. CT and MRI may also be helpful. Complications include progression to sepsis and death. Treatment consists of appropriate antibiotics with drainage or surgical treatment as necessary.

Imaging findings include cystic collections containing complex material, primarily within the transitional and central zones of the prostate. The anatomy of the gland may be distorted. The differential diagnosis would include prostatic cysts or neoplasm. Multiplanar imaging with CT or MRI helps to determine the extent of disease, especially beyond the genitourinary tract and into adjacent muscles of the pelvic floor. The seminal vesicles should be symmetric and have gracile septa, unlike in this case where the septa are thick and the ejaculatory duct obstructed.

Notes

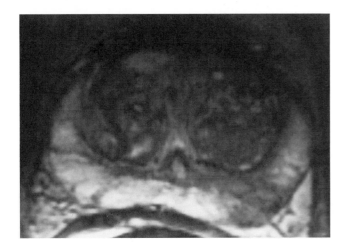

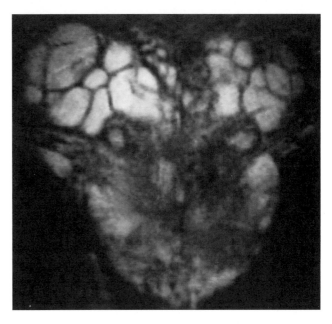

1. What is the differential diagnosis for a focal area of hypointense signal in the peripheral zone on a T2W image of the prostate?

2. True or false: For MRI of the prostate in which an endorectal surface coil is used, contrast-enhanced MRI is usually unnecessary.

3. True or false: MRI is as sensitive for the detection of central zone cancers as it is for peripheral zone adenocarcinoma.

4. True or false: Some peripheral zone cancers have high signal intensity on T2W images.

Prostate and Seminal Vesicles: MRI of the Prostate

1. Adenocarcinoma, hyperplasia (fibrous, fibromuscular, muscular, and atypical adenomatous types), prostatitis, and hemorrhage after biopsy.

2. True. In most cases enhanced MRI is of no added benefit.

3. False. Central zone cancers are often undetectable with MRI.

4. True. Mucinous or signet-ring adenocarcinoma.

Reference

Schiebler ML, Schnall MD, Pollack HM, et al: Current role of MR imaging in the staging of adenocarcinoma of the prostate, *Radiology* 189:339–352, 1993.

Cross-Reference

Zagoria RJ, *Genitourinary Radiology: THE REQUISITES,* 2nd ed, pp 332–333.

Comment

First, some comments about a few standard techniques and sequences for endorectal MRI (erMRI) of the prostate: This study is most often performed with the intent of staging prostate cancer. Intravenous glucagon 1 mg should be administered to reduce artifact resulting from bowel peristalsis. After a digital rectal examination is performed, the endorectal coil is positioned directly behind the prostate gland, and the coil balloon is inflated with about 100 ml of air. Transverse axial fast or turbo spin-echo T2W images with thin (3-mm) slices form the cornerstone of prostate erMRI; supplemental fast spin-echo T2W images in the coronal (as in this case) or sagittal plane may be performed as needed to confirm the diagnosis based on evaluation of the transaxial images. A transaxial T1W sequence through the prostate gland is also performed before the endorectal coil is removed. Finally, transaxial T1W images of the pelvis and lower abdomen are performed to evaluate for pelvic-retroperitoneal lymphadenopathy and metastases to the bone marrow. The routine use of contrast material is not necessary.

On fast spin-echo T2W images the majority of prostate adenocarcinomas appear as focal areas of decreased signal in the normally hyperintense peripheral zone. Mucinous adenocarcinoma, which occurs in about 5% of cases, may be of high signal intensity on T2W images and is the major exception to this rule. Hemorrhage from a recent biopsy also may result in a hypointense focus in the peripheral zone. Hemorrhage after biopsy usually appears as a focal area of increased signal on the T1W image and corresponds in location to the hypointense area on the T2W image. Tumor surrounded by hemorrhage resulting from a recent biopsy should be suspected if only a rim of hyperintensity is visible around the suspicious focus on the T1W image. Alternatively, to avoid confusion, the clinician may delay the staging study until 3 or 4 weeks after prostate biopsy.

Notes

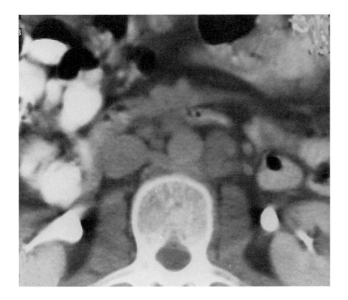

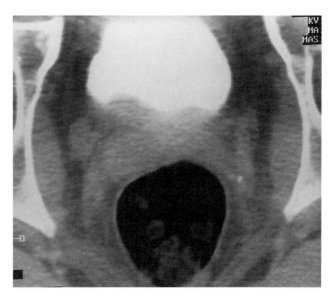

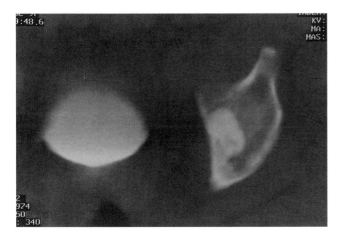

1. What is the most likely diagnosis?

2. What stage of neoplasm would this patient have?

3. What neoplasms are associated with osteoblastic bone metastases?

4. Would it be surprising if this patient had a prostate-specific antigen level of 10 ng/mL?

Prostate and Seminal Vesicles: Staging of Prostate Cancer

1. Prostate cancer metastatic to lymph nodes and to bone.

2. Using the Hopkins modification of the Whitmore-Jewett staging system, stage D.

3. Prostate, breast, bladder, lymphoma, lung, carcinoid, and medulloblastoma.

4. Yes, the likelihood of bone metastases with a prostate-specific antigen level of less than or equal to 10 ng/mL is less than 2%.

References

Hittelman AB, Purohit RS, Kane CJ: Update of staging and risk assessment for prostate cancer patients, *Curr Opin Urol* 14:163–170, 2004.

Perez CA: Carcinoma of the prostate: a model for management under impending health care system reform. 1994 RSNA annual oration in radiation oncology, *Radiology* 196:309–322, 1995.

Cross-Reference

Zagoria RJ, *Genitourinary Radiology: THE REQUISITES,* 2nd ed, pp 336–342.

Comment

The staging of prostate cancer has important implications for treatment. Microscopic and nonpalpable tumors (T1 and A on the TNM and Whitmore-Jewett staging systems, respectively) are usually found in transurethral prostatectomy specimens or by needle biopsy as a result of elevated serum prostate-specific antigen (PSA) levels. Tumors that are confined to the gland (stage T2 or B) may be either palpable or identified by imaging. Tumors that have already penetrated the prostatic capsule (stage T3a or C1) and invaded surrounding tissues (stage T3b or C2) have high rates of recurrence and morbidity. For this reason, an important staging threshold for treatment is between stages T2 (tumor confined to the prostate gland) and T3b (gross or bilateral extracapsular tumor). Patients with stage T2 or B disease are offered curative radical prostatectomy; there is some research suggesting that patients with microscopic extracapsular tumor (T3a) also should be candidates for this surgery. Patients with stage T3b cancer or more advanced disease are treated with external beam radiation, hormonal ablation, or both, with a palliative intent.

Patients undergo staging after the diagnosis of prostate cancer has been made, often after ultrasound-guided prostate biopsy. The serum PSA level and histologic grade (Gleason score) of the tumor may be helpful in predicting the likelihood of extraprostatic spread. For example, 75% of patients with serum PSA levels less than 4 ng/mL have prostate-confined cancer, whereas this value falls to 50% for those with PSA levels between 4 and 10 ng/mL and is only 2% when the patient's PSA level exceeds 30 ng/mL. The likelihood of lymph node metastases in prostate cancer also is correlated with the clinical T stage. For example, the chance that a patient with a poorly differentiated stage T3 tumor has lymph node metastases is 68% to 93%, but is 0% in the patient with a stage T1a tumor.

Historically, imaging modalities have been used for both detection and staging of prostate cancer. Serum PSA and ultrasound-guided biopsy are primarily used for diagnosing prostatic cancer. Serum PSA is also useful to stage prostatic cancer as described above. Currently CT is generally used to confirm extraprostatic disease in patients with markedly elevated serum PSA levels (greater than 20 ng/mL).

Notes

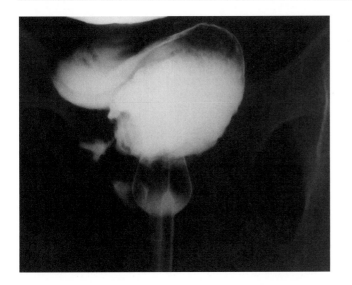

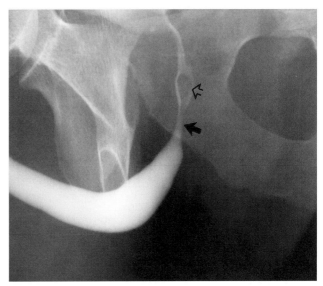

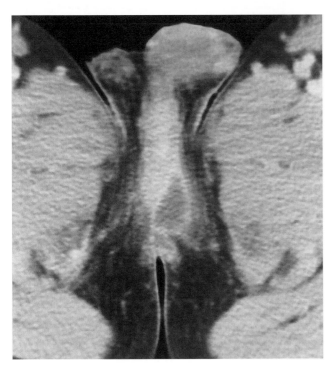

1. This patient has rectal Crohn's disease, pelvic pain, and irritative voiding symptoms. What is the diagnosis?

2. True or false: The *solid arrow* points to a posterior urethral stricture.

3. What is the filling defect (*open arrow*) in the posterior urethra?

4. What type of renal stones may form because of ileal Crohn's disease and fat malabsorption?

Scrotum: Perineal Abscess Caused by Crohn's Colitis

1. Perineal abscess.

2. False. It points to the normal caliber membranous urethra.

3. Verumontanum.

4. Oxalate stones.

References

Furukawa A, Saotome T, Yamasaki M, et al: Cross-sectional imaging in Crohn disease, *Radiographics* 24:689–702, 2004.

Shield DE, Lytton B, Weiss RM, Schiff M Jr: Urologic complications of inflammatory bowel disease, *J Urol* 115:701–706, 1976.

Cross-Reference

Zagoria RJ, *Genitourinary Radiology: THE REQUISITES,* 2nd ed, pp 78–79, 191–194, 222–223.

Comment

Shield and colleagues report urologic complications in 23% of 233 patients with Crohn's ileitis. Granulomatous enterocolitis may cause genitourinary tract disease because of the local extension of Crohn's disease, metabolic aberrations secondary to malabsorption and dehydration, or secondary local or systemic disease associated with the chronic inflammatory process (e.g., amyloidosis).

Genitourinary tract involvement by Crohn's disease is most often caused by direct extension of granulomatous enterocolitis. Regional enteritis may cause obstruction of the ureter (typically the right ureter); bladder wall lesions ("herald lesions"); or fistulas to the ureter, bladder, urethra, or vagina. Retroperitoneal fibrosis and amyloidosis caused by long-standing Crohn's disease also may have manifestations in the genitourinary tract. Of patients with Crohn's disease, 10% develop renal calculus disease. Intestinal fat, which is malabsorbed because of ileal disease, binds calcium and leads to excessive absorption of dietary oxalate. This process in turn leads to hyperoxaluria and the formation of oxalate stones. Uric acid stones may form because of dehydration and hyperuricosuria in patients with ileostomies.

This patient had rectal Crohn's disease and irritative voiding symptoms caused by a perineal abscess. Although not demonstrated in this case, fistulas to the bladder, vagina, and urethra may complicate rectal Crohn's disease.

Notes

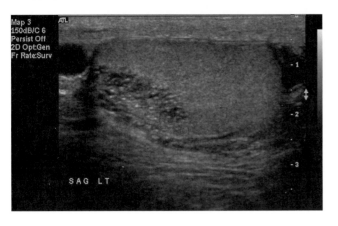
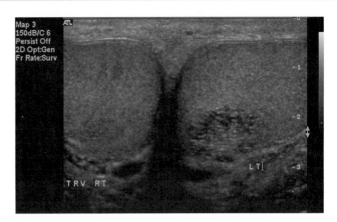

1. Is this a benign or malignant entity?

2. What is the differential diagnosis?

3. What abnormality of the epididymis is associated with this testicular finding?

4. What should be done next?

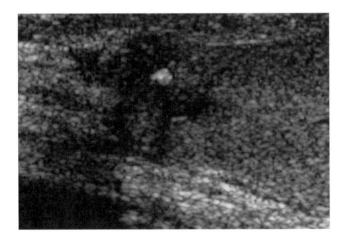
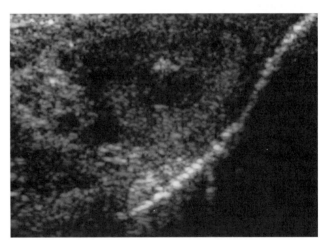

1. Two images from an ultrasound examination of the testicle are shown. What is the most likely diagnosis?

2. Name three nonmalignant causes of calcified testicular masses.

3. What is the most common extragonadal site associated with a burned-out primary testicular cancer?

4. True or false: All testicular tumors with calcification have an associated discrete mass separate from the calcification or calcifications.

C A S E   1 7 6

Scrotum: Tubular Ectasia of the Rete Testis

1. This is a benign process—tubular ectasia of the rete testis.

2. There is no differential diagnosis.

3. Cysts.

4. No further imaging follow-up is needed.

Reference

Weingarten BJ, Kellman GM, Middleton WD, et al: Tubular ectasia within the mediastinum testis, *J Ultrasound Med* 11:349–353, 1992.

Cross-Reference

Zagoria RJ, *Genitourinary Radiology: THE REQUISITES,* 2nd ed, pp 313–314.

Comment

Tubular ectasia is often incidentally discovered in middle-aged or elderly men undergoing evaluation for scrotal pathology. The etiology is uncertain but is thought to be due to obstruction of efferent ducts (vasa efferentia). Appearance is that of branching tubular anechoic structures with gracile walls located in the mediastinum testis. Occasionally the ducts become more dilated, simulating cysts. Because there is no vascular supply, no Doppler flow is detectable. There is an association with epididymal cysts that may involve the head, body, or tail.

It is critical that this abnormality be recognized as benign so as to avoid surgical exploration and possible orchiectomy. While some testicular tumors may appear hypoechoic to adjacent parenchyma, they are always solid. Focal orchitis may be hypoechoic but will often expand the testicle and almost always demonstrates increased blood flow. Infarcts are also hypoechoic, usually well defined, and show no blood flow, but lack the anechoic spaces and branching pattern. Varicoceles are located external to the testis and demonstrate obvious blood flow within them.

Notes

C A S E   1 7 7

Scrotum: Calcified Testicular Mass

1. Calcified primary testicular neoplasm, probably a nonseminomatous germ cell tumor.

2. Epidermoid cyst, resolved infection, hematoma, and infarction.

3. Most often, a regressed germ cell testicular tumor coexists with a retroperitoneal mass.

4. False.

Reference

Comiter CV, Renshaw AA, Benson CB, Loughlin KR: Burned-out primary testicular cancer: sonographic and pathological characteristics, *J Urol* 156:85–88, 1996.

Cross-Reference

Zagoria RJ, *Genitourinary Radiology: THE REQUISITES,* 2nd ed, pp 322–325.

Comment

This is a case of a teratocarcinoma of the testis containing a small focus of calcification. In contrast to seminomas, nonseminomatous germ cell tumors are more likely to be of mixed echogenicity. Teratomas and teratocarcinomas are often heterogeneous and may have well-formed multilocular cysts that contain bone, cartilage, keratin, muscle, hair, mucous glands, or neural tissue. These tumors are more common in children.

Typically a calcified testicular tumor appears as a hypoechoic mass with focal areas of shadowing hyperechogenicity. Uncommonly a focus of calcification dominates the appearance of the tumor. Two examples are burned-out primary testicular cancer and large-cell calcifying Sertoli tumors of the testis. These lesions may have greater color Doppler signal around the focus of calcification, suggesting the coexistence of a vascularized mass. Burned-out primary tumors may be associated with extragonadal germ cell tumors that typically present as ipsilateral retroperitoneal lymphadenopathy. In contrast, the majority of mediastinal and central nervous system germ cell tumors are believed to represent primary extragonadal lesions.

The differential diagnosis of calcified testicular masses includes primary malignant or benign neoplasm, either de novo or treated; burned-out neoplasm; testicular microlithiasis; and resolved infection, traumatic hematoma, or segmental infarction.

Notes

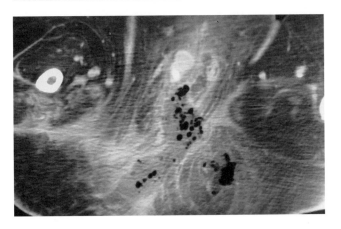 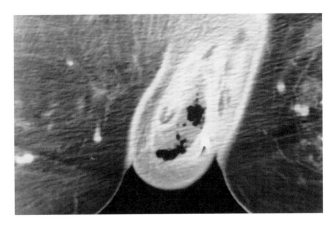

1. CT images of the scrotum and perineum are shown. True or false: The alpha toxin produced by clostridial bacteria, especially *Clostridium perfringens*, is the most common cause of this disease.

2. In women, where does this disease most often originate?

3. What are some of the findings of this disease on scrotal sonography?

4. True or false: This disease is a surgical emergency.

C A S E   1 7 8

Scrotum: Fournier's Gangrene

1. False. Fournier's gangrene is usually a polymicrobial necrotizing fasciitis caused by gram-negative rods or streptococcal, staphylococcal, and anaerobic streptococcal organisms.

2. From abscesses of the vulva or Bartholin's gland.

3. Thickened scrotal wall containing gas and presence of peritesticular fluid; testes and epididymides often are unaffected.

4. Absolutely true.

Reference

Rajan DK, Scharer KA: Radiology of Fournier's gangrene, *Am J Roentgenol* 170:163–168, 1998.

Cross-Reference

Zagoria RJ, *Genitourinary Radiology: THE REQUISITES,* 2nd ed, pp 321–322.

Comment

Fournier's gangrene is a polymicrobial necrotizing fasciitis of the perineum. This disease is a surgical emergency because of the rapidity with which the fasciitis can spread to the anorectum and the lower genital, anterior abdominal, and pelvic retroperitoneal spaces. Surgical débridement within 24 hours of presentation reduces the mortality rate from 76% to 12%. Clinically the typical patient seeks treatment days after the onset of perineal pain, pruritus, and fever and appears toxic; the genitalia may be gangrenous. Crepitus is detected in 19% to 64% of patients at the time of diagnosis. The cause of Fournier's gangrene is usually an invasive infection from the perianal or colorectal area and may be preceded by regional trauma or surgery. An infectious obliterative endarteritis is responsible for the rapidly progressive necrotizing fasciitis. Diabetes is a risk factor.

The diagnosis usually is established clinically, and imaging is often unnecessary. Ultrasound and CT have been performed to confirm the clinical diagnosis and to reveal the full extent of disease. Sonography of the scrotum may demonstrate hyperechoic foci with posterior acoustical shadowing, typical of gas, in swollen scrotal and perineal soft tissues. CT may reveal an infected pelvic or abdominal fluid collection, perianal abscess, fistulous tract, incarcerated inguinal hernia, or other potential source for the necrotizing infection.

Notes

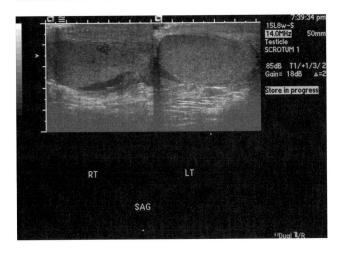 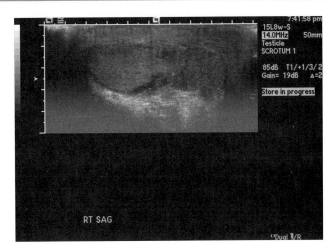

1. What is the cause of this abnormality?

2. Is the tunica of the testicle intact?

3. What would you expect color Doppler to show?

4. What is the appropriate treatment?

Scrotum: Testicular Rupture

1. Blunt trauma to the scrotum.

2. No, this is testicular rupture, not fracture.

3. No flow in the extruded portion of the testicle.

4. Emergent surgery.

Reference

Ragheb D, Higgins Jr JL: Ultrasonography of the scrotum: technique, anatomy, and pathologic entities, *J Ultrasound Med* 21:171–185, 2002.

Cross-Reference

Zagoria RJ, *Genitourinary Radiology: THE REQUISITES,* 2nd ed, p 327.

Comment

A testicular fracture appears as a linear hypoechoic band that extends across the testicular parenchyma and represents a break in the normal testicular architecture. The overall contour remains smooth because the testicular shape and the tunica albuginea are maintained. Normal blood flow is also usually preserved. A hematocele may be seen. Conservative therapy with preservation of the testicle is the rule. In this case of testicular rupture due to blunt trauma, the hyperechoic band of the tunica albuginea is disrupted. There is hemorrhage and extrusion of testicular contents into the inferior portion of the scrotal sac. No distinct fracture line is identified. Doppler signal was absent.

With rupture, the portion of the testicle remaining within the tunica often shows focal alterations in parenchymal echogenicity corresponding to areas of hemorrhage or infarction. Associated findings include scrotal wall thickening and hematocele. Doppler signal is present but often decreased. Treatment is surgical.

Notes

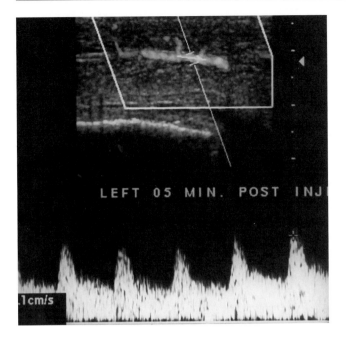 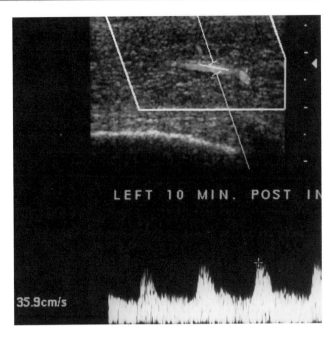

1. Two images from a Doppler ultrasound examination of the penis are shown. Spectral analysis reveals a peak systolic velocity of 36 cm/second and an end-diastolic velocity of 16 cm/second. What vessel is being investigated?

2. Is there an abnormal finding? What is it?

3. Name four causes of erectile dysfunction.

4. What are the two main causes of vasculogenic erectile dysfunction?

Penis: Vasculogenic Erectile Dysfunction

1. One of the two cavernosal arteries.

2. Yes. Abnormally high diastolic flow.

3. Etiologies of erectile dysfunction include endocrinologic, neurogenic, pharmacologic, psychogenic, or vasculogenic.

4. Arterial inflow disease and venous incompetence.

References

Bacar MM, Batislam E, Altinok D, et al: Sildenafil citrate for penile hemodynamic determination: an alternative to intracavernosal agents in Doppler ultrasound evaluation of erectile dysfunction, *Urology* 57:623–626, 2001.

Kaufman JM, Borges FD, Fitch WP 3rd, et al: Evaluation of erectile dysfunction by dynamic infusion cavernosometry and cavernosography (DICC). Multi-institutional study, *Urology* 41:445–451, 1993.

Rosen M, Schwartz A, Levine F, et al: Radiologic assessment of impotence: angiography, sonography, cavernosography and scintigraphy, *Am J Roentgenol* 157: 923–931, 1991.

Cross-Reference

Zagoria RJ, *Genitourinary Radiology: THE REQUISITES,* 2nd ed, pp 345–350.

Comment

Erection of the penis occurs when smooth muscle of the cavernosal arteries and sinusoids relaxes, causing distention of both corpora cavernosa. This distention leads to compression of the draining emissary veins, which limits venous outflow. The combination of increased arterial inflow and limited venous outflow results in penile erection.

Vasculogenic causes have been estimated to account for up to 37% of cases of erectile dysfunction. For Doppler ultrasound examination of the penis, the diameter and velocities of flow in both cavernosal arteries are measured. Then, 30 mg of papaverine is injected into one of the corpus cavernosa with a 27-gauge needle. Papaverine is a smooth muscle relaxant that causes dilation of the cavernosal arteries and sinusoids of the corpus cavernosa. Injection of this medication usually results in an erection. The diameter of the cavernosal arteries and the arterial and venous velocities are measured every 5 minutes for up to 20 minutes after the injection of papaverine. A normal response is an increase in the diameter of the cavernosal artery by more than 75% compared with the baseline size and a peak systolic velocity of 35 to 60 cm/second. A peak systolic velocity of less than 25 cm/second indicates arterial inflow disease. The peak diastolic velocity should be less than 3 cm/second. As illustrated in this case, diastolic velocity exceeding 3 cm/second in the presence of adequate arterial inflow reflects malfunction of the venous occlusive mechanism. Patients with arterial inflow disease may undergo selective angiography of the pudendal artery to determine whether atherosclerotic disease or a focal (often post-traumatic) stenosis can be treated with angioplasty or vascular surgery.

The pharmacologic agent sildenafil (Viagra) causes smooth muscle relaxation of the cavernosal arteries, which increases blood flow to the corpora cavernosa resulting in an erection. The introduction of sildenafil and related pharmacologic agents has resulted in decreased indications for Doppler examinations of the penis in the past decade.

Notes

Challenge

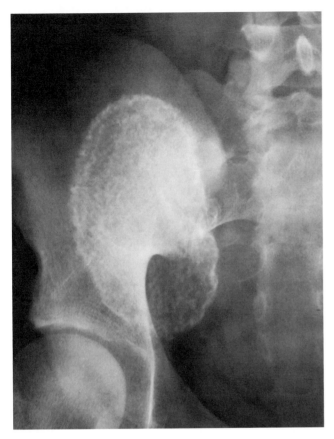

1. What part of the renal parenchyma is calcified in this kidney?

2. What are the major causes of this pattern of renal calcification?

3. What are the common causes of medullary nephrocalcinosis?

4. What causes calcification in patients with this pattern of nephrocalcinosis?

Kidney: Cortical Nephrocalcinosis

1. Cortex.

2. Chronic renal failure, acute cortical necrosis, oxalosis, Alport's syndrome, and chronic transplant rejection.

3. Hypercalcemia, medullary sponge kidney, and renal tubular acidosis.

4. Dystrophic calcification of necrotic renal cortex.

Reference

Davidson AJ, Hartman DS, eds: *Radiology of the Kidney and Urinary Tract,* 2nd ed, Philadelphia, 1994, Saunders, pp 177–189.

Cross-Reference

Zagoria RJ, *Genitourinary Radiology: THE REQUISITES,* 2nd ed, p 147.

Comment

Unlike medullary nephrocalcinosis, which usually results from precipitation of calcium products within tubules or in normal renal tissue, cortical nephrocalcinosis results from dystrophic calcification secondary to a prior insult, usually ischemia. The major causes of this pattern of renal calcification have in common cortical necrosis caused by either ischemia or inflammation.

Cortical nephrocalcinosis is easily recognized by its eggshell pattern of calcification. At the edges of the kidney, where it is seen in profile, the calcification tends to have a "tram track" pattern, as seen in this image of a transplant kidney. As is also illustrated by this patient with chronic transplant rejection, most patients with cortical nephrocalcinosis have global atrophy of the kidney, causing small, smooth kidneys and chronic renal insufficiency.

Notes

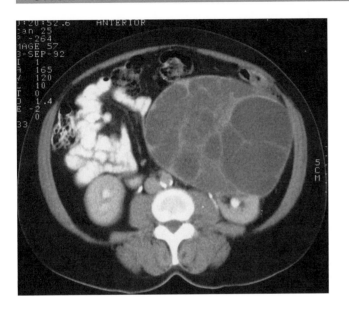
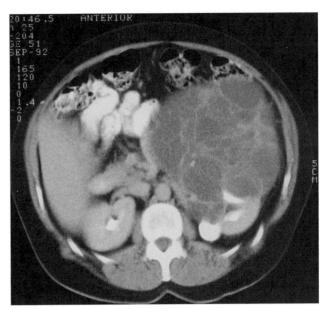

1. What are the characteristic features of this neoplasm?

2. What is the differential diagnosis?

3. Is this a benign or malignant process?

4. What is the appropriate management?

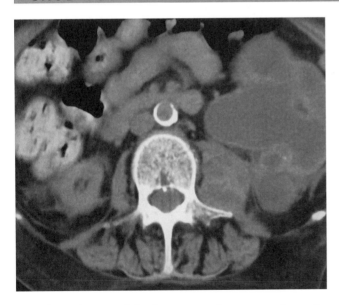
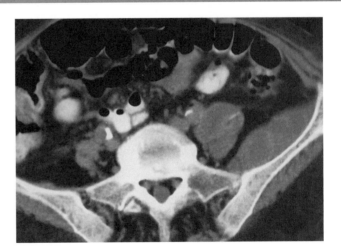

1. What abnormal findings are shown on these images?

2. What group of patients is typically afflicted by this disease?

3. What is the classic urographic triad seen in these patients?

4. What complications are associated with this disease?

Kidney Multilocular Cystic Nephroma

1. Multiple cysts separated by septa and a thick fibrous capsule.

2. In an adult, cystic renal cell carcinoma and multilocular cystic nephroma.

3. Multilocular cystic nephroma is a benign process.

4. Nephrectomy—definitive diagnosis is not possible using imaging.

Reference

Lowe LH, Isuani BH, Heller RM, et al: Pediatric renal masses: Wilms' tumor and beyond, *Radiographics* 20:1585–1603, 2000.

Cross-Reference

Zagoria RJ, *Genitourinary Radiology: THE REQUISITES,* 2nd ed, pp 101–103.

Comment

Multilocular cystic nephroma is an uncommon, benign tumor of the kidney. It is always unilateral and unifocal. There is a bimodal distribution in age and sex, with one peak occurring in young male children and the other in middle-aged women. Patients may be asymptomatic or present with an abdominal mass, particularly in children. Hematuria is uncommon. On contrast-enhanced CT, the tumor is usually large and composed of cysts separated by septa of variable thickness. The cysts are usually of water density and the septa may visibly enhance. A nearly universal finding is that of a thick fibrous capsule. Calcification occasionally occurs and hemorrhage is rare. Herniation of the mass into the renal pelvis is common. This may obstruct adjacent calyces and distort the collecting system. The renal cortex and urothelium are normal. In the child, the differential diagnosis is a cystic Wilms' tumor and in the adult a cystic renal cell carcinoma. For this reason, these tumors are removed.

Notes

Kidney: Xanthogranulomatous Pyelonephritis Complicated by Iliopsoas Abscess

1. Enlargement of the left kidney, left ureteral stone, and enlargement and hypodensity of left psoas and iliacus muscles.

2. Middle-aged (45–65 years) women with a history of repeated urinary tract infections.

3. Nephromegaly, markedly diminished or absent renal function, and nephrolithiasis.

4. Extrarenal extension and renal-cutaneous or renal-enteric fistula formation.

Reference

Eastham J, Ahlering T, Skinner E: Xanthogranulomatous pyelonephritis: clinical findings and surgical considerations, *Urology* 43:295–299, 1994.

Cross-Reference

Zagoria RJ, *Genitourinary Radiology: THE REQUISITES,* 2nd ed, pp 118–121, 139–141.

Comment

Xanthogranulomatous pyelonephritis (XGP) is an uncommon form of renal inflammation in which a chronically infected and obstructed kidney is infiltrated with lipid-laden macrophages. A renal calculus is present in at least 80% of patients. In addition to the urographic findings described, diffuse XGP has typical imaging features on both ultrasonography and CT. Ultrasonography usually demonstrates a renal pelvic calculus, reniform enlargement of the kidney, and generalized loss of corticomedullary differentiation. On CT the kidney is enlarged; has a thin rim of enhancing parenchyma; contains multiple hypoattenuating, cystic areas (attributed to necrosis rather than to hydronephrosis); and has a central calculus. The appearance of the last two CT features listed has been likened to a bear's paw print. Another useful finding is fragmentation of the staghorn calculus, referred to as the fractured calculus sign. On the basis of the CT examination, correct preoperative diagnosis can be made in 87% of patients.

Extrarenal extension of XGP is common and is accurately identified on CT. Extension into the perinephric fat, Gerota's fascia, and the ipsilateral psoas muscle is common. Renal-cutaneous and renal-enteric fistulas rarely develop.

Focal or tumefactive XGP accounts for only 15% of the total number of cases. This form is difficult to differentiate from a renal tumor because the imaging findings are less specific. Both the focal and diffuse forms are irreversible and therefore are managed with surgery.

Notes

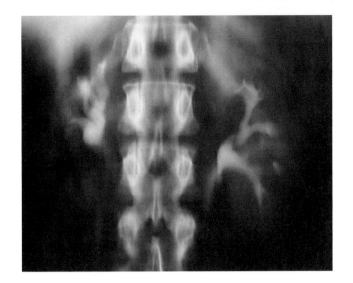
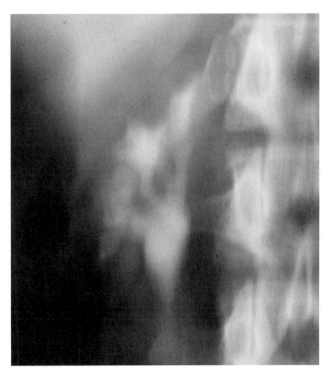

1. What is the differential diagnosis for a unilateral small, smooth kidney?

2. Which cause of a unilateral small, smooth kidney also typically causes dilated calyces?

3. What causes a unilateral small, irregular kidney?

4. What is the lower limit of normal size for either kidney?

Kidney: Renal Hypoplasia

1. Chronic ischemia (e.g., caused by renal artery stenosis or chronic renal vein thrombosis), postobstructive atrophy, renal hypoplasia, chronic subcapsular hematoma, and previous radiation treatment.

2. Postobstructive atrophy.

3. Reflux nephropathy, analgesic nephropathy, or renal segmental arterial occlusions as seen in some diseases associated with preferential small vessel atherosclerosis, such as diabetes mellitus.

4. Each kidney should be no less than three normal lumbar vertebrae and intervening interspaces (L1–L3) in height. A height equal to four vertebral bodies and their interspaces is the upper limit of normal.

Reference

Daneman A, Alton DJ: Radiographic manifestations of renal anomalies, *Radiol Clin North Am* 29:351–363, 1991.

Cross-Reference

Zagoria RJ, *Genitourinary Radiology: THE REQUISITES,* 2nd ed, pp 128–132.

Comment

Unilateral renal atrophy has many causes. It is best to limit the possible diagnoses by classifying according to the pattern of atrophy. A common cause, reflux nephropathy, also called chronic atrophic pyelonephritis, usually causes atrophy with marked irregularity of the cortical margin and underlying clubbed calyces. A unilateral small, smooth kidney usually is the result of renal artery stenosis, and in this case the calyces appear normal. Other findings of renal underperfusion, including delay in opacification of the kidney and calyces, also may be present in patients with renal artery stenosis. A diagnosis of renal hypoplasia should be made when there is a unilateral small, smooth kidney that excretes contrast and has normal-appearing but few calyces. When there are five or fewer calyces and all other features of a hypoplastic kidney are present, as in this case, the diagnosis should be made. The etiology of hypoplastic kidney is unknown, but it is hypothesized that in utero ischemia leads to this pathologic condition. Renal arteriography demonstrates a small but unobstructed renal artery supplying the kidney.

As illustrated in this case, compensatory hypertrophy of the contralateral kidney is a common associated finding in cases of unilateral renal atrophy. Compensatory hypertrophy can occur well into adulthood, until the sixth or seventh decade of life, and does not necessarily indicate a congenital or childhood abnormality of the other kidney.

Notes

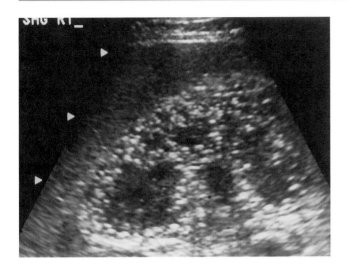

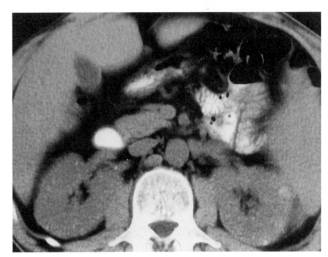

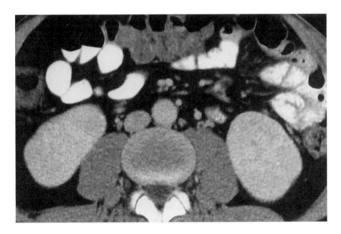

1. In an immunocompromised patient, infection with what organisms may manifest as punctate calcifications in the kidneys?

2. How can a diagnosis be established?

3. Infection in what other organs is commonly caused by this organism?

4. Do calcifications imply healed inactive disease?

Kidney: *Pneumocystis carinii* Infection of the Kidney

1. *Pneumocystis carinii, Mycobacterium avium-intracellulare*, and cytomegalovirus.

2. Percutaneous biopsy of involved organ.

3. Lung, liver, spleen, lymph nodes, and bone marrow.

4. No.

References

Kawashima A, LeRoy AJ: Radiologic evaluation of patients with renal infections, *Infect Dis Clin North Am* 17: 433–456, 2003.

Miller FH, Parikh S, Gore RM, et al: Renal manifestations of AIDS, *Radiographics* 13:587, 1993.

Cross-Reference

Zagoria RJ, *Genitourinary Radiology: THE REQUISITES,* 2nd ed, p 148.

Comment

A wide variety of renal abnormalities are described in patients with AIDS. The most common renal abnormality in this patient population is HIV nephropathy, which is diagnosed when there is renal insufficiency, nephritic syndrome, and glomerulonephropathy.

Patients with AIDS have an increased incidence of opportunistic infection with agents such as *Pneumocystis carinii, Mycobacterium avium-intracellulare, Mycobacterium tuberculosis,* cytomegalovirus (CMV), and others. When the CD4 count is low (less than 200), prophylaxis against *P. carinii* infection is recommended, and oral trimethoprim-sulfamethoxazole is most often administered. Aerosolized pentamidine provides therapeutic levels of pentamidine to the lung (the most commonly affected organ) and does not cause systemic side effects. However, an adverse consequence of the use of aerosolized pentamidine is more frequent infection in other organs, such as the liver, spleen, lymph nodes, and bone marrow, because of subtherapeutic systemic levels of the medication. Thus, prophylactic aerosolized pentamidine is rarely used today.

The imaging findings of renal pneumocystosis include echogenic foci in the renal cortex on ultrasonography and small punctuate calcifications on noncontrast CT. The calcifications are often obscured with intravenous contrast on CT as in this case (third image). Calcifications are evident in both active and inactive forms of renal pneumocystic infection. Although most commonly associated with pneumocystic infections, these calcifications may also occur with *M. avium-intracellulare* and CMV infection. Diagnosis can be made by percutaneous biopsy.

In the case presented, a splenic biopsy demonstrated multiple pneumocystic organisms.

Notes

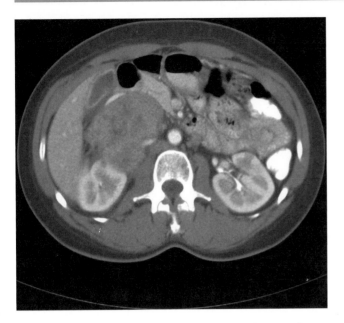 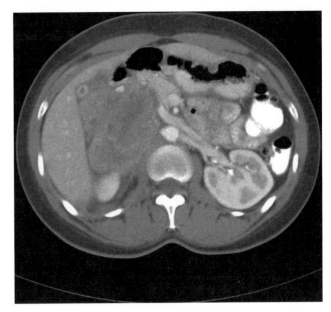

1. What are the three main differential considerations for the above renal mass?

2. Does the location of the tumor help with its identification?

3. Can benign renal leiomyoma be differentiated from a small primary renal leiomyosarcoma?

4. True or false: Renal leiomyosarcomas arise from the transitional epithelium of the medullary collecting ducts.

C A S E   1 8 6

Kidney: Renal Leiomyosarcoma

1. Renal cell carcinoma, oncocytoma, and renal sarcoma.

2. Originating from the capsule suggests sarcoma.

3. Not with confidence.

4. False.

References

Shirkhoda A, Lewis E: Renal sarcoma and sarcomatoid renal cell carcinoma: CT and angiographic features, *Radiology* 162:353–357, 1987.

Srinivas V, Sogani PC, Hajdu SI, et al: Sarcomas of the kidney, *J Urol* 132:13–16, 1984.

Cross-Reference

Zagoria RJ, *Genitourinary Radiology: THE REQUISITES,* 2nd ed, pp 81–83.

Comment

Primary sarcoma of the kidney is a rare entity, accounting for 1.1% of all malignant renal tumors. Many subtypes of renal sarcoma have been reported, including leiomyosarcoma, fibrosarcoma, liposarcoma, rhabdomyosarcoma, primary osteosarcoma, chondrosarcoma, malignant neurilemmoma, clear cell sarcoma, angiosarcoma, and sarcomatoid carcinoma. Of these, leiomyosarcoma is the most common primary renal sarcoma. Renal leiomyosarcoma generally occurs in patients between the ages of 40 and 70, similar to the age distribution for renal cell carcinoma (RCC). The most common presenting symptoms are pain and a palpable mass. Hematuria may be a presenting symptom, but is less common.

Primary renal leiomyosarcomas originate from smooth muscle located in the renal capsule, the renal pelvis, or blood vessels in the renal parenchyma. When these tumors arise from blood vessels, they cannot be differentiated from RCC, due to their parenchymal location. In the series reported by Srinivas et al, renal leiomyosarcomas tend to be large at diagnosis, ranging in size from 10 to 15 cm. On CT they tend to appear as large heterogeneously enhancing renal masses. According to the case series of Shirkhoda and Lewis, the CT signs that suggest primary renal sarcoma as a diagnosis are (1) origination from the renal capsule or sinus (2) lack of extracapsular extension, and (3) fat density (in the case of liposarcoma).

Notes

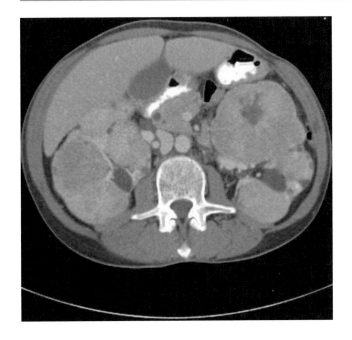
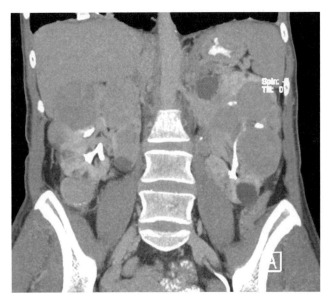
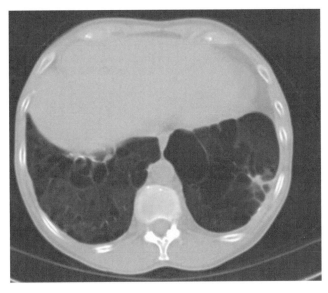

1. What are the cutaneous manifestations and pulmonary complications of this syndrome? (This patient does not have intracranial lesions.)

2. Which three types of renal neoplasms are most common in this disorder?

3. Name three other hereditary renal neoplastic disorders.

4. Describe several general differences between sporadic and hereditary renal neoplasms.

Kidney: Birt-Hogg-Dubé Syndrome

1. Fibrofolliculomas (white papules) and acrochordons ("skin tags"); spontaneous pneumothoraces (25%).

2. Chromophobe and clear cell renal carcinomas and oncocytomas.

3. Tuberous sclerosis, von Hippel-Lindau disease, hereditary renal oncocytoma, hereditary papillary renal cancer, hereditary leiomyoma renal cell carcinoma, and medullary carcinoma.

4. Hereditary neoplasms: bilateral/multiple, younger patients, lack of predominance among males and females.

References

Choyke PL, Glenn GM, Walthier MM, et al: Hereditary renal cancers, *Radiology* 226:33–46, 2003.

Pavlovich CP, Walthier MM, Eyler RA, et al: Renal tumors in the Birt-Hogg-Dubé syndrome, *Am J Surg Pathol* 26:1542–1552, 2002.

Cross-Reference

Zagoria RJ, *Genitourinary Radiology: THE REQUISITES*, 2nd ed, pp 111–112.

Comment

The images show cystic lung lesions and multiple solid kidney tumors. One tumor shown has a stellate scar, suggesting it is an oncocytoma. Birt-Hogg-Dubé (BHD) syndrome includes the constellation of fibrofolliculomas, pulmonary cysts, and renal neoplasms. It represents an autosomal-dominant familial renal neoplasia syndrome. The abnormal gene has been identified on chromosome 17. In patients who develop renal neoplasms at a young age, one must consider the possibility of a hereditary condition. Physical examination and other imaging for staging can often indicate the components of a particular syndrome and allows differentiation between the major syndromes. Historically, 4% of patients with renal cancer have been found to have a syndrome, but the true percentage is most likely greater.

Pavlovich et al identified multiple types of renal neoplasms in individual families with BHD and also identified individuals with BHD who harbored different types of renal neoplasms. The most common renal neoplasms identified include chromophobe and clear cell carcinomas as well as hybrid tumors that contained oncocytes and chromophobe cancer cells. Benign tumors included oncocytes. The incidence of renal cancer in these patients is approximately 15% to 25%. As opposed to patients with BHD, with sporadic renal cell carcinoma, clear cell represents the majority of tumors. Clear cell is also the most common type of renal cancer in patients with von Hippel-Lindau disease and tuberous sclerosis.

Imaging of patients with BHD often demonstrates multiple solid renal masses. Oncocytomas may demonstrate a central scar which can calcify, but this appearance is not universal. Pulmonary cysts, seen in 70% of patients, can sometimes be identified in the lung bases on abdominal imaging.

Once families are identified who carry hereditary renal neoplastic syndromes such as BHD, screening imaging of family members is often performed. CT or MRI is preferred over ultrasonography.

Notes

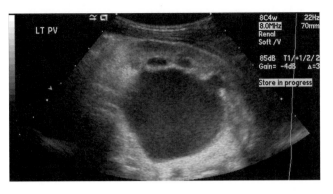
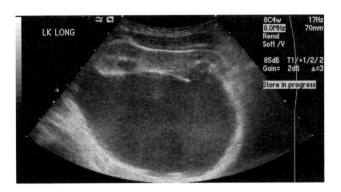

1. What are the two major renal abnormalities?

2. How can the sonographer confirm the presence of debris within the collecting system?

3. What is the debris composed of?

4. What is the appropriate management?

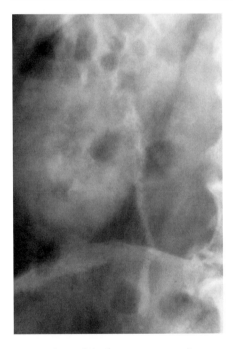
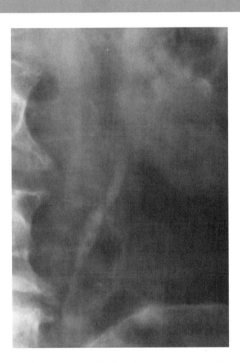

1. In this elderly patient with recurrent urinary tract infections, what is the most likely diagnosis for the abnormality shown?

2. In what percentage of patients does transitional cell carcinoma involve the upper tracts bilaterally?

3. What multifocal ureteral lesions are closely associated with recurrent urinary tract infections?

4. Between cystitis cystica and cystitis glandularis, which inflammatory bladder lesion is believed to be premalignant?

CASE 188

Pelvicalices and Ureter: Pyonephrosis with Ureteropelvic Junction Obstruction

1. Hydronephrosis, especially involving the pelvis, and pyonephrosis.

2. Reposition the patient and demonstrate movement of the debris into a dependent position.

3. Usually either white or red cells.

4. Decompression and drainage.

Reference
Paterson A: Urinary tract infection: an update on imaging strategies, *Eur Radiol* 14:89–100, 2004.

Cross-Reference
Zagoria RJ, *Genitourinary Radiology: THE REQUISITES,* 2nd ed, pp 152–153.

Comment
Ultrasonography is the test of choice in evaluating renal failure and suspected urosepsis in both children and adults. Separation of diffuse parenchymal disease from postrenal obstruction is critical in determining treatment.

This case demonstrates two common findings in children with renal disease: hydronephrosis and pyonephrosis. The massively dilated renal pelvis suggests that the obstruction is at the ureteropelvic junction. In children, this is usually a functional obstruction that is repaired either endoscopically or with an open pyeloplasty. The identification of debris within a dilated collecting system suggests the presence of either pus or blood. Care must be taken to accurately locate the focal zone of the ultrasound beam to avoid reverberation artifact, which may mimic debris. Positioning of the patient in the supine and left or right lateral decubitus positions will also help in identifying settling of debris into a dependent position. Once the diagnosis is confirmed, the pus must be drained either using a ureteral stent or, more commonly, a percutaneous nephrostomy tube. Failure to identify pyonephrosis can lead to severe urosepsis, kidney failure, and death.

Notes

CASE 189

Pelvicalices and Ureter: Pyeloureteritis Cystica

1. Pyeloureteritis cystica.

2. 1% to 2%.

3. Pyeloureteritis cystica and malacoplakia.

4. Cystitis glandularis.

Reference
Banner MP: Genitourinary complications of inflammatory bowel disease, *Radiol Clin North Am* 25:199–209, 1987.

Cross-Reference
Zagoria RJ, *Genitourinary Radiology: THE REQUISITES,* 2nd ed, p 196.

Comment
This case demonstrates poor excretion of contrast material from both kidneys and numerous filling defects within the ureter and marginal irregularity of the ureter and renal pelvis. There are numerous causes of multifocal radiolucent filling defects, most of which are unilateral. In addition, the history of recurrent urinary tract infections suggests the diagnosis of pyeloureteritis cystica. Malacoplakia is extremely rare but is associated with recurrent urinary tract infections. This condition could have a similar appearance, but its rarity in comparison with pyeloureteritis cystica makes it much less likely.

Pyeloureteritis cystica is analogous to cystitis cystica, which occurs in the bladder. Both result from chronic or recurrent urinary tract infections that cause encystment of submucosal glands. These cysts are usually multifocal and small. Rarely they can be unifocal and may be several centimeters in diameter. These filling defects can persist for months after resolution of the infection, but they have no known malignant potential. A similar-appearing abnormality in the bladder is cystitis glandularis. Unlike cystitis cystica, which is always associated with urinary tract infections, cystitis glandularis often occurs without bacterial infection. In addition, cystitis glandularis is believed to be premalignant. Multifocal, bilateral transitional cell carcinoma can have a similar appearance, but it is quite rare and is unrelated to recurrent urinary tract infections.

Notes

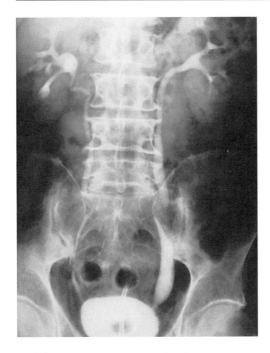 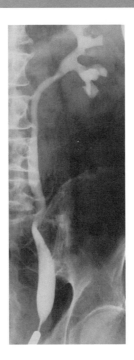

1. The pattern seen on the intravenous urogram and the retrograde pyelogram is typical of what diagnosis?

2. Is this disease usually unilateral or bilateral?

3. Is this disease more akin to Hirschsprung's disease or achalasia of the gastrointestinal tract?

4. Is there a gender predilection for this disease?

Pelvicalices and Ureter: Primary Megaureter

1. Primary megaureter.

2. Unilateral.

3. Achalasia.

4. Yes. Men are more commonly affected than are women.

Reference

Pfister RC, Papanicolaou N, Yoder IC: The dilated ureter, *Semin Roentgenol* 21:224–235, 1986.

Cross-Reference

Zagoria RJ, *Genitourinary Radiology: THE REQUISITES*, 2nd ed, pp 176–180, 184.

Comment

When the ureter is dilated to more than 10 mm in diameter, it is by definition a megaureter. If there is an identifiable cause for the megaureter, such as chronic ureteral obstruction, vesicoureteral reflux, diabetes insipidus, or psychogenic polydipsia, then the diagnosis is secondary megaureter. Idiopathic cases are classified as primary megaureter. Typically, primary megaureter is a unilateral process that occurs more frequently on the left and in men. Typically, primary megaureter presents with marked dilation, predominantly of the lowest one third of the ureter, as in this case. Careful evaluation of the upper tracts in this case demonstrates no evidence of increased pressure; that is, the calyces and upper ureter are not dilated. This pattern strongly suggests primary megaureter. Other causes of megaureter typically affect the entire ureter and also lead to blunting and dilation of the calyces. The intravenous urogram in this case shows completely normal, unobstructed calyceal anatomy. The etiology of primary megaureter is insufficient musculature in the segment of ureter near the ureterovesical junction and below the dilated segment. This deficiency leads to diminished peristalsis through this segment. Innervation is completely normal throughout the ureter. Therefore it is easier to understand the pathologic findings of this disease as being similar to those in patients with achalasia than those in patients with Hirschsprung's disease of the colon. The aperistaltic segment of the ureter causes delayed passage of urine and chronically increased volume just above that segment, which then results in ureteral dilation without significantly increased pressure in the ureter.

Rarely, primary megaureter can involve the entire length of the ureter and the calyces. In such cases it is difficult to distinguish this entity from ureteral obstruction.

Notes

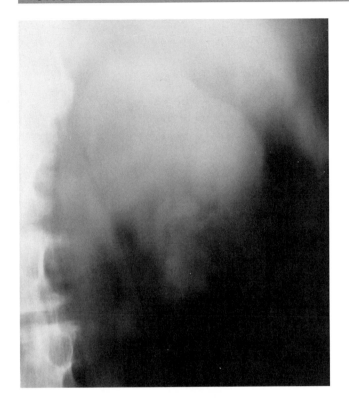

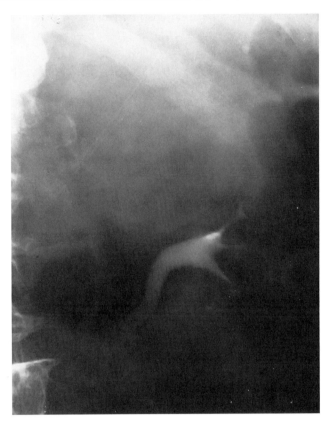

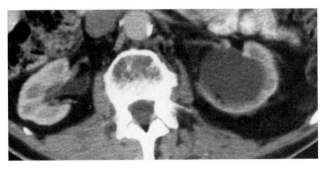

1. What is the likely lesion in this 80-year-old patient with gross hematuria?

2. What is the fluid-containing structure filling the left renal sinus on the CT scan?

3. What term describes the opacified lower pole calyces in this and similar cases?

4. What associated congenital anomalies usually cause obstruction in this type of case?

Pelvicalices and Ureter: Duplication Anomaly

1. Duplication anomaly.

2. Obstructed upper pole pyelocalyceal system.

3. "Drooping lily" sign.

4. Ectopic ureterocele and extravesical ectopic insertion of the ureter.

Reference

Fernbach SK, Feinstein KA, Spencer K, Lindstrom CA: Ureteral dilatation and its complications, *Radiographics* 17:109–127, 1997.

Cross-Reference

Zagoria RJ, *Genitourinary Radiology: THE REQUISITES,* 2nd ed, pp 163, 165.

Comment

This patient has obstruction of the upper pole moiety of a duplicated system with resulting hydronephrosis, nonopacification of the upper pole calyces, and deviation of the lower pole calyces inferiorly. Note that a line drawn through the most medial opacified calyces of the left kidney would point to the ipsilateral shoulder. This is usually caused by nonvisualization of an upper collecting system or by lateral deviation of the upper pole of the kidney by a mass. The axis of this kidney is normal, suggesting that a mass is not deviating the kidney. Otherwise the lower pole calyces appear normal. The two congenital causes of upper pole obstruction include ectopic ureterocele and extravesical ectopic insertion of the ureter. These anomalies are usually discovered during childhood. When the ureter inserts ectopically within the bladder, its abnormal course and position in the bladder wall may lead to formation of an obstructing ectopic ureterocele. Because the upper moiety ureter is the ectopic ureter, it may insert inferior to the bladder. Its abnormal insertion may lead to obstruction because of limited outflow from its insertion site or fibrosis. If the ureter inserts in a site such as the female urethra or vagina, chronic infection can lead to stenosis of its orifice and resulting obstruction.

Duplication anomalies are commonly associated with other malformations. Approximately 30% of patients have other significant congenital urinary tract anomalies, such as renal agenesis or ureteropelvic junction stricture. Also, duplicated systems are susceptible to all of the pathologic problems that may occur in a single system. This 80-year-old patient with gross hematuria developed a transitional cell carcinoma of the ureter draining the upper pole moiety. This carcinoma was the cause of the hydronephrosis.

Notes

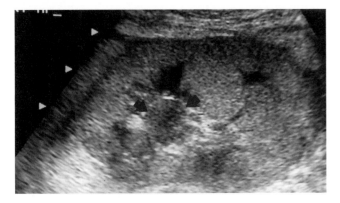

1. A sagittal sonogram of a transplanted kidney is shown. To what do the *arrows* point?

2. What is the differential diagnosis for this mass?

3. List several factors that can predispose an individual to fungal infections of the kidney.

4. How are fungal infections of the urinary tract treated?

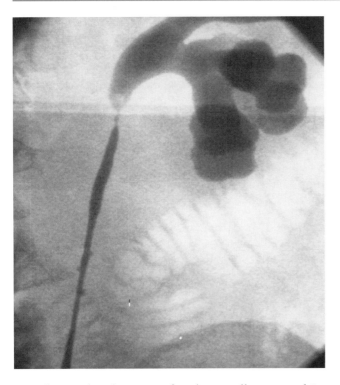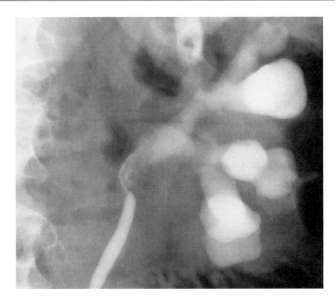

1. What is the diagnosis for the small outpouchings from the ureter?

2. Do these outpouchings represent a benign or malignant abnormality?

3. What is the significance of these outpouchings?

4. What is the most likely diagnosis for the filling defect in the upper pole calyx and the narrowing at the ureteropelvic junction?

Pelvicalices and Ureter: Fungal Infection in a Transplanted Kidney

1. Mass in the renal collecting system.

2. Blood clot, fungus ball, neoplasm, and lymphoproliferative disease.

3. Immunosuppression, diabetes, neurogenic bladder, use of an indwelling catheter for long periods, and long-term antibiotic or steroid use.

4. Systemic antifungal agents, bladder irrigation with antifungal agents, and percutaneous extraction.

Reference

Kennedy CA, Panosian CB: Infectious complications of kidney transplantation. In Danovitch GM, ed: *Handbook of Kidney Transplantation,* Boston, 1992, Little, Brown.

Cross-Reference

Zagoria RJ, *Genitourinary Radiology: THE REQUISITES,* 2nd ed, p 194.

Comment

Immunosuppressive therapy has contributed to the long-term success of renal transplantation, but with it come many associated problems. Chief among these problems is a susceptibility to opportunistic infections. Urinary tract infection is the most common infection after organ transplantation, occurring in approximately 40% of renal allograft recipients. This incidence has been reduced to around 10% since the institution of prophylactic therapy with trimethoprim-sulfamethoxazole. Gram-negative organisms, such as *Escherichia coli* and *Klebsiella* species, are the most common causative agents (76%), followed by gram-positive bacteria (22%) and fungi (1%). The most common fungal pathogens are *Candida* and *Aspergillus* species. Predisposing factors for posttransplantation urinary tract infection include extensive manipulation during surgery, placement of indwelling urinary catheters, anatomic abnormalities resulting in urostasis, and neurogenic bladder. Infection most commonly occurs in the first 6 months after transplantation. After this time, infection is usually related to impaired allograft function.

Renal parenchymal fungal infection usually occurs via hematogenous dissemination. In contrast, infection in the lower urinary tract usually occurs via an ascending route from the bladder. Fungus balls are found in the urinary bladder more often than in the upper collecting system. Detection of a fungus ball relies on signs and symptoms of obstruction coupled with funguria. Hydronephrosis may or may not be present. The fungus ball is an echogenic, weakly shadowing mass within the collecting system.

Notes

Pelvicalices and Ureter: Ureteral Pseudodiverticula

1. Ureteral pseudodiverticula.

2. Benign.

3. They indicate increased risk for synchronous or metachronous transitional cell carcinoma.

4. Transitional cell carcinoma.

Reference

Wasserman NF, Zhand G, Posalaky IP, Reddy PK: Ureteral pseudodiverticula: frequent association with uroepithelial malignancy, *Am J Roentgenol* 157:69–72, 1991.

Cross-Reference

Zagoria RJ, *Genitourinary Radiology: THE REQUISITES,* 2nd ed, p 185.

Comment

Ureteral pseudodiverticula are uncommon but not rare. They represent intramural outpouchings from the ureteral lumen. In and of themselves, ureteral pseudodiverticula are completely benign and represent invagination of the urothelium into hyperplastic nests of cells in the ureteral wall. These pouches are visible on both retrograde pyelograms and intravenous urograms, although they are most commonly identified on retrograde studies because of the pressure of injection. The significance of these diverticula is their association with transitional cell carcinoma (TCC). Up to one fourth of patients with ureteral pseudodiverticula have a coexisting TCC, as does this patient, or will develop a TCC within several years. The TCC can occur ipsilateral to the pseudodiverticula or within the bladder. It has been postulated that pseudodiverticula result from chronic ureteral inflammation, which also may predispose these patients to development of urothelial neoplasms. When ureteral pseudodiverticula are evident, careful evaluation of the entire urothelium should be performed to exclude coexisting TCC. If none is found, follow-up imaging is recommended semiannually.

Notes

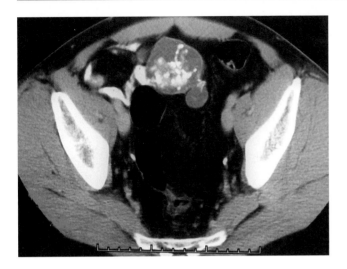
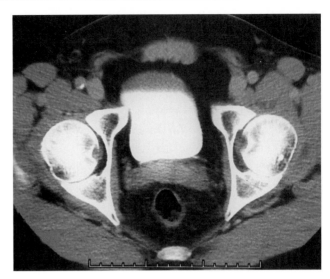

1. What is the differential diagnosis for this pelvic mass?

2. In which anatomic space is this mass located? Is it intra- or extraperitoneal?

3. In what percentage of bladder transitional cell carcinomas is calcification identified?

4. True or false: The prognosis for patients with urachal carcinoma is better than those with nonurachal bladder malignancies.

C A S E 1 9 4

Bladder: Urachal Adenocarcinoma

1. Benign (e.g., hemangioma) or malignant bladder tumor, urachal adenocarcinoma, ovarian metastasis, and peritoneal metastasis from a gastrointestinal tumor.

2. Space of Retzius. Extraperitoneal; the urachus is bordered anteriorly by the transversalis fascia and posteriorly by the peritoneum.

3. 1% to 7%.

4. False.

References

Siefker-Radtke AO, Gee J, Shen Y, et al: Multimodality management of urachal carcinoma: the M. D. Anderson Cancer Center experience, *J Urol* 169:1295–1298, 2003.

Thali-Schwab CM, Woodward PJ, Wagner BJ: Computed tomographic appearance of urachal adenocarcinomas: review of 25 cases, *Eur Radiol* 15:79–84, 2005.

Cross-Reference

Zagoria RJ, *Genitourinary Radiology: THE REQUISITES,* 2nd ed, p 241.

Comment

The urachus is an epithelium-lined fibrous cord (median umbilical ligament) connecting the bladder apex to the umbilicus. It is the remnant of the fetal communication between the fetal bladder and allantois and normally closes spontaneously by the middle of the second trimester. Urachal cancer accounts for less than 0.5% of all bladder cancers and arises in the extraperitoneal space from the juxtavesical segment of the urachus in 90% of patients. In general, any adenocarcinoma arising at or near the bladder dome should be considered to be of urachal origin. Two thirds of patients are men between the ages of 40 and 70 years. Of urachal cancers, 85% are mucinous adenocarcinoma, although squamous cell carcinoma, transitional cell carcinoma, and sarcoma have been reported. The prognosis for urachal adenocarcinoma is worse than that for bladder carcinoma because the tumor grows to a large size in a clinically occult space; the 5-year survival rate is approximately 10%. Painless hematuria is the most common presenting symptom.

The diagnosis of urachal carcinoma is usually suggested on CT where it appears as a midline soft tissue mass arising near the superior aspect of the bladder extending anterosuperiorly to the umbilicus. These masses usually are large (6 cm in diameter), and calcification is recognized in 72% of cases on CT. Approximately 50% of patients have metastases at the time of original diagnosis. Urachal carcinoma has a propensity to invade the abdominal wall, peritoneum, or small bowel. Treatment includes surgical resection and chemotherapy in patients who present with metastases.

Notes

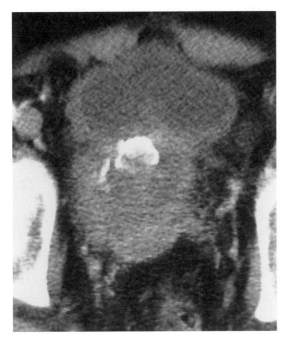 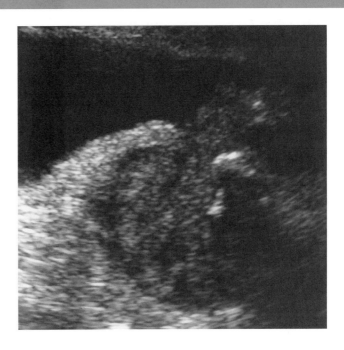

1. Explain the abnormal shape of the urinary bladder.

2. Worldwide, what is the most common cause of bladder wall calcification?

3. What is alkaline encrustation cystitis?

4. What is the most likely diagnosis in this case?

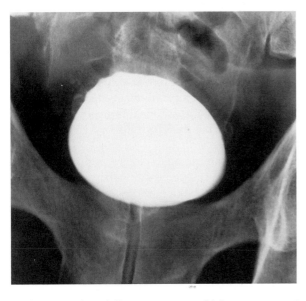 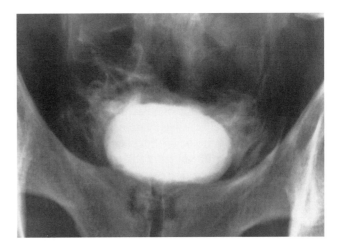

1. What are the different types of blunt traumatic bladder injury?

2. In what percentage of traumatic injuries of the anterior pelvic ring does bladder injury occur?

3. What are some causes of spontaneous bladder rupture?

4. This patient has chronic renal failure and is being evaluated for renal transplantation. What is the diagnosis?

Bladder: Carcinoma Arising in a Bladder Diverticulum

1. There is a large bladder diverticulum.

2. Bilharzial cystitis.

3. A form of cystitis where inflamed or devitalized mucosa is covered by a layer of calcium phosphate, the precipitation of which is enhanced by alkaluria.

4. Carcinoma arising from a bladder diverticulum.

Reference

Dondalski M, White EM, Ghahremani GG, Patel SK: Carcinoma arising in urinary bladder diverticula: imaging findings in six patients, *Am J Roentgenol* 161:817–820, 1993.

Cross-Reference

Zagoria RJ, *Genitourinary Radiology: THE REQUISITES,* 2nd ed, pp 177, 229.

Comment

In this case, a transitional cell carcinoma (TCC) is growing from the lateral wall of a bladder diverticulum, and the diverticulum neck arises from the posterior wall of the urinary bladder. The ultrasound study shows that a papillary component of the TCC has grown through the neck of the diverticulum and into the lumen of the bladder.

Stasis of urine or long-standing infection may incite inflammatory changes in the mucosa of bladder diverticula, and neoplasm develops in 2% to 7%. In 80% of cases the histologic tumor type is TCC, but squamous cell carcinoma, adenocarcinoma, and mixed carcinoma have been reported. Carcinoma arising within bladder diverticula has a poorer prognosis than cancers of the native bladder because of early transmural spread. In the case presented, note the thickened lateral wall of the diverticulum and the strands of tumor in the perivesical fat that indicate transmural spread (stage C or T3b).

Cystography and cross-sectional imaging are more reliable than excretory urography and cystoscopy for the evaluation of complications of bladder diverticula. Cystoscopy is a reliable method for diagnosing most mucosal bladder tumors, but those arising in diverticula may be inaccessible to the cystoscope. A diverticular bladder neoplasm may appear as an intraluminal filling defect, mass, or focus of mucosal irregularity. Incomplete contrast opacification of a diverticulum, and failure of a previously identified diverticulum to fill are additional signs.

Notes

Bladder: Extravasation in an Unused Urinary Bladder

1. Mural contusion, partial-thickness laceration, and full-thickness bladder laceration. Full thickness laceration can result in intraperitoneal, extraperitoneal, or combined ruptures.

2. 7% to 10%.

3. Lesions that thin or weaken the bladder wall, bladder outlet obstruction, neurogenic bladder, cystitis, radiation treatment, tumor, and perivesical inflammation.

4. Extraperitoneal rupture of an unused bladder.

Reference

Caroline DF, Pollack HM, Banner MP, Schneck C: Self-limiting extravasation in the unused urinary bladder, *Radiology* 155:311–313, 1985.

Cross-Reference

Zagoria RJ, *Genitourinary Radiology: THE REQUISITES,* 2nd ed, pp 231–234.

Comment

Full-thickness rupture of the bladder most often occurs after pelvic trauma and is generally accompanied by local (pain, tenderness, and guarding) and systemic (fever and malaise) symptoms. However, bladder rupture can be spontaneous or iatrogenic. Isolated extraperitoneal rupture (prevalence 50%–85%) is more common than either isolated intraperitoneal rupture (prevalence 15%–45%) or combined intraperitoneal and extraperitoneal rupture (prevalence 5%–10%). Although intraperitoneal bladder lacerations are less commonly associated with traumatic osseous pelvic injury, between 80% and 95% of traumatic extraperitoneal ruptures are associated with fractures of the anterior pubic ring or diastasis of the pubic symphysis.

Although complications are rare, mucosal tears and self-limited contrast extravasation have been reported in unused urinary bladders during cystourethrography. Over time, the nonfunctioning bladder becomes hypertonic and less compliant. These changes are likely to be intrinsic properties of the unused detrusor muscle because they develop independent of infection, inflammation, denervation, or fibrosis. Unused bladders are studied to evaluate bladder capacity, vesicoureteral reflux, or urethral anatomy. Acute distention of the bladder beyond its normal capacity during cystourethrography may cause small rents in the mucosa. Contrast dissects within the bladder wall, and extravasation may be visible. However, it never extends much further than the immediate perivesical space.

Notes

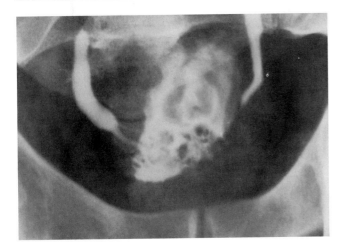
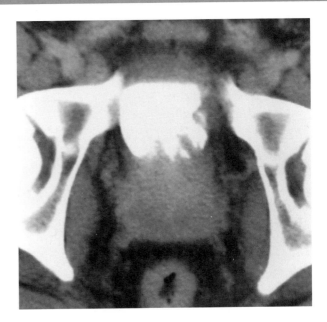

1. Given the clinical history of gross hematuria, what is the differential diagnosis for the bladder lesion(s)?

2. Name three types of chronic proliferative cystitis that can mimic a papillary or invasive bladder neoplasm.

3. True or false: The majority of patients with malacoplakia are immunocompromised.

4. Cystitis cystica, eosinophilic cystitis, and squamous cell carcinoma are associated with which bladder infection?

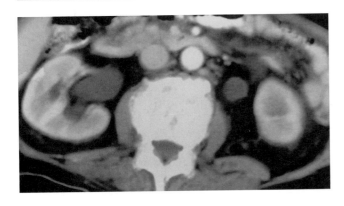
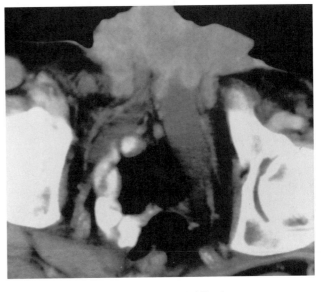

1. This patient has a congenital anomaly of the lower urinary tract. What is the fluid-filled structure entering the mass in the lower abdominal wall?

2. What abnormality of the pubic bones may accompany this congenital anomaly?

3. An unusual configuration of the distal ureters in this anomaly mimics the shape of a stick used in an Irish game. What name is given to this configuration?

4. What complication of this anomaly is illustrated by this case?

Bladder: Cystitis Glandularis

1. Bladder carcinoma, focal proliferative cystitis, and adherent blood clots.

2. Cystitis cystica, cystitis glandularis, malacoplakia, bullous cystitis, follicular cystitis, Hunner's ulcer, and eosinophilic cystitis.

3. True.

4. Bilharziasis (*Schistosoma haematobium* bladder infection).

Reference

Hochberg DA, Motta J, Brodherson MS: Cystitis glandularis, *Urology* 51:112–113, 1998.

Cross-Reference

Zagoria RJ, *Genitourinary Radiology: THE REQUISITES,* 2nd ed, p 212.

Comment

The urothelium retains the potential to form numerous epithelial variants, such as mucus-producing glandular epithelium and squamous epithelium, because of its complex embryonal derivation. In the initial stages of bladder inflammation, Brunn's nests are found with increasing frequency in the lamina propria. These nests are nodular proliferations of urothelium that grow inward into the submucosa. If the centers of these urothelial cell nests degenerate, fluid-filled cysts (cystitis cystica) may result. Intestinal or vaginal glandular metaplasia of Brunn's nests in the lamina propria results in cystitis glandularis (CG). Parenthetically, squamous metaplasia probably occurs with a different sequence of events because it is not preceded by the formation of Brunn's nests. Follicular cystitis is characterized by the presence of reactive lymphoid follicles in the lamina propria and is more common in children with chronic urinary tract infections.

The metaplastic submucosal glands of CG may enlarge such that they present as multiple discrete nodules, clusters of lobulated nodules, or a discrete papillary mass. Thus, CG may mimic a papillary bladder carcinoma, bullous cystitis or edema, or a bladder-invasive prostate or cervical cancer. This process has a predilection for the bladder neck and trigone and has been associated with the passage of mucus.

Although adenocarcinoma presents in 10% to 42% of cases, it is not clear whether CG is a premalignant condition. The association with adenocarcinoma has been reported only in patients with the intestinal type of CG, not in patients with the much more common, typical variant of CG.

Notes

Bladder: Bladder Exstrophy Complicated by Adenocarcinoma

1. A dilated left ureter.

2. The pubic bones are separated more than 1 cm at the symphysis. Also note the everted left pubic bone in this case.

3. Hurley stick appearance.

4. Bladder carcinoma.

Reference

Vik V, Gerharz EW, Woodhouse CRJ: Invasive carcinoma in bladder exstrophy with transitional, squamous and mucus-producing differentiation, *Br J Urol* 81:173–174, 1998.

Cross-Reference

Zagoria RJ, *Genitourinary Radiology: THE REQUISITES,* 2nd ed, p 207.

Comment

Exstrophy of the bladder and epispadias represent the two ends of a spectrum of abdominal wall defects caused by abnormal cloacal membrane closure. Bladder exstrophy (which means "turned inside out") occurs in 1 of every 30,000 to 40,000 live births, is twice as common in men, and is three times more common than epispadias. In exstrophy the ventral bladder wall and the remaining bladder are everted and protrude through a defect in the lower anterior abdominal wall. A short penis, epispadias, and chordee are present. Affected girls may have vaginal stenosis or müllerian anomalies of uterovaginal fusion, but the uterus, tubes, and ovaries are usually unaffected. Characteristically the pubic bones are widely separated at the pubic symphysis, the iliac bones are rotated outward along the fulcrum of the sacroiliac joints, and each pubic bone is rotated outward at its junction with the ilium and ischium.

The mucosa of the bladder may be normal, metaplastic, or ulcerated. Squamous metaplasia may be found at the apex, or glandular metaplasia (cystitis glandularis) may occur at the bladder base. The risk for developing carcinoma is increased 200-fold. Adenocarcinoma has been found in 70 of the 82 reported cases of carcinoma complicating bladder exstrophy. The pathogenesis of this unusual type of bladder cancer may be glandular metaplasia, ectopic rectal mucosa displaced during cloacal division, or proliferation of an uncommitted epithelial stem cell.

Notes

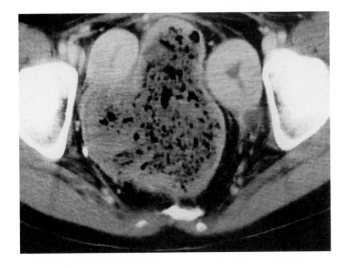

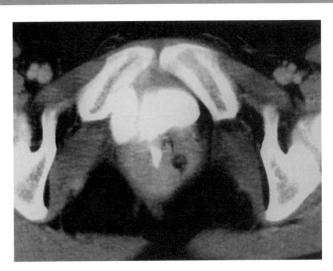

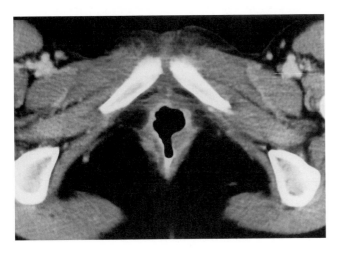

1. What are the abnormal findings on these images? What is the most likely diagnosis?

2. What is the most common cause of morbidity in these patients?

3. Which radiologic test usually is performed initially?

4. What is the meaning of the word *cloaca*?

Bladder: Cloaca

1. Duplicated uterus, dilated rectum, and a common cavity for the urethra, vagina, and rectum are the abnormal findings. Cloacal malformation is the most likely diagnosis.

2. Renal failure resulting from obstruction, vesicoureteral reflux, or chronic infection.

3. Instillation of water-soluble contrast through the perineal orifice under fluoroscopy. This test is useful to determine the anatomic relationship between the bladder, urethra, vagina, and rectum. Cross-sectional imaging is less useful initially because of the variable and often complicated anatomy.

4. Latin for "sewer."

Reference

Jaramillo D, Lebowitz RL, Hendren WH: Cloacal malformation: radiologic findings and imaging recommendations, *Radiology* 177:441–448, 1990.

Cross-Reference

Zagoria RJ, *Genitourinary Radiology: THE REQUISITES,* 2nd ed, p 202.

Comment

Cloacal malformation occurs exclusively in females and is a congenital anomaly in which the urinary, genital, and intestinal tracts empty into a single orifice in the perineum, the cloaca. A cloaca exists in fish, birds, and amphibians, as well as the normal human embryo at 4 weeks' gestation. This congenital anomaly is believed to result from incomplete separation of the rectum and urogenital sinus by the urorectal septum. This anomaly is heterogeneous in that there are many variations in the connections between the bladder, vagina, and rectum. The rectum and vagina may empty into the ureter, the ureter and vagina may drain into the rectum, or the ureter and rectum may empty into the vagina.

Cloacal malformation is associated with a number of complications and anomalies. One large series reported uterine duplication in 55% of affected women, vaginal duplication in 46%, sacral agenesis in 40%, and bladder diverticula in 20%. The primary complications of this anomaly are renal failure resulting from obstruction, vesicoureteral reflux, or both, and repeated urinary tract infections caused by contamination from the fecal stream.

The role of radiologic studies is to facilitate surgical correction of this disorder by precisely defining the complex anatomic relationships between the lower genital, urinary, and gastrointestinal tracts.

Notes

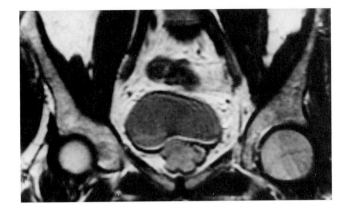

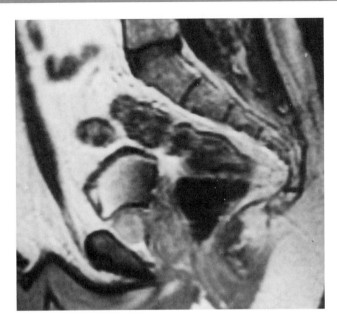

1. What is the pulse sequence shown on the sagittal image?

2. This patient complained of diaphoresis during and after micturition. What other clinical symptoms might be expected in this patient?

3. In what other sites may this tumor occur?

4. What precautions should be taken before the lesion is surgically removed?

Bladder: Bladder Paraganglioma (Pheochromocytoma)

1. Proton density-weighted spin echo (the fat is bright, the urine in the bladder is bright, and the cerebrospinal fluid is dark).

2. Headache, palpitations, and other symptoms related to catecholamine excess.

3. Adrenal glands (in 90% of patients), the paravertebral sympathetic plexus, and the organ of Zuckerkandl (paraganglion cells along the lower abdominal aorta from the inferior mesenteric artery to the iliac arteries).

4. The patient should be pretreated with alpha-adrenergic blockers, such as phenoxybenzamine, to prevent a hypertensive crisis.

References

Atiyeh BA, Baraket AJ, Abumrad NN: Extra-adrenal pheochromocytoma, *J Nephrol* 10:25–29, 1997.

Elsayes KM, Narra VR, Leyendecker JR, et al: MRI of adrenal and extraadrenal pheochromocytoma, *Am J Roentgenol* 184:860–867, 2005.

Cross-Reference

Zagoria RJ, *Genitourinary Radiology: THE REQUISITES,* 2nd ed, p 215.

Comment

The images show a T2-bright mass (pheochromocytoma) adjacent to, or arising from, the bladder base. Extraadrenal pheochromocytoma arises from the paraganglion chromaffin cells of the sympathetic nervous system. These abnormalities occur most commonly in the paraadrenal area, followed by the region of aortic bifurcation (organ of Zuckerkandl). Other sites include the bladder, mediastinum, and heart. Extraadrenal pheochromocytomas are estimated to occur in 10% of adults and up to 40% of children. These lesions are larger, more likely to recur, and more likely to metastasize than their adrenal counterparts. The work-up for a suspected pheochromocytoma consists of measurement of urinary catecholamine levels and noncontrast CT of the abdomen and pelvis. Treatment is surgical excision. Radiation therapy and chemotherapy are ineffective. Follow-up after resection should include annual measurement of urinary catecholamine levels and, if these levels are elevated, repeat cross-sectional imaging. MRI and adrenomedullary scintigraphy with metaiodobenzylguanidine iodine 131 are adjunctive examinations if CT is not diagnostic.

Notes

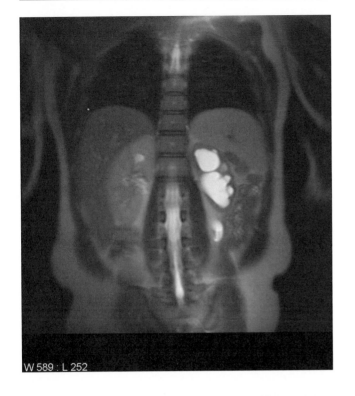

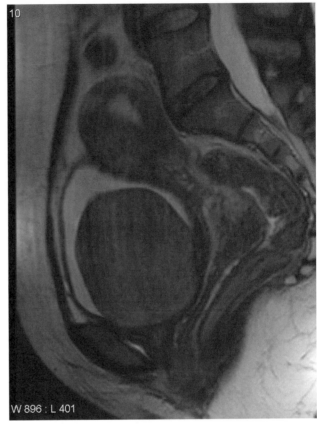

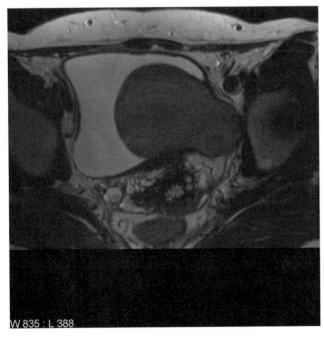

1. What is the likely origin of this mass?

2. Is malignant transformation of this lesion common?

3. What is the differential diagnosis of a bladder wall mass?

4. Where else in the urinary tract can this lesion arise?

Bladder: Bladder Leiomyoma

1. Submucosal bladder wall.

2. No.

3. Transitional cell carcinoma, leiomyosarcoma, leiomyoma, pheochromocytoma, and hamartoma.

4. Anywhere, but the most common location is the renal capsule.

References

Betts MT, Huo EJ, Miller FH: Pictorial essay: gastrointestinal and genitourinary smooth muscle tumors, *Am J Roentgenol* 181:1349–1354, 2003.

Cornella JL, Larson TR, Lee RA, et al: Leiomyoma of the female urethra and bladder: report of twenty-three patients and review of the literature, *Am J Obstet Gynecol* 176:1278–1285, 1997.

Cross-Reference

Zagoria RJ, *Genitourinary Radiology: THE REQUISITES,* 2nd ed, p 205.

Comment

The MRIs show a large tumor in the bladder obstructing the left ureter. The mass is smooth, and homogeneous without evidence of extravesical spread, which would be unusual for a malignancy of this size. Leiomyomas account for less than 1% of bladder tumors. They may arise elsewhere in the urinary tract, including the renal capsule and urethra. Pathologically they are smooth muscle and connective tissue tumors and are similar to uterine leiomyomas. They are most commonly submucosal endovesical lesions, but may also be intramural or extravesical. Endovesical lesions may cause symptoms of bladder irritation, flank pain, and hematuria. Large, pedunculated lesions may cause bladder outlet obstruction and hydronephrosis. A mass may be palpable on bimanual pelvic examination. After resection, recurrence is rare, and malignant transformation has not been reported.

On cystography or excretory urography, bladder leiomyomas appear as well-defined, smooth intramural masses that form sharp angles with the bladder wall. A smooth, homogeneous solid mass may be demonstrated by ultrasonography. It may be difficult to distinguish between extravesical bladder leiomyomas and other pelvis masses, particularly uterine fibroids. On T1- and T2-weighted MRIs, leiomyomas are isointense to the bladder wall. Some enhance homogeneously after contrast administration, while others exhibit peripheral enhancement. Leiomyomas and leiomyosarcomas may have a similar appearance; however, large size, irregular margins, and heterogeneity favor a diagnosis of leiomyosarcoma. A submucosal location can help differentiate a leiomyoma from the more common transitional cell carcinoma. The differential diagnosis of an intramural bladder mass includes leiomyoma, leiomyosarcoma, hamartoma, and pheochromocytoma.

Notes

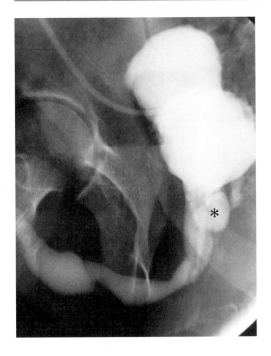
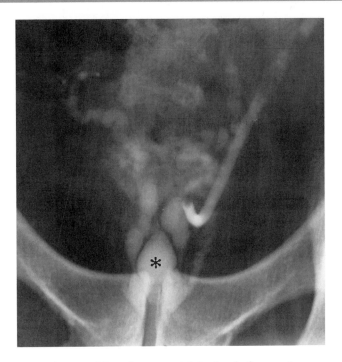

1. What is the most likely cause of the structure denoted by the *asterisk* in both figures?

2. Name two congenital anomalies associated with this structure.

3. What genital ducts are opacified in the image on the right?

4. What is the most likely explanation for the abnormal appearance of the anterior urethra?

Urethra: Large Prostatic Utricle

1. Prostatic utricle.

2. Hypospadias, ambiguous genitalia, undescended testis, and congenital urethral polyp.

3. Ductus deferens, vas deferens, and ejaculatory ducts.

4. Hypospadias repair.

Reference

Ikoma F, Shima H, Yabumoto H: Classification of enlarged prostatic utricle in patients with hypospadias, *Br J Urol* 57:334–337, 1985.

Cross-Reference

Zagoria RJ, *Genitourinary Radiology: THE REQUISITES,* 2nd ed, pp 254, 336.

Comment

Before or after surgical correction, boys with hypospadias are not routinely evaluated radiologically. However, suspected postoperative complications, such as urethrocutaneous fistula or urethral obstruction, often are investigated with contrast urethrography. In this case the patient was evaluated because of recurrent epididymitis after hypospadias repair of the anterior urethra.

Although all males have a small prostatic utricle (utriculus masculinus), it is visible on cystourethrography only in those individuals with hypospadias, ambiguous genitalia, undescended testis, or congenital urethral polyps. Four types of congenitally large prostatic utricles are recognized and have been assigned grades 0 to III. Grades 0, I, and II utricles open in the center of the verumontanum. The grade 0 utricle does not extend above the verumontanum, the grade I utricle extends above the verumontanum but below the bladder neck, and the grade II utricle extends above the bladder neck. The grade III congenitally large utricle arises from the bulbous urethra. In this case a grade I utricle communicates with the ejaculatory ducts, which explains the patient's recurrent epididymitis. Other complications of a prostatic utricle include stone formation and recurrent infections. Also note that the prostatic utricle has a dome-shaped fundus. A filling defect in the fundus of the diverticulum suggests vagina masculina (i.e., a cervix or uterus is attached).

In patients with hypospadias, the prostatic utricle is more likely to be large, as in this case. The grade of the utricle is related to the severity of the hypospadias. For instance, patients with penile hypospadias usually have utricles of grade 0 or I, whereas those with perineal hypospadias usually have grade III prostatic utricles.

Notes

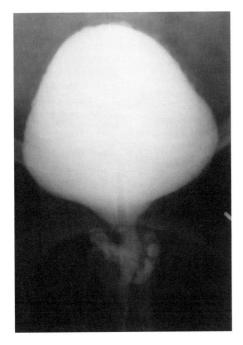 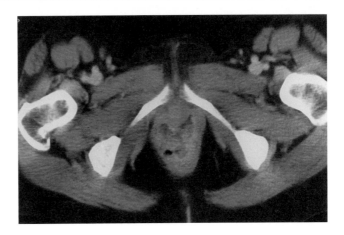

1. What imaging studies were performed?

2. What is the differential diagnosis for the abnormal urethra?

3. What should be recommended next to further evaluate this finding?

4. Name three complications of urethral diverticula.

Urethra: Adenocarcinoma Arising from a Urethral Diverticulum

1. Voiding cystourethrography and CT.

2. Neoplasm, abscess, and ureteral tear with contrast extravasation.

3. Depends on the clinical history. If a mass is palpable, aspiration or biopsy could be performed.

4. Infection, stone formation, and neoplasia.

References

Rajan N, Tucci P, Mallouh C, Choudhury M: Carcinoma in female urethral diverticulum: case reports and review of management, *J Urol* 150:1911–1914, 1993.

Seballos RM, Rich RR: Clear cell adenocarcinoma arising from a urethral diverticulum, *J Urol* 153:1914–1915, 1995.

Cross-Reference

Zagoria RJ, *Genitourinary Radiology: THE REQUISITES*, 2nd ed, pp 250, 254.

Comment

Urethral diverticula may be complicated by infection and calculus formation, and an association with benign and malignant neoplasms has been reported. The development of malignancy in a urethral diverticulum is rare; fewer than 100 cases have been reported. The average age at diagnosis is 40 years, and the development of hematuria and irritative voiding symptoms usually brings the patient to medical attention. Dyspareunia is reported in only 5% of patients, although it is a common symptom in women with uncomplicated urethral diverticula. On physical examination a tender, suburethral mass may be palpable. Further evaluation may include urethroscopy, MRI, cystourethrography, or double-balloon urethrography. Urethrography may demonstrate a paraurethral mass displacing the urethra or an irregular filling defect within a diverticulum, as in this case.

Although the most common primary urethral malignancy is a squamous cell carcinoma, adenocarcinoma and transitional cell carcinoma account for two thirds of the malignancies that arise from within a urethral diverticulum. This finding is consistent with the theory that diverticula result from inflammation of obstructed paraurethral glands. Transitional cell carcinoma is more common in the proximal third of the urethra.

The prognosis for these carcinomas is poor, and failures can be both local and systemic. Diverticulectomy alone is inadequate; anterior exenteration with total urethrectomy, wide excision of the vaginal wall, and postoperative radiation are recommended.

Notes

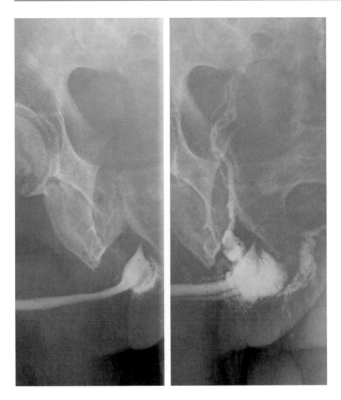

1. On this retrograde urethrogram, what are the tubular structures filling vertically in the pelvis on the second image?

2. Which segment of the urethra is opacified, anterior or posterior?

3. Does this type of injury usually result from blunt trauma or iatrogenic causes?

4. What is the typical symptom associated with this pathology?

Urethra: Anterior Urethral Tear

1. Pelvic veins draining the penis.

2. The anterior urethra only.

3. Usually iatrogenic.

4. Gross hematuria.

Reference
Pierce JM: Disruptions of the anterior urethra, *Urol Clin North Am* 16:329–340, 1989.

Cross-Reference
Zagoria RJ, *Genitourinary Radiology: THE REQUISITES,* 2nd ed, p 247.

Comment
The two images from a retrograde urethrogram show filling of only the anterior urethra and extravasation of contrast material. The extravasated contrast material drains via the pelvic veins. This is the typical appearance for a laceration of the anterior urethra. Contrast material communicates with the corpora cavernosa adjacent to the urethra and then drains via pelvic veins. Due to the low resistance of this pathway it is often impossible to overcome the tone of the external sphincter and opacify the posterior urethra in the presence of a tear of the anterior urethra. These tears can be caused by direct blunt trauma, most commonly a straddle injury, or more likely from iatrogenic trauma. In the hospital setting these tears usually result from trauma caused by insertion of a catheter. Gross hematuria inevitably occurs with anterior urethral tears. Even though the radiologic findings can be dramatic, treatment typically only requires careful insertion of a transurethral bladder catheter and usually results in spontaneous healing without sequela.

Notes

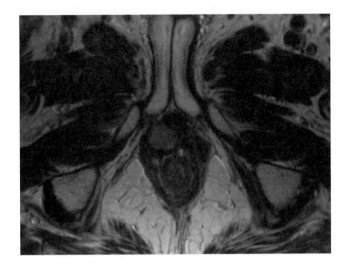

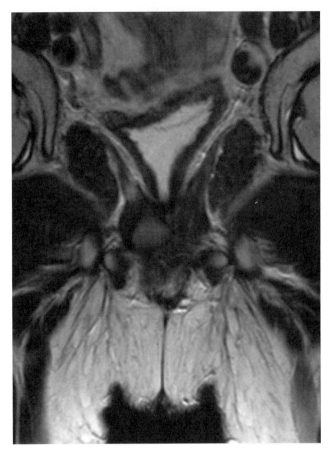

1. What is the differential diagnosis for this periurethral mass?

2. What is atypical about these images for urethral diverticula?

3. Periurethral injection of collagen is an established means of treating what disorder?

4. What is the most common complication of injectable collagen?

Urethra: Periurethral Collagen

1. Periurethral bulking agent, urethral diverticulum, periurethral infection, or neoplasm.

2. Signal intensity and location.

3. Urethral intrinsic sphincter dysfunction with urinary incontinence.

4. Migration to other sites.

References

Bridges M, Petrou S, Lightner D: Urethral bulking agents, *Am J Roentgenol* 185:257–264, 2005.

Hahn W, Israel G, Lee V: MRI of female urethral and periurethral disorders, *Am J Roentgenol* 182:677–682, 2004.

Cross-Reference

Zagoria RJ, *Genitourinary Radiology: THE REQUISITES,* 2nd ed, pp 244–246.

Comment

Clinical use of urethral bulking agents continues to expand. Although classically used to treat female incontinence resulting from intrinsic sphincter dysfunction, men who experience postprostatectomy urinary incontinence have also been treated with periurethral bulking agents. Radiologists will be expected to recognize the various imaging appearances of the different urethral bulking agents and be able to distinguish them from periurethral pathology.

Agents most commonly used at the current time include cross-linked bovine collagen (Contigen, Bard) and carbon-coated beads (Durasphere, Carbon Medical Technologies). On computed tomography collagen has a density similar to that of soft tissue, and contrast must be used to distinguish the periurethral tissue, which will enhance. When recently injected, collagen will be hyperintense on T2-weighted images and may mimic urethral diverticulum. As degradation of the collagen occurs, it may become isointense on T2-weighted images and mimic a solid mass. Contrast-enhanced T1-weighted images will help in this situation because the bulking agent will not take up gadolinium-based agents. Carbon-coated microbeads and even more recently graphite-coated microbeads both lack mobile protons and are hypointense on T1- and T2-weighted images.

Location can be of value in distinguishing between periurethral pathology and bulking agents. Periurethral injection of bulking agents is aimed at the immediate periurethral tissue at the junction with the urinary bladder base. Urethral diverticula tend to be located in the mid-urethra at the level of the pubic symphysis and are usually posterolateral in location. Periurethral cystic masses located more distally, near the external urethral meatus, are more likely to represent cysts or abscesses of Skene's gland.

Notes

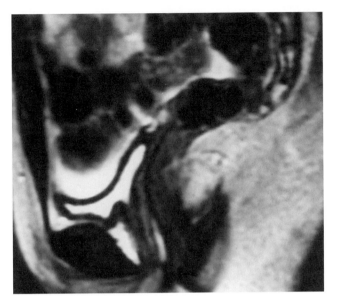
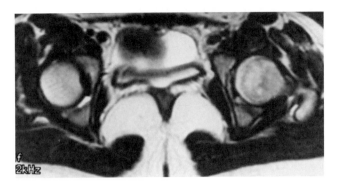

1. What is the most common cause of primary amenorrhea?

2. What is the role of imaging with regard to the selection of appropriate surgery for the lesion shown?

3. What renal anomalies have been reported in patients with Mayer-Rokitansky-Kuster-Hauser syndrome?

4. True or false: Patients with Mayer-Rokitansky-Kuster-Hauser syndrome have ovaries.

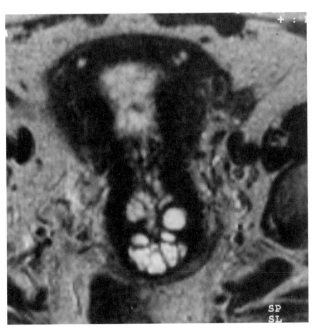
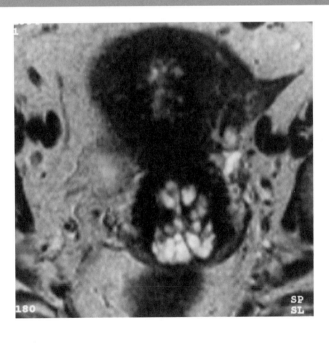

1. What is the differential diagnosis for the endocervical mass visible on these turbo spin-echo T2W MRIs?

2. What clinical symptom is characteristic of this rare tumor?

3. This lesion may be associated with two other diseases. Name one of them.

4. True or false: This is a benign-appearing malignancy with an excellent prognosis.

Ob/Gyn: Vaginal Atresia

1. Vaginal agenesis.

2. To determine whether there is a normal, patent cervix and an endometrial canal.

3. Pelvic kidney and renal agenesis.

4. True.

Reference

Reinhold C, Hricak H, Forstner R, et al: Primary amenorrhea: evaluation with MR imaging, *Radiology* 203: 383–390, 1997.

Cross-Reference

Zagoria RJ, *Genitourinary Radiology: THE REQUISITES,* 2nd ed, pp 261–266.

Comment

Primary amenorrhea is defined as the absence of menarche by the age of 16 years. The most common cause is congenital absence of the vagina, which occurs in approximately 1 in every 4000 to 5000 women; other causes of primary amenorrhea include müllerian duct anomalies, congenital disorders of sexual differentiation, ovarian dysfunction or failure, and hormonal abnormalities caused by hypothalamic or pituitary disorders. Patients with Mayer-Rokitansky-Kuster-Hauser syndrome have vaginal hypoplasia or agenesis and normal fallopian tubes and ovaries. There are variable associated anomalies of the uterus, urinary tract, and musculoskeletal system, but these patients are endocrinologically normal, are phenotypically female, and have complete gonadal development.

Transperineal sonography and MRI are effective in the evaluation of patients with vaginal agenesis. The primary role of imaging in these patients is to evaluate the length of the atretic segment and the patency of the endometrial canal and cervix. Vaginal agenesis with a functioning uterus and cervix can be treated with vaginoplasty. The distance between the agenetic vaginal segment and the introitus has implications for the particular type of vaginoplasty (primary anastomosis versus skin grafting). If the cervix is absent but there is functioning endometrial tissue, hysterectomy usually is performed because a surgically formed uterovaginal fistula or an artificial cervix often closes and cannot sustain a pregnancy. Closure of the uterovaginal fistula results in endometriosis.

Notes

Ob/Gyn: Adenoma Malignum

1. Cystic endometrial hyperplasia, deep nabothian cysts, and adenoma malignum.

2. Profuse, watery vaginal discharge.

3. Peutz-Jeghers syndrome or mucinous tumor of the ovary.

4. Unfortunately, false.

Reference

Doi T, Yamashita Y, Yasunaga T, et al: Adenoma malignum: MR imaging and pathologic study, *Radiology* 204:39–42, 1997.

Cross-Reference

Zagoria RJ, *Genitourinary Radiology: THE REQUISITES,* 2nd ed, pp 308–309.

Comment

Adenocarcinoma accounts for about 10% of all cases of cervical carcinoma; adenoma malignum or minimally differentiated adenocarcinoma of the cervix makes up about 3% of all cervical adenocarcinomas. This malignancy may be associated with Peutz-Jeghers syndrome, and an association with mucinous tumor of the ovary also has been described. The most common presenting symptom is watery cervical discharge; vaginal bleeding is uncommon.

Macroscopically this neoplasm presents as a multicystic mass; cysts range from microscopic to several centimeters in diameter. Even solid and enhancing areas on MRI are composed of minute cysts with edematous cervical tissue. Although the gross appearance is deceptively benign, this tumor deeply invades the cervical stroma. The walls of these cysts are lined with a single layer of mucin-secreting columnar cells, which resemble normal cervical glands. For the pathologist the diagnosis of malignancy may be difficult because tumor cells usually are well differentiated. Despite this difficulty, the clinical course of adenoma malignum is characterized by early dissemination, poor response to treatment, and a dismal long-term prognosis.

The differential diagnosis of adenoma malignum includes cystic endometrial hyperplasia and deeply invasive nabothian cervical cysts. Contrast-enhancing solid tissue should not be associated with nabothian cysts, and stromal invasion is not present in cases of cystic endometrial hyperplasia.

Notes

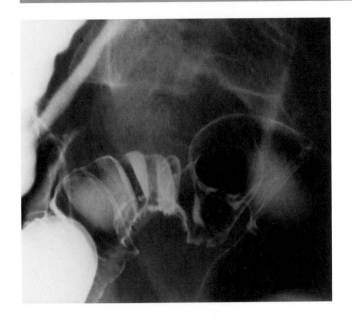

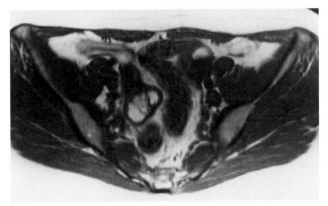

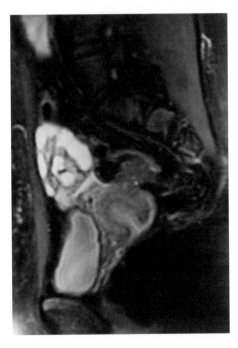

1. What is the differential diagnosis for the abnormal finding on the air-contrast barium enema?

2. What are the abnormal findings on MRI?

3. What primary malignancies are associated with colonic serosal metastases?

4. Could the diagnosis be made by colonoscopic biopsy in this case?

Ob/Gyn: Endometriosis of the Sigmoid Colon

1. Polyp or other submucosal tumor.

2. The T1W and fat-saturated T2W images show a right adnexal mass; the fat saturated T2W image shows a mass, similar in signal intensity to myometrium, involving the rectosigmoid colon.

3. Ovarian carcinoma and melanoma.

4. Probably not; mucosa looks intact.

Reference

Weed JC, Ray JE: Endometriosis of the bowel, *Obstet Gynecol* 69:727–730, 1987.

Cross-Reference

Zagoria RJ, *Genitourinary Radiology: THE REQUISITES,* 2nd ed, pp 267–270.

Comment

Endometriosis most commonly involves the ovaries, uterosacral ligaments, Douglas cul-de-sac, serosal surface of the uterus, and fallopian tubes. However, it has been estimated that 50% of patients with severe endometriosis have some degree of bowel involvement. Progressive endometriosis of the alimentary or lower urinary tract may produce fibrotic masses that can mimic a serosal or submucosal mass, or postoperative or postinflammatory adhesions.

Endometriosis of the alimentary tract most often affects the rectosigmoid colon, ileum, or appendix. Although multiple symptoms have been reported (diarrhea, constipation, rectal bleeding, abdominal distention, and partial or complete bowel obstruction), virtually all are cyclic, coinciding with menstrual function. Because the serosa is involved first, a stricture-forming lesion or an eccentric mural filling defect is most often visible on barium enema examination. In some cases endometriosis may encircle the bowel and mimic an "apple core" carcinoma. Deep penetration of endometriosis may even result in mucosal destruction, but this finding is unusual. Unlike rectosigmoid endometriosis, colon cancer is generally painless and causes intermittent rather than cyclic bleeding. Endometriosis of the bowel may require implant or bowel resection if medical treatments (i.e., medroxyprogesterone acetate, combined estrogen and progestin oral contraceptives, androgen derivatives, or gonadotropin-releasing hormone agonist) are unsuccessful.

Notes

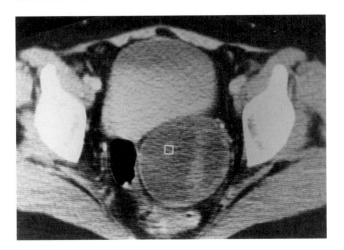 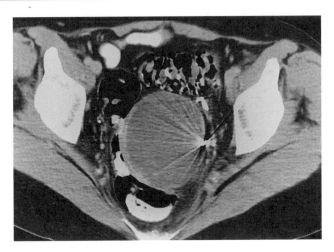

1. What are the four most common histologic types of ovarian cancer?

2. The CT image on the left was obtained 15 years before the image on the right. Does this time course suggest a particular type of ovarian tumor?

3. Hormone production is a characteristic of which pathologic type of ovarian neoplasm?

4. Name several clinical presentations of hormone-producing ovarian tumors.

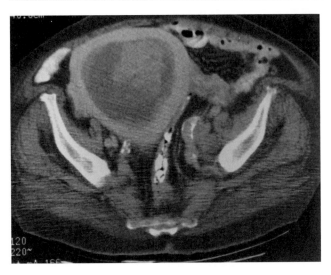 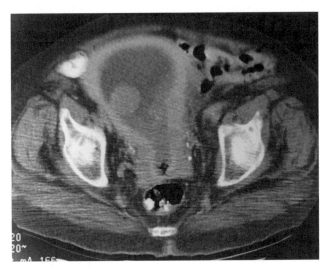

1. What is the most likely diagnosis in this 81-year-old woman?

2. True or false: Excessive estrogen is linked to most risk factors associated with endometrial carcinoma.

3. True or false: Leiomyosarcoma is the most common nonepithelial endometrial malignancy.

4. True or false: Prior pelvic radiation has been linked to endometrial sarcoma.

Ob/Gyn: Ovarian Stromal Tumor (Granulosa Cell Tumor)

1. Epithelial, germ cell, stromal sex cord, and metastatic disease.

2. Yes. A benign, solid neoplasm, such as a stromal tumor or a benign germ cell tumor.

3. Stromal.

4. Menstrual abnormalities, sexual precocity, vaginal bleeding (estrogen production), and virilization or hirsutism (androgen production).

References

Hines JF, Khalifa MA, Moore JL, et al: Recurrent granulosa cell tumor of the ovary 37 years after initial diagnosis: a case report and review of the literature, *Gynecol Oncol* 60:484–488, 1996.

MacSweeney JE, King DM: Computed tomography, diagnosis, staging and follow-up of pure granulosa cell tumor of the ovary, *Clin Radiol* 49:241–245, 1994.

Cross-Reference

Zagoria RJ, *Genitourinary Radiology: THE REQUISITES,* 2nd ed, pp 287–288.

Comment

Ovarian neoplasm has four main histologic types with various subtypes. Epithelial ovarian neoplasms are the most common, accounting for 65% of ovarian malignancies. Approximately 65% of epithelial neoplasms are benign.

The two least common tumors of the ovary are sex cord stromal tumors and metastatic disease to the ovary. Each accounts for approximately 5% of ovarian neoplasms. Sex cord stromal tumors have three subtypes: fibroma-thecoma, granulosa cell tumor, and Sertoli-Leydig tumor (listed in descending order of frequency). The fibroma-thecoma is a benign fibrous tumor that may be associated with ascites and a right effusion, or Meigs' syndrome. Granulosa cell tumors originate from the ovarian stroma and can secrete estrogen; 66% occur in postmenopausal women, may lead to endometrial hyperplasia or endometrial carcinoma, and can present with postmenopausal bleeding. In younger patients the estrogen production may cause precocious puberty. This case is typical of granulosa cell tumors in that the tumor responds to surgical therapy but can recur up to 20 years after the original resection. Patients with this tumor have a good prognosis; the 10-year survival rate is greater than 85%.

Notes

Ob/Gyn: Malignant Mixed Müllerian Tumor of the Uterus

1. Endometrial carcinoma.

2. True.

3. False.

4. True.

Reference

Costa MJ, Khan R, Judd R: Carcinosarcoma (malignant mixed müllerian [mesodermal] tumor) of the uterus and ovary: correlation of clinical, pathologic, and immuno-histochemical features in 29 cases, *Arch Pathol Lab Med* 115:583–590, 1991.

Cross-Reference

Zagoria RJ, *Genitourinary Radiology: THE REQUISITES,* 2nd ed, pp 298–301.

Comment

Only about 3% of uterine cancers are sarcomas, but of these the malignant mixed müllerian tumor (MMMT or triple MT) is the most common. These tumors are considered biphasic neoplasms of the female genital tract because they are composed of both carcinomatous and sarcomatous elements (carcinosarcoma). Recall that the paramesonephric ducts are formed by mesenchyme of the urogenital ridge and are lined by coelomic epithelium. The epithelial component of the MMMT is typically an adenocarcinoma of the endometrioid type, and the most common mesenchymal components are fibrosarcoma and endometrial stromal sarcoma.

Because MMMT is uncommon and the clinical and radiologic presentations are not specific, a prebiopsy diagnosis of this tumor is a real homerun. These tumors are associated with a clinical history of pelvic radiation treatment. In one study, 9.5% of patients had a history of radiotherapy, and the median latent period between pelvic radiation and the diagnosis of MMMT was 16 years. MMMT is known for its very aggressive clinical course and poor prognosis. Even with stage I disease the 5-year survival rate is not greater than 35%; 85% of recurrences and metastases occur within the first 2 years of follow-up. Prognostic factors are similar to those for endometrial carcinomas and include depth of myometrial invasion (when the tumor is confined to the uterus), stage of disease, presence of lymphatic or vascular space invasion, and size of the resected tumor. As many as half of all cases are in an advanced stage (stage III or IV) at the time of diagnosis.

Notes

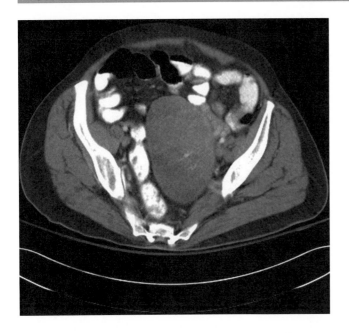

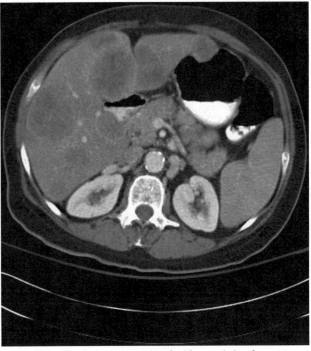

Upper left and right images reprinted with permission from Lee JKT, Sagel SS, Stanley RJ, Heiken P, *Computed Body Tomography with MRI Correlation*, ed 4, Philadelphia: Lippincott Williams and Wilkins, 2006.

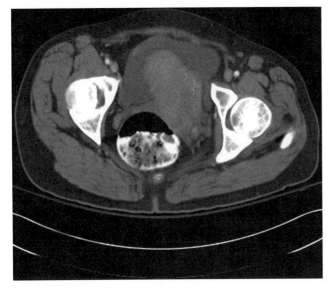

1. What is the differential diagnosis for the provided images, assuming that the finding in the first image arises from the uterus?

2. Can any imaging modality determine whether this uterine mass is benign or malignant?

3. Assuming a malignant entity, what are the most common sites of distant metastasis?

4. True or false: All uterine leiomyosarcomas arise from malignant degeneration of leiomyomas.

Ob/Gyn: Uterine Leiomyosarcoma

1. Degenerating leiomyoma with unrelated liver metastases or leiomyosarcoma with liver metastases.

2. There is no reliable way to differentiate leiomyoma from leiomyosarcoma based on imaging, due to the heterogeneous nature of cellular and degenerative forms of benign leiomyomas that can mimic the typical appearance of leiomyosarcoma.

3. After local invasion, the most common sites of distant metastasis are liver and lung.

4. False. Uterine leiomyosarcomas may arise de novo from uterine myometrium.

References

Kido A, Togashi K, Koyama T, et al: Diffusely enlarged uterus: evaluation with MR imaging, *Radiographics* 23:1423, 2003.

Sahdev A, Sohaib SA, Jacobs I, et al: MR imaging of uterine sarcomas, *Am J Roentgenol* 177:1307–1311, 2001.

Cross-Reference

Zagoria RJ, *Genitourinary Radiology: THE REQUISITES,* 2nd ed, pp 276–282.

Comment

Uterine leiomyosarcomas are rare malignant tumors that can arise either de novo from smooth muscle cells within the uterine myometrium, or from malignant degeneration of an existing uterine leiomyoma. Although the benign leiomyoma is the most common uterine neoplasm (seen in approximately 20% of women over age 30), the rate of sarcomatous degeneration is very small, estimated at only 0.1% to 0.8%.

The most common presentation of leiomyosarcoma is a large uterine mass, and these lesions are best characterized by MRI. In contradistinction to the homogeneously decreased T2 signal and well-circumscribed nature of the typical nondegenerated benign leiomyoma, leiomyosarcomas are characterized by a greater degree of heterogeneity. MRI usually reveals areas of intense T2 signal corresponding to foci of cystic degeneration. Precontrast T1 imaging may reveal hyperintense foci corresponding to regions of hemorrhagic necrosis. Following contrast administration, enhancement of solid components is typical.

It should be emphasized, however, that each of these imaging findings may be observed in either cellular or degenerating benign leiomyomas. To date, no imaging modality can reliably differentiate these variants of leiomyomas from leiomyosarcoma. Studies have questioned rapid enlargement and poor definition of borders as possible indicators of malignancy, although these have not proven reliable in differentiation. Nonetheless, features such as local invasion and rapid growth of a leiomyoma in a postmenopausal patient remain highly suspicious.

The typical pattern of disease spread is through local invasion of adjacent pelvic vasculature and lymphatics. The most common sites of distant metastasis are liver and lung.

The typical differential diagnosis is that of a cellular or degenerating leiomyoma. Endometrial stromal sarcomas and malignant mixed müllerian tumors may have similar appearances. Rarely, the tumor is indistinguishable from endometrial carcinoma or adenomyosis. Primary uterine lymphoma and metastatic disease are uncommon, although they can present as large heterogeneous uterine masses.

Notes

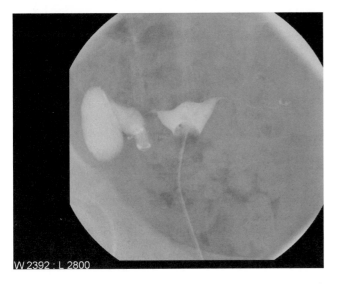

W 2392 : L 2800

1. What are the four segments of the fallopian tube?

2. What portion of the tube is obstructed?

3. What is the etiology of the obstruction?

4. What is the appropriate immediate treatment following hysterosalpingography?

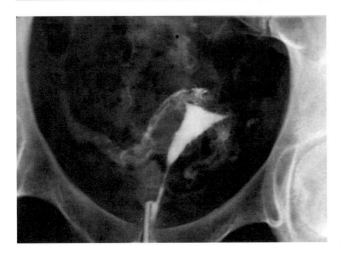

1. What is the most likely diagnosis?

2. What other entity can have a similar appearance?

3. What are the risks of hysterosalpingography?

4. What other findings at hysterosalpingography indicate a higher likelihood for this to occur?

Ob/Gyn: Hydrosalpinx

1. Interstitial, isthmic, ampullary, and infundibular.

2. Ampullary.

3. Sequela of pelvic inflammatory disease.

4. Oral antibiotics.

Reference

Thurmond AS: Imaging of female infertility, *Radiol Clin North Am* 41:757–767, 2002.

Cross-Reference

Zagoria RJ, *Genitourinary Radiology: THE REQUISITES*, 2nd ed, pp 13–15.

Comment

The fallopian tube connects the uterus to the ovary. It measures approximately 12 cm in length and is divided into four sections: the interstitial, isthmic, ampullary, and infundibular. Obstruction of the fallopian tubes is one of the most common causes of infertility, and tubal patency is still best assessed using hysterosalpingo-graphy (HSG). Obstruction of the proximal portions of the tube—interstitial and isthmic—is usually due to the presence of debris, chronic inflammation, obliterative fibrosis, and salpingitis isthmica nodosa. Dilation of the ampullary and infundibular portions of the tube without spill of contrast material into the peritoneal cavity is diagnostic of hydrosalpinx. This is usually a sequela of previous inflammatory disease, either sexually transmitted infectious processes or inflammatory bowel disease. Fallopian tubes may also become obstructed due to adhesions following surgery in the lower abdomen. Degree of dilation does not correlate well with surgical results. A minimally dilated tube may have an extremely thick, rigid wall that cannot be easily resected or repaired. The presence of rugal folds is thought to imply a better surgical prognosis. Once hydrosalpinx is identified on HSG, patients should be placed on oral antibiotics, usually doxycycline, for several days following the procedure to avoid infection.

Notes

Ob/Gyn: Venous Intravasation on Hysterosalpingography

1. Venous intravasation during hysterosalpingography.

2. Intravasation into the lymphatic system.

3. Patients may develop cramping from uterine disten-tion, which can be severe. Pelvic infection is uncommon, but patients with hydrosalpinx are at increased risk and may need prophylactic antibiotic therapy. Uterine rupture and contrast reaction are extremely rare.

4. Patients with proximal fallopian tubal obstruction as the contrast has no other outlet from the uterine cavity during instillation.

Reference

Dalfo AR, Ubeda B, Ubeda A, et al: Diagnostic value of hysterosalpingography in the detection of intrauterine abnormalities: a comparison with hysteroscopy, *Am J Roentgenol* 183:1405–1409, 2004.

Cross-Reference

Zagoria RJ, *Genitourinary Radiology: THE REQUISITES*, 2nd ed, p 403.

Comment

Hysterosalpingography (HSG) is used in the routine eval-uation of infertile couples. Indications for HSG also include women with uterine or fallopian tube surgery or a history of recurrent miscarriages. It is a minimally invasive examination providing imaging of the uterine cavity and fallopian tube lumen and assessment of fallopian tube patency. HSGs are typically performed 7 to 10 days after the patient's last menstrual period (when she has finished menstruating and has not ovulated yet and thus cannot be pregnant). The procedure is performed by using a specu-lum to insert a 5-French catheter into the endocervical canal. A balloon may be inflated in the endocervical canal depending on radiologist preference. Water-based contrast agents are injected while performing spot fluoroscopic images to assess for uterine and fallopian tube filling and free spill into the peritoneal cavity. At the author's institu-tion, antibiotics are not routinely administered prophylac-tically, but are given to patients who have the finding of a hydrosalpinx to prevent infection of the distended tube.

Lymphatic or venous intravasation of contrast occurs in less than 5% of examinations. Predisposing factors include tubal disease or obstruction, uterine adhesions, and malformations. Intravasation may also occur from injection of contrast material with excessive pressure or inappropriate placement of the HSG catheter tip. Water-soluble contrast material usually disperses quickly once intravasation occurs. Systemic reaction to contrast also occurs very rarely.

Notes

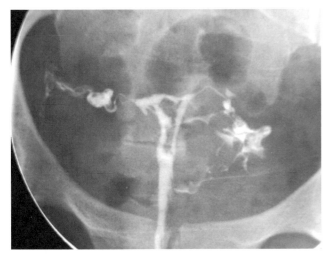
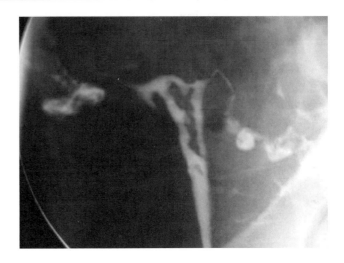

1. If the patient is presenting with infertility, what is the most likely diagnosis?

2. What is the differential diagnosis?

3. What other imaging studies can detect this abnormality?

4. At what part of the menstrual cycle should hysterosalpingography be performed?

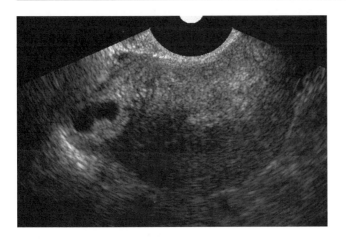
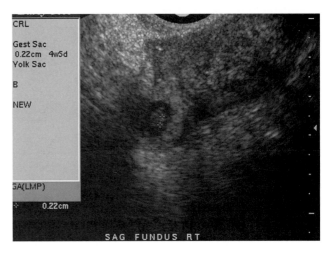

1. What is the most likely diagnosis?

2. What laboratory test could be ordered for confirmation?

3. Does a normal ultrasound result exclude ectopic pregnancy?

4. What is the leading cause of pregnancy-related death in the first trimester?

Ob/Gyn: Asherman's Syndrome

1. Asherman's syndrome.

2. Diethylstilbestrol exposure, genital tuberculosis.

3. MRI and sonohysterography can also detect this finding.

4. Hysterosalpingography should be performed after menstruation and prior to ovulation, approximately days 7 to 10 in the menstrual cycle.

Reference

Dalfo AR, Ubeda B, Ubeda A, et al: Diagnostic value of hysterosalpingography in the detection of intrauterine abnormalities: a comparison with hysteroscopy, *Am J Roentgenol* 183:1405–1409, 2004.

Cross-Reference

Zagoria RJ, *Genitourinary Radiology: THE REQUISITES,* 2nd ed, pp 265–266.

Comment

Hysterosalpingography (HSG) is the most commonly used technique for the evaluation of female infertility. It provides the best imaging assessment of the fallopian tubes and also provides a method to evaluate the endometrial cavity. Uterine abnormalities are the cause of infertility in 10% to 15% of women. HSG demonstrates a high sensitivity (60%–98%) but a low specificity (15%–80%) for intrauterine lesions, which are demonstrated as filling defects. The differential diagnosis for intrauterine filling defects includes polyps, hyperplasia, fibroids, synechiae, and septa. False-positive findings can be caused by air bubbles, mucus, and blood.

Scar tissue creates adhesions, also known as synechiae, in the uterine cavity. Scarring results from endometrial trauma or infection, and is most commonly caused by dilatation and curettage. The scar tissue can obliterate the uterine cavity, leading to infertility. Asherman's syndrome refers to the association of infertility and uterine synechiae.

On HSG, the synechiae appear as well-defined, linear, irregular filling defects and may lead to a small or obliterated uterine cavity. Treatment is hysteroscopic lysis of adhesions.

Notes

Ob/Gyn: Interstitial Ectopic Pregnancy

1. Right-sided interstitial ectopic pregnancy.

2. Serum beta human chorionic gonadotropin level.

3. No.

4. Ectopic pregnancy.

References

Ackerman TE, Levi CS, Dashefsky SM, et al: Interstitial line: sonographic finding in interstitial (cornual) ectopic pregnancy, *Radiology* 189:83–87, 1993.

Tulandi T, Al-Jaroudi D: Interstitial pregnancy: results generated from the Society of Reproductive Surgeons Registry, *Obstet Gynecol* 103:47–50, 2004.

Cross-Reference

Zagoria RJ, *Genitourinary Radiology: THE REQUISITES,* 2nd ed, p 259.

Comment

The interstitial section of the fallopian tube is the portion that is contained within the myometrium of the uterus. A pregnancy implanted in this portion of the fallopian tube is called an interstitial pregnancy. Because of this unique location of implantation, early diagnosis may be difficult. Transvaginal ultrasonography is the most useful diagnostic test, with a sensitivity of 80% and a specificity of 99%. Ultrasonographic diagnosis relies on detection of an eccentric location of the gestational sac within the uterus and thinning of the surrounding myometrium.

History of ipsilateral salpingectomy, previous ectopic pregnancy, and in vitro fertilization are associated with interstitial ectopic pregnancy. This is a rare type of ectopic pregnancy, accounting for 2% to 3% of all ectopic pregnancies. However, it carries a mortality rate more than twice as high as other tubal pregnancies. Uterine rupture may occur, leading to catastrophic hemorrhage.

Traditional treatment has been open hysterectomy or cornual resection. However, more conservative therapies including methotrexate administration or laparoscopic resections have also been successful. Despite concerns that the cornual part of the uterus might be weakened after surgery for interstitial pregnancy, subsequent pregnancies can be possible without complication.

Notes

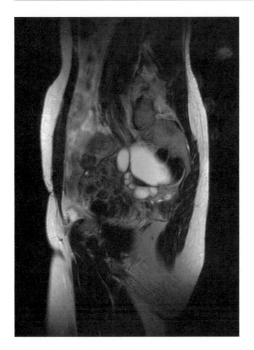

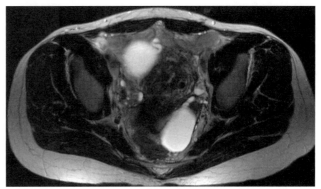

Upper left and right images reprinted with permission from Lee JKT, Sagel SS, Stanley RJ, Heiken P, *Computed Body Tomography with MRI Correlation*, ed 4, Philadelphia: Lippincott Williams and Wilkins, 2006.

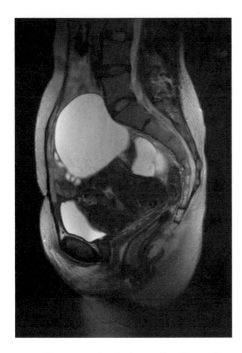

1. What are the bilateral adnexal masses?

2. What is the most common cause of this disorder?

3. How would the masses appear on T1-weighted images?

4. How can this mass be differentiated from the ovary?

Ob/Gyn: Hydrosalpinges

1. Hydrosalpinges.

2. Pelvic inflammatory disease.

3. In the case of simple fluid, low T1 signal.

4. Absence of follicles.

Reference

Outwater EK, Siegelman ES, Chiowanich P, et al: Dilated fallopian tubes: MR imaging characteristics, *Radiology* 208:463–469, 1998.

Cross-Reference

Zagoria RJ, *Genitourinary Radiology: THE REQUISITES,* 2nd ed, p 272.

Comment

T2-weighted MRIs show bilateral cystic pelvic structures. These are separate from the normal follicle-containing ovaries and the leiomyomatous uterus.

Hydrosalpinges or dilation of the fallopian tubes is most often the sequelae of pelvic inflammatory disease. Other etiologies include fibroids, scarring of the endometrial canal secondary to instrumentation, and radiation. The distalmost portion of the ampullary tube adjacent to the fimbria dilates to the greatest degree, and on hysterosalpingography, usually no intraperitoneal spill of contrast material is identified.

Using MRI, the hydrosalpinx appears as a low T1 and high T2 signal ovoid mass. It is necessary to use all three planes of imaging to clearly diagnose the mass as a tubular structure and exclude the presence of an ovarian mass such as an endometrioma or hemorrhagic cyst. The proximal isthmic portion of the tube may be dilated or of normal caliber, in which case it is usually tortuous. Debris or high T1 signal within the dilated tube may indicate pyo- or hematosalpinx. It is also important to clearly identify both ovaries in order to exclude them as the origin of the mass. Ovaries should be visible in virtually all women of menstrual age and appear as ovoid soft tissue signal intensity structures that contain numerous low T1, high T2 signal follicles. A dilated fallopian tube may also mimic a bowel loop, but careful assessment of the origin and lack of valvulae conniventes should exclude this diagnosis.

Notes

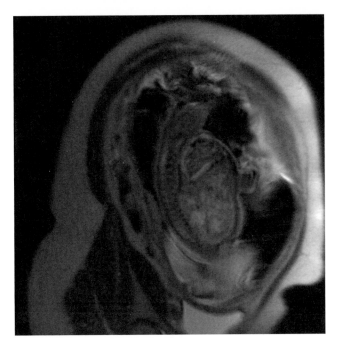 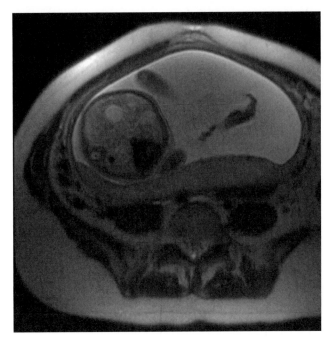

1. In the image on the left, the mixed solid and cystic mass is located in which fetal organ?

2. True or false: Fetal hydrops associated with the above lesion has a poor prognosis.

3. Give three differential diagnoses for a prenatal chest mass.

4. What neonatal complication is most likely to arise from this lesion?

Ob/Gyn: Congenital Cystic Adenomatoid Malformation In Utero

1. Right lung (assuming normal left-sided heart and descending aorta).

2. True.

3. Congenital diaphragmatic hernia, congenital cystic adenomatoid malformation, and bronchopulmonary sequestration.

4. Respiratory distress from pulmonary hypoplasia.

References

Barnes NA, Pilling PW: Bronchopulmonary foregut malformations: embryology, radiology and quandary, *Eur Radiol* 13:2659–2673, 2003.

Hubbard AM, Adzick NS, Crombleholme TM, et al: Congenital chest lesions: diagnosis and characterization with prenatal MR imaging, *Radiology* 212:43–48, 1999.

Comment

The most common prenatal chest masses are diaphragmatic hernia, congenital cystic adenomatoid malformation (CCAM), and bronchopulmonary sequestration. Hubbard and co-workers have demonstrated the utility of prenatal fetal MRI in diagnosing fetal chest lesions using ultra-fast T2-weighted acquisition techniques in orthogonal planes to the fetal spine.

CCAM of the lung is a rare lesion that is characterized by a mixed solid and cystic mass composed of abnormal disorganized distal components of the respiratory tract. The lesion usually communicates with the bronchial tree and receives its blood supply from pulmonary vasculature, in contrast to bronchopulmonary sequestration. CCAM is categorized into three types: (1) predominant cyst greater than 2 cm in diameter with surrounding smaller cysts; (2) multiple small cysts less than 2 cm and greater than 0.5 cm in diameter; and (3) "microcystic" bulky mass, with no cysts larger than 5 mm, containing bronchiole-like structures and alveolar ducts.

On T2-weighted MRIs, type 1 and type 2 CCAM lesions appear as masses with very high signal intensity that is significantly greater than adjacent normal lung and almost equal to that of amniotic fluid. Type 3 CCAM lesions are relatively homogeneous masses on T2-weighted MRIs with greater signal intensity than normal lung but less than that of amniotic fluid. A disrupted diaphragm and anomalous systemic vascular supply are useful features to help identify congenital diaphragmatic hernia and bronchopulmonary sequestration, respectively.

The clinical course of prenatal CCAM lesions is variable. Larger lesions are more frequently associated with mediastinal shift, pulmonary hypoplasia, vascular compromise, and fetal hydrops. Hydrops associated with CCAM has a poor prognosis. Surgical excision of large CCAM lesions in utero may reduce morbidity and mortality associated with pulmonary hypoplasia. Compression of the esophagus by a large CCAM lesion may lead to polyhydramnios. CCAM lesions can involute in utero, which is believed to result from differential growth rates of the thorax and the mass. Complications of CCAM in childhood and adulthood include recurrent pulmonary infections, pneumothorax, and malignancy. Rhabdomyosarcoma and bronchoalveolar carcinoma have been reported to arise from CCAM lesions. Although large (greater than 3 cm) and symptomatic CCAM lesions in infants are surgically resected with good outcomes, surgical treatment of asymptomatic and smaller CCAM lesions remains a controversial topic.

Notes

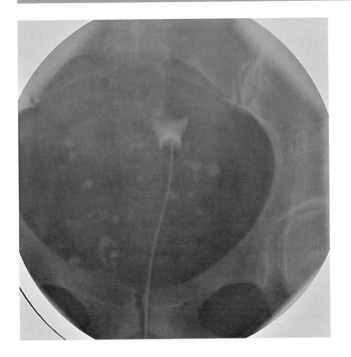

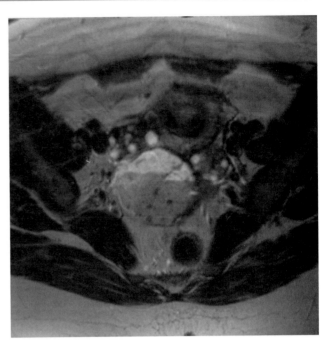

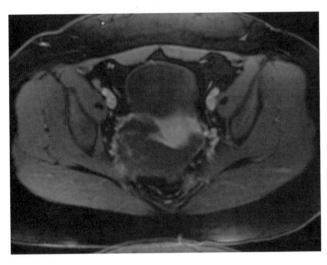

1. Were the multiple, rounded, and irregular radiodensities in the pelvis present prior to contrast administration? What is the diagnosis?

2. What is the classical clinical presentation of this condition?

3. What are factors that help to determine treatment?

4. True or false: This condition will always preclude further pregnancies.

Ob/Gyn: Cavernous Hemangioma and Arteriovenous Malformations of the Uterus

1. Yes, these represent calcifications. Cavernous hemangioma of the uterus.

2. Marked vaginal bleeding.

3. Desire for pregnancy, size of lesion, type of arteriovenous malformation.

4. False.

References

Hoffman MK, Meilstrup JW, Shackelford DP, Kaminski P: Arteriovenous malformations of the uterus: an uncommon cause of vaginal bleeding, *Obstet Gynecol Surv* 52:736–740, 1997.

Kobayashi T, Yamazaki T, Takahashi M, et al: Characteristic radiologic findings for cavernous hemangioma of the uterus, *Am J Roentgenol* 172:1147–1148, 1999.

Cross-Reference

Zagoria RJ, *Genitourinary Radiology: THE REQUISITES,* 2nd ed, pp 257, 258.

Comment

Cavernous hemangiomas and arteriovenous malformations (AVMs) are both vascular lesions that require a high index of suspicion for diagnosis. They are rare, but can have disastrous outcomes if undiagnosed. The most common clinical presentation is abnormal, increased vaginal bleeding, which can be life threatening. Often, patients present with hemorrhage after an invasive procedure such as dilatation and curettage. Congestive heart failure is rare. Patients are usually in the third to fourth decade of life, but the age range at presentation is broad. Traditionally, AVMs of the uterus are described as congenital or acquired. Acquired AVMs are associated with trauma from surgical procedures or malignancies such as carcinoma and gestational trophoblastic disease. These lesions have also been reported following infections involving the endometrium/myometrium. Hoffman et al report that elevated hormones, such as during pregnancy, may cause congenital lesions to grow.

Imaging findings will vary depending on the type of malformation. Findings on hysterosalpingography such as multiple phleboliths can be suggestive of a cavernous hemangioma. For AVMs, Doppler ultrasonography can demonstrate hypoechoic areas with increased or turbulent blood flow. Cavernous hemangiomas demonstrate minimal flow on Doppler, however. MRI demonstrates enlargement of the uterus and typical findings of vascular malformations such as flow voids. Calcifications in hemangiomas can mimic flow voids on MRI. Angiography is diagnostic but invasive. While acquired AVMs often involve single abnormal connections, congenital AVMs tend to demonstrate multiple abnormal arteriovenous connections and be more extensive.

With improved percutaneous interventional techniques, embolization can sometimes be performed to attempt to preserve fertility. Therapy is based on the size of the lesion and the severity of hemorrhage. The most common treatment is hysterectomy. Successful postembolization pregnancies have been reported.

Notes

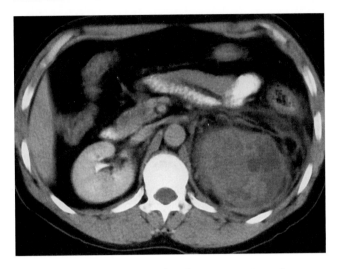 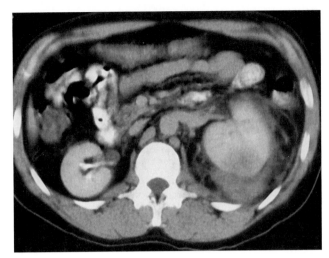

1. In what organ does this lesion originate?

2. What is the differential diagnosis?

3. What percentage of these tumors present with metastases at the time of diagnosis?

4. Does imaging-guided biopsy play a role in this patient's treatment?

Adrenal: Adrenocortical Carcinoma

1. Left adrenal gland or possibly the upper pole of the left kidney.

2. Primary differential diagnosis is an adrenal carcinoma and an exophytic renal cell carcinoma; less likely possibilities include adrenal metastasis and hemorrhage (given the lesion's large size, low density, and the lack of other lesions).

3. Up to 50%.

4. Only if the patient has a known primary neoplasm or other site of disease. If there is only one lesion and the patient has no known primary neoplasm, biopsy probably is unnecessary and the treatment of choice would be surgical resection.

References

Mayo-Smith WW, Boland GW, Noto RB, Lee MJ: State of the art adrenal imaging, 21:995–1012, 2001.

Szolar DH, Korobkin M, Reittner P, et al: Adrenocortical carcinomas and adrenal pheochromocytomas: mass and enhancement loss evaluation at delayed contrast-enhanced CT, *Radiology* 234:479–485, 2005.

Wooten MD, King DK: Adrenal cortical carcinoma: epidemiology and treatment with mitotane and a review of the literature, *Cancer* 72:3145–3155, 1993.

Cross-Reference

Zagoria RJ, *Genitourinary Radiology: THE REQUISITES*, 2nd ed, pp 365–366.

Comment

Adrenocortical carcinoma is a relatively rare primary adrenal neoplasm; only about 2000 cases have been reported in the English-language medical literature. The disease has a bimodal age distribution, with peak occurrence in the first and fifth decades. There is a slight female predominance (59%), and 68% of patients have advanced nonresectable disease. Hyperfunctioning tumors are more common in children; 85% of adrenocortical carcinomas in children and 15% in adults are hyperfunctioning. Hyperfunctioning tumors present at an earlier stage than their nonfunctional counterparts, and the most sensitive biochemical assay for hormonal hyperfunction is measurement of urinary 17-ketosteroid levels. The most common clinical presentation for functioning tumors is Cushing's syndrome, whereas for nonfunctioning adrenal carcinomas it is pain resulting from local invasion and mass effect. Sites of metastases include lung, liver, regional lymph nodes, bone, and extension into the adrenal veins or inferior vena cava.

Adrenocortical carcinomas do not have specific imaging characteristics, although most nonhyperfunctional tumors tend to exceed 6 cm in diameter. Hemorrhage, necrosis, and heterogeneous enhancement are visible on enhanced CT, and the margins of the tumor are often irregular as in this example. Thirty percent of adrenal cortical carcinomas may calcify. The MRI characteristics overlap with those of metastases and chronic adrenal hemorrhage. There is a limited role for percutaneous biopsy because the pathologic diagnosis can be difficult to make and the treatment for nonmetastatic disease is surgical resection.

Notes

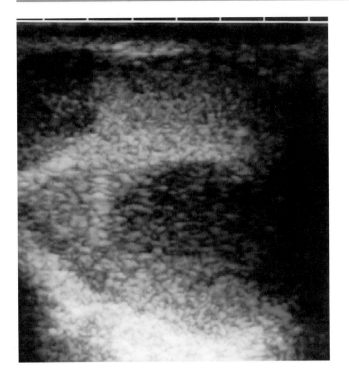

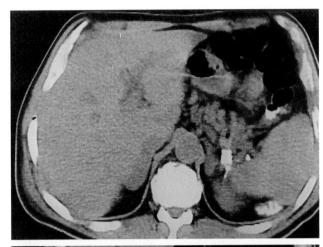

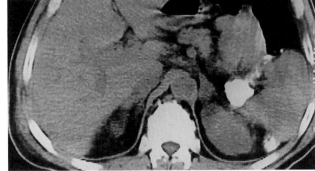

1. A sagittal sonogram of the testes and an abdominal CT in a 57-year-old man are shown. What is the most likely diagnosis?

2. What is the differential diagnosis for bilateral adrenal masses?

3. Given the clinical history of bronchogenic carcinoma, what is the most likely cause of bilateral adrenal masses?

4. True or false: Adrenal insufficiency is a common presentation of this disease.

Adrenal: Adrenal Lymphoma

1. Lymphoma or leukemia (based primarily on the testicular findings).

2. Adenomas, metastases (including lymphoma), hemorrhage, tuberculosis, and histoplasmosis.

3. Bilateral adenomas.

4. False.

References

Iwamizu-Watanabe S, Asai T, Mori N: Bilateral adrenal lymphoma with hypercalcemia: an autopsy case report with review of the literature, *J Clin Exp Hematopathol* 43:29–34, 2003.

Wang J, Sun NCJ, Rensio R, et al: Clinically silent primary adrenal lymphoma: a case report and review of the literature, *Am J Hematol* 58:130–136, 1998.

Cross-Reference

Zagoria RJ, *Genitourinary Radiology: THE REQUISITES*, 2nd ed, pp 367–368.

Comment

The adrenal glands are affected in approximately 25% of cases of widespread lymphoma. Adrenal gland infiltration by lymphoma most often occurs with retroperitoneal or ipsilateral renal lymphoma. Adrenal involvement occurs more frequently with non-Hodgkin's lymphoma than with Hodgkin's disease.

Because adrenal adenomas are common (estimated to occur in up to 1.5% of the population), an isolated adrenal mass in a patient with lung carcinomas is more likely an adenoma than a metastasis. A patient with lung cancer and isolated bilateral adrenal masses may have either bilateral adenomas or metastases. In this circumstance, further investigation with either imaging (PET, CT, or MRI characterization) or image-guided biopsy should be performed for definite characterization.

Primary lymphoma of the adrenal gland (PLA), a distinct entity, is thought to arise from intrinsic hematopoietic tissue and is exceedingly rare; only about 70 cases have been reported. It tends to affect older men and there is a high incidence of immunodeficiency and other cancers in these patients. Diffuse large cell non-Hodgkin's B-cell lymphoma is the most common histologic subtype. Chemotherapy or surgical extirpation may be attempted, but prognosis for patients with PLA is poor; most patients died as a result of tumor, intercurrent diseases, or infection within 1 year.

Notes

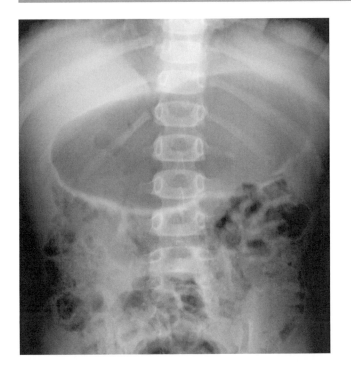
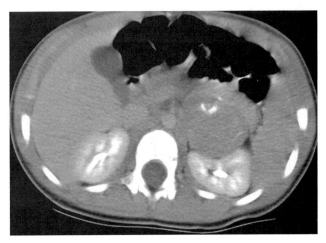
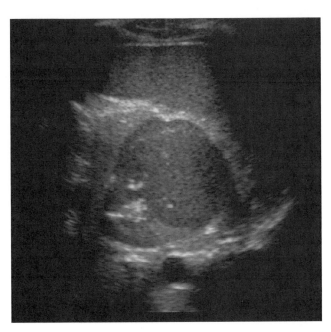

1. What is the differential diagnosis for an adrenal mass in a pediatric patient?

2. Which adrenal masses are associated with hormonal abnormalities?

3. What vascular structures can be involved with extension of an adrenal neoplasm?

4. How are pediatric adrenal masses treated?

Adrenal: Adrenocortical Neoplasm in a Pediatric Patient

1. Adrenal hemorrhage, neuroblastoma, adrenocortical neoplasm, and pheochromocytoma.

2. Adrenocortical neoplasm (adenoma and adrenocortical carcinoma).

3. Adrenal vein, interior vena cava, and even right atrium.

4. Surgical resection. Even incidental adrenal masses are excised in the pediatric population.

References

Agrons GA, Lonergan GJ, Dickey GE, Perez-Monte JE: From the archives of the AFIP: adrenocortical neoplasms in children, *Radiographics* 19:989–1008, 1999.

Masiakos PT, Gerstle JT, Cheang T, et al: Is surgery necessary for incidentally discovered adrenal masses in children? *J Pediatr Surg* 39:754–758, 2004.

Wieneke JA, Thompson LD, Heffess CS: Adrenal cortical neoplasms in the pediatric population: a clinicopathologic and immunophenotypic analysis of 83 patients, *Am J Surg Pathol* 27:867–881, 2003.

Cross-Reference

Zagoria RJ, *Genitourinary Radiology: THE REQUISITES*, 2nd ed, pp 355–369, 379.

Comment

The differential diagnosis of pediatric adrenal masses varies with the patient's age. In neonates, adrenal hemorrhage and neuroblastoma are most common. Follow-up ultrasonography often will help distinguish the two, because hemorrhage will resolve and neuroblastoma will enlarge. The average age of diagnosis for neuroblastoma is 2 years.

Adenomas and adrenocortical carcinomas are often difficult to distinguish at pathology in pediatric patients; thus, the term *adrenocortical neoplasm* is often applied to include both entities. Adenomas are encapsulated, less than 10 cm in diameter, weigh less than 50 g, and have fewer than 15 mitoses per high-power field on microscopy. Prognosis is good if there is complete surgical excision. Adrenocortical neoplasms are most common in young children, slightly more common in girls, and have been associated with hemihypertrophy, Beckwith-Wiedemann, and Li Fraumeni syndromes.

Pediatric adrenocortical neoplasms are most often hormonally active, which is rare in adults. Children often present with virilization. Vascular invasion can involve the adrenal vein, inferior vena cava, and right atrium and is best evaluated with contrast CT or MRI. If there is extension into the chest, surgery requires a thoracic and abdominal approach.

Pheochromocytoma is the rarest pediatric adrenal neoplasm, and is often active on PET and meta-iodobenzylguanidine (MIBG) scans. Even incidental pediatric adrenal masses are resected because of the 30% risk of malignancy. This case involves a 2-year-old girl who had prominent virilization compared with her male twin. She had an abnormal biochemical profile and this mass on plain radiograph, ultrasonography, and CT. The mass was resected and the pathology showed adrenocortical neoplasm. She returned to normal after the resection.

Notes

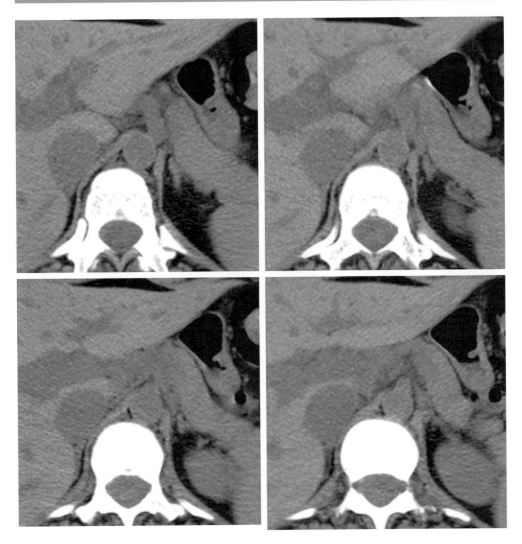

1. What is the most likely diagnosis?

2. How is the diagnosis made?

3. What are the common imaging findings?

4. What is the treatment?

Adrenal: Addison's Disease

1. The diagnosis may be difficult to make independently on CT without history, but the adrenal glands do appear small in this patient with recently diagnosed adrenocortical insufficiency (Addison's disease).

2. Adrenocorticotropic hormone stimulation test.

3. If the adrenocortical insufficiency is secondary to an autoimmune cause (which is the most common etiology and is true for this case), both adrenal glands will appear small. If it is secondary to another cause, such as tuberculosis, or replacement by tumor, the glands are enlarged.

4. Glucocorticoid replacement, correction of metabolic and electrolyte abnormalities, and correction of hypovolemia.

References

Mayo-Smith WW, Boland GW, Noto RB, Lee MJ: State-of-the-art adrenal imaging, *Radiographics* 21:995–1012, 2001.

Ten S, New M, Maclaren N: Clinical review 130: Addison's disease 2001 [Review], *J Clin Endocrinol Metab* 86: 2909–2922, 2001.

Cross-Reference

Zagoria RJ, *Genitourinary Radiology: THE REQUISITES*, 2nd ed, pp 377–379.

Comment

Addison's disease, or primary adrenocorticoinsufficiency, is hypofunctioning of the adrenal cortex resulting in decreased production of cortisol and aldosterone. Greater than 90% of the gland must be involved before signs of adrenal insufficiency appear. Primary adrenocorticoinsufficiency may be secondary to autoimmune causes, granulomatous processes such as tuberculosis, coccidioidomycosis, or histoplasmosis, or replacement by neoplasm, hemorrhage, or infection. The diagnosis is based on clinical and biochemical findings, and is not reliably established by imaging. The diagnosis is made following an adrenocorticotropic hormone (ACTH) stimulation test: the normal response following the injection of ACTH is a rise in serum and urine cortisol levels; an abnormal response is if serum cortisol levels fail to rise. On cross-sectional imaging, if adrenocortical insufficiency is secondary to an autoimmune cause, both adrenal glands are small in size (as in this case). If it is secondary to another cause, such as tuberculosis, or replacement by tumor, the gland may appear enlarged. Signs and symptoms include weight loss, loss of appetite, muscle weakness, fatigue, hypotension, and hyperpigmentation. Hyponatremia may result due to aldosterone deficiency. Despite being described over 150 years ago, the disease is still underdiagnosed, most likely due to the nonspecific nature of the symptoms. Treatment includes glucocorticoid replacement, correction of metabolic and electrolyte abnormalities, and correction of hypovolemia.

Notes

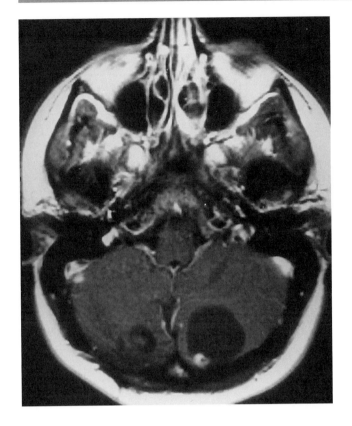
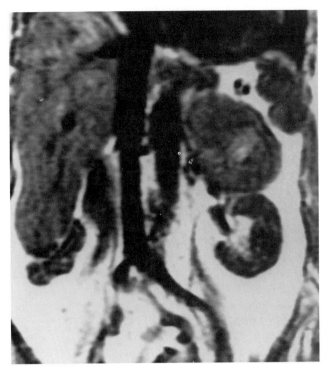
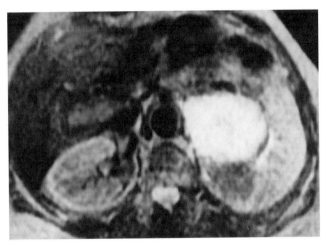

1. In patients with von Hippel-Lindau disease, what pancreatic lesion is most frequently associated with the development of pheochromocytoma?

2. In patients with von Hippel-Lindau disease, what percentage of pheochromocytomas are multiple or bilateral?

3. In patients with multiple endocrine neoplasia syndromes, what adrenomedullary pathologic condition may precede the development of a pheochromocytoma?

4. Name two other syndromes or diseases in which a pheochromocytoma may occur.

Adrenal: Pheochromocytoma in von Hippel-Lindau Disease

1. Islet cell tumor.

2. 50% to 80% (as opposed to approximately 10% of sporadic tumors).

3. Medullary hyperplasia of the adrenal gland.

4. Sturge-Weber syndrome, tuberous sclerosis, and Carney's syndrome (pulmonary chondromas and gastric stromal neoplasms).

References

Choyke PL, Glenn GM, Walter MM, et al: Von Hippel-Lindau disease: genetic, clinical, and imaging features, *Radiology* 194:629–642, 1995.

Couch V, Lindor NM, Karnes PS, Michels VV: Von Hippel-Lindau disease [Review], *Mayo Clin Proc* 75:265–272, 2000.

Cross-Reference

Zagoria RJ, *Genitourinary Radiology: THE REQUISITES,* 2nd ed, pp 358–365.

Comment

Pheochromocytomas can be associated with a number of syndromes and diseases. Medullary carcinoma of the thyroid and pheochromocytoma are associated with both multiple endocrine neoplasia syndromes IIA (Sipple's syndrome) and IIB/III (ganglioneuromatosis and multiple mucosal neuromas). Approximately 10% of pheochromocytomas are inherited; the majority are inherited in an autosomal-dominant pattern. About 1% of patients with neurofibromatosis develop pheochromocytomas.

The case presented is that of pheochromocytoma in a patient with von Hippel-Lindau disease (VHL). VHL is an autosomal-dominant "tumor predisposition syndrome" characterized by the presence of benign and malignant tumors. The most commonly affected organs and tumors are retinal angiomas, hemangioblastomas of the cerebellum and spinal cord, and renal cell carcinomas. Less common manifestations include cystic tumors of the kidneys, pancreas, and epididymis, and adrenal pheochromocytomas.

Notes

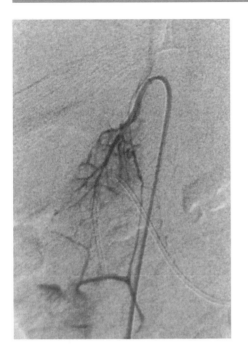

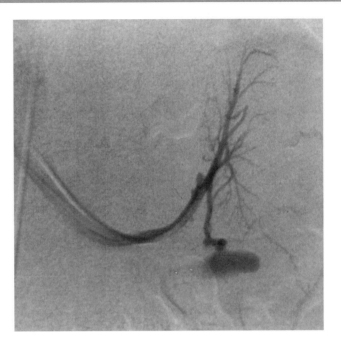

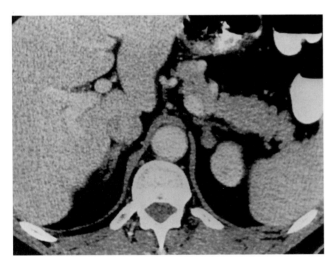

1. What are the causes of primary aldosteronism?

2. Why is it important to distinguish between the various causes?

3. When is CT alone diagnostic?

4. What is the most common complication of adrenal venography and venous sampling?

Adrenal: Primary Aldosteronism

1. Autonomous adrenocortical adenoma (80%), adrenal hyperplasia (20%), and adrenocortical carcinoma (less than 1%).

2. Unilateral adrenalectomy cures a hyperfunctional adenoma, whereas hyperplasia is managed medically.

3. When a unilateral hypodense adrenal mass that is smaller than 4 cm in diameter and a normal or atrophic contralateral adrenal gland are identified.

4. Adrenal venous extravasation occurs in about 4% of cases and often results in loss of function. It is an absolute contraindication to contralateral adrenal venography and venous sampling.

References

Al Fehaily M, Duh QY: Clinical manifestation of aldosteronoma, *Surg Clin North Am* 84:887–905, 2004.

Doppman JL, Gill JR: Hyperaldosteronism: sampling the adrenal veins, *Radiology* 198:309–312, 1996.

Hokotate H, Inoue H, Baba Y, et al: Aldosteronomas: experience with superselective adrenal arterial embolization in 33 cases, *Radiology* 227:401–406, 2003.

Mayo-Smith WW, Dupuy DE: Adrenal neoplasms: CT-guided radiofrequency ablation—preliminary results, *Radiology* 231:225–230, 2004.

Cross-Reference

Zagoria RJ, *Genitourinary Radiology: THE REQUISITES*, 2nd ed, pp 376–377.

Comment

About 1% of patients with hypertension have primary aldosteronism. Clinically, patients present with polyuria, diastolic hypertension, hypernatremia, hypokalemia, and an elevated plasma aldosterone level. The best diagnostic test is the plasma aldosterone concentration to plasma renin activity ratio.

In primary aldosteronism, the stimulus for overproduction originates in the adrenal gland, whereas secondary aldosteronism is due to stimulation of the adrenal from an extraadrenal source (via the renin-angiotensin system). The causes of primary hyperaldosteronism are unilateral adrenal adenoma in 80% of patients and bilateral adrenal hyperplasia in 20% of patients. Distinction between these etiologies is critical as the treatment for a unilateral adenoma is surgical resection and the treatment for bilateral hyperplasia is medical therapy. The radiologist's task is to detect the appropriate cause to guide the appropriate treatment. Thin-section CT (2–3 mm collimation) is the initial modality of choice. It is 98% sensitive for nodules that are larger than 1 cm in diameter. However, it is difficult to distinguish between a smaller adenoma and adrenal hyperplasia on CT. Therefore, when CT demonstrates normal adrenal glands, bilateral hyperplasia, or a nodule with contralateral hyperplasia, adrenal function must be evaluated by iodine 131-6β-iodomethyl-19-norcholesterol (NP-59) scintigraphy or adrenal venous sampling because a significant number of patients will have a small unilateral aldosteronoma.

Despite being nearly 100% accurate, selective adrenal venous sampling is performed infrequently because of a failure to sample the right adrenal vein in 30% of cases. However, subselective sampling is acceptable because measuring the aldosterone/cortisol ratio in the venous blood can correct for dilution. An aldosterone/cortisol ratio that increases significantly after corticotropin stimulation and is at least five times greater than the contralateral adrenal indicates an aldosteronoma. Suppressed aldosterone levels and a blunted response to corticotropin from the contralateral adrenal gland are the best predictors for the success of unilateral adrenalectomy. Treatment for unilateral aldosteronomas is surgical, but newer experimental treatments including embolization and tumor ablation have been reported.

Notes

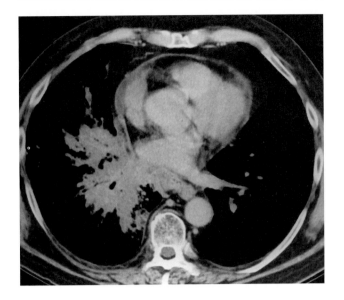
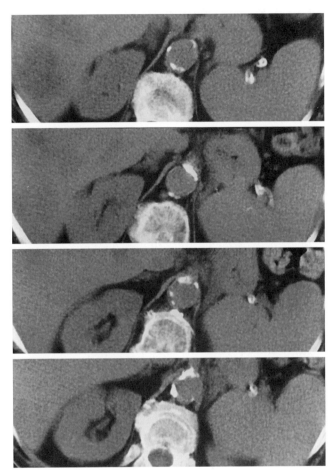

1. CT scans of a patient with Cushing's syndrome are shown. What is the most likely cause of the endocrinopathy in this patient?

2. What is the most common cause of ectopic corticotropin-releasing hormone syndrome?

3. What are the most common causes of corticotropin-independent Cushing's syndrome?

4. Name another common cause of Cushing's syndrome.

Adrenal: Cushing's Syndrome: Ectopic Corticotropin Syndrome

1. Small cell carcinoma of the lung.

2. Bronchial carcinoid tumor.

3. Adrenocortical tumors and, rarely, nodular adrenal hyperplasia.

4. Exogenous steroids taken by the patient.

References

Orth DN: Cushing's syndrome, *N Engl J Med* 332: 791–803, 1995.

Lindsay JR, Nieman LK: Differential diagnosis and imaging in Cushing's syndrome, *Endocrinol Metab Clin North Am* 34:403–421, 2005.

Cross-Reference

Zagoria RJ, *Genitourinary Radiology: THE REQUISITES*, 2nd ed, pp 374–376.

Comment

Cushing's syndrome is the result of excess production of cortisol by the adrenal gland. In 20% of patients, this is due to a primary adrenal tumor and in 80% it is due to excess stimulation of the adrenal by corticotropin, usually from the pituitary gland. Certain neoplasms can produce ectopic corticotropin, which results in stimulation of both adrenal glands. Acute ectopic corticotropin syndrome is associated with small cell carcinoma of the lung in 75% of cases and results in hypertension, edema, hypokalemia, and glucose intolerance. The chronic ectopic corticotropin syndrome is clinically indistinguishable from Cushing's disease and is caused by various neuroendocrine tumors, including carcinoid tumors of the bronchus, thymus, or pancreas and medullary carcinomas of the thyroid. These same tumors also can cause Cushing's syndrome by the excessive production of corticotropin-releasing hormone (CRH). CRH is normally synthesized in the hypothalamus and is the most potent regulator of corticotropin secretion by the anterior pituitary. Excluding exogenous corticosteroid administration, overproduction of cortisol or cortisol precursors from an adrenal tumor is the main cause of corticotropin-independent Cushing's syndrome.

Notes

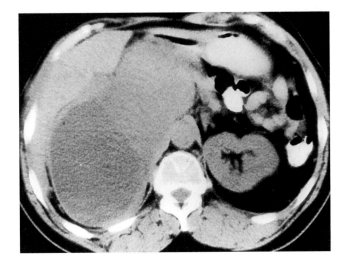

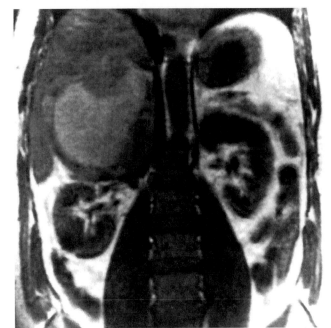

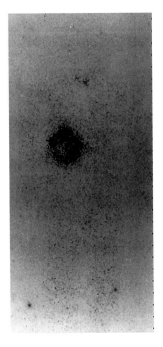

1. What is the differential diagnosis for this right adrenal mass?

2. What is the finding on the nuclear medicine study? What type of radiopharmaceutical was administered?

3. True or false: Aspiration of cyst fluid should be recommended next.

4. True or false: The majority of adrenocortical carcinomas are larger than 6 cm in diameter, contain areas of cystic necrosis, and may have foci of calcification.

Adrenal: Cystic Pheochromocytoma

1. Chronic hematoma (pseudocyst), necrotic metastasis, "cystic" pheochromocytoma, adrenocortical carcinoma, adrenal cyst, and parasitic cyst.

2. Coronal anteroposterior image from a meta-iodobenzylguanidine (MIBG) iodine 123 scan shows increased uptake in the right adrenal mass.

3. False.

4. True.

References

Belden CJ, Powers C, Ros PR: MR demonstration of a cystic pheochromocytoma, *J Magn Reson Imaging* 5:778–780, 1995.

Blake MA, Kalra MK, Maher MM, et al: Pheochromocytoma: an imaging chameleon, *Radiographics* 24(Suppl):87–99, 2004.

McCorkell SJ, Niles NL: Fine-needle aspiration of catecholamine-producing adrenal masses: a possibly fatal mistake, *Am J Roentgenol* 145:113–114, 1985.

Cross-Reference

Zagoria RJ, *Genitourinary Radiology: THE REQUISITES,* 2nd ed, pp 358–365, 374.

Comment

Rarely, pheochromocytoma may present as a large cystic adrenal mass because of central necrosis. Biochemical screening (measurement of unconjugated catecholamines and vanillylmandelic acid levels in a 24-hour urine collection) to exclude a pheochromocytoma should precede aspiration or biopsy of an isolated enlarged adrenal mass. If the biochemical tests suggest pheochromocytoma, surgical resection should be performed. If the biochemical screening for pheochromocytoma is negative, there is no history of known malignancy, and the chest, abdomen, and pelvic CT are negative, the presumptive diagnosis in this case would be necrotic adrenocortical carcinoma and surgical resection should be performed.

Percutaneous needle aspiration or biopsy of a pheochromocytoma may result in potentially fatal complications. During adrenal angiography, catecholamine storm leading to hypertensive crisis has been reported in up to half of patients with unsuspected pheochromocytomas, and a similar risk has been postulated for needle biopsy.

Sympathomedullary imaging has been made possible with meta-iodobenzylguanidine (MIBG), an analog of norepinephrine. MIBG iodine 123 is useful for detecting extraadrenal and metastatic pheochromocytomas because the whole body can be evaluated. It is also useful in the patient who has a suspected recurrence of pheochromocytoma after adrenalectomy because surgical clips or distorted anatomy may reduce the accuracy of CT or MRI. A significant number of medications may interfere with the accumulation of MIBG. Tricyclic antidepressants, labetalol, and cocaine are just a few of the medications that can decrease MIBG uptake by sympathomedullary tissues.

Notes

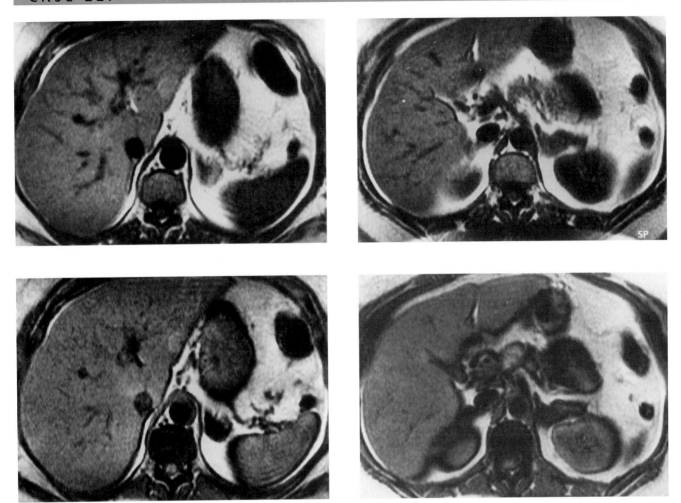

1. The top two photographs are contiguous axial MR images. The bottom two photographs are contiguous axial MR images through the same levels. What pulse sequences were used for these image pairs?

2. What is a collision tumor?

3. What are the two most common histologic tumor types found in an adrenal collision tumor?

4. What are the implications for biopsy of an adrenal collision tumor?

Adrenal: Collision Tumor of the Adrenal Gland

1. In-phase and opposed-phase T1W gradient-echo images of a left adrenal mass.

2. A mass that contains two coexistent but independent neoplasms without substantial histopathologic admixture. In this example, the medial rounded component of the tumor is the adenoma (loses signal on lower, out-of-phase images). The serpiginous lateral component does not lose signal and is a metastatic focus.

3. Adenoma and metastasis.

4. The component of the tumor that is more likely to be malignant should be biopsied.

References

Mayo-Smith WW, Boland GW, Noto RB, Lee MJ: State-of-the-art adrenal imaging, 21:995–1012, 2001.

Otal P, Escourrou G, Mazerolles C, et al: Imaging features of uncommon adrenal masses with histopathologic correlation, *Radiographics* 19:569–581, 1999.

Schwartz LH, Macari M, Huvos AG, Panicek DM: Collision tumors of the adrenal gland: demonstration and characterization at MR imaging, *Radiology* 201: 757–760, 1996.

Cross-Reference

Zagoria RJ, *Genitourinary Radiology: THE REQUISITES,* 2nd ed, pp 355–358.

Comment

Rarely, adrenal masses may consist of more than one histologic type. Adrenal adenomas are very common (up to 1.5% on one autopsy series) and the adrenal is also a common site of metastases. Because of this, a metastasis could occur to an adrenal with a preexisting adenoma. When this occurs, it is called a collision tumor.

In the adrenal gland, collision tumors consisting of an adenoma and metastasis have been reported. As illustrated in this case, in- and opposed-phase T1W gradient-echo pairs show a focal area of the tumor that loses signal on the opposed-phase image (suggesting a fat-containing adenoma) and another part of the tumor that does not demonstrate signal loss (and is more suspicious for metastasis). As suggested by Schwartz and co-workers, collision tumors of the adrenal gland should be suspected when (1) there has been growth of a known adrenal adenoma or (2) the signal intensities of two adjacent adrenal lesions show distinctly different characteristics on MRI. In addition, collision tumors may be suspected on CT when an enlarged adrenal has two separate but distinct densities, one low density (the adenoma) and one higher density (the metastasis). This appearance differs from a myelolipoma, which has variable density but is a single mass. Needle biopsy of the more suspicious component of the mass (i.e., the mass that shows no signal loss on the opposed-phase, T1W gradient-echo image or the denser portion of the mass on CT) should be considered.

Notes

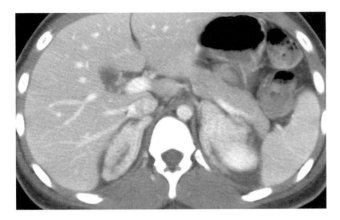

1. What is the normal thickness of the adrenal gland?

2. What is causing the diffuse enlargement of both adrenal glands in this adolescent?

3. What are two possible causes of this appearance?

4. What syndrome is associated with this appearance?

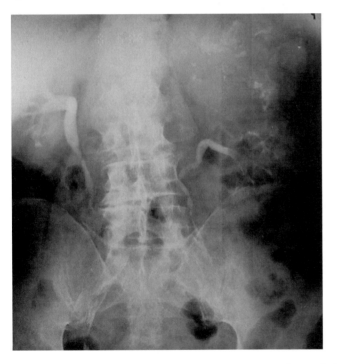
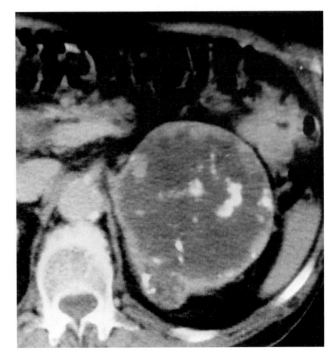

1. What is the differential diagnosis for this large left suprarenal mass?

2. To make a management recommendation, is knowledge about adrenal hyperfunction necessary?

3. Are these masses associated with altered adrenal function?

4. What are phleboliths?

Adrenal: Adrenal Hyperplasia

1. Each normal adrenal limb measures from 4 to 9 mm in width.

2. Adrenal hyperplasia.

3. Adrenal hyperplasia may be primary (idiopathic) or can be caused by excess adrenocorticotropic hormone production. Diffuse smooth adrenal enlargement can also be caused by acute infection and lymphoma.

4. Cushing's, Conn's, and adrenogenital syndromes can be seen with hyperplasia.

Reference

Lockhart ME, Smith JK, Kenney PJ: Imaging of adrenal masses, *Eur J Radiol* 41:95–112, 2002.

Cross-Reference

Zagoria RJ, *Genitourinary Radiology: THE REQUISITES,* 2nd ed, pp 352–380.

Comment

These contrast-enhanced CT images show smooth, marked enlargement of both adrenal glands. They maintain their normal shape. This is a typical, albeit an exaggerated, appearance of adrenal hyperplasia. Less often adrenal hyperplasia can be nodular with the appearance of multiple small nodules throughout both adrenal glands. Adrenal hyperplasia indicates an increased number of adrenal cortical cells. It can be unilateral, but more often is bilateral. The most common cause of adrenal hyperplasia is overproduction of adrenocorticotropic hormone (ACTH). This may be due to pathology in the pituitary gland or hypothalamus, or from ectopic ACTH production. Ectopic production of ACTH is usually seen from tumors such as bronchial carcinoids, and from bronchogenic carcinomas. Adrenal hyperplasia can cause Cushing's syndrome and, less commonly, Conn's syndrome with hypertension and hypokalemia. This teenager has congenital adrenal hyperplasia.

The appearance of adrenal hyperplasia can be mimicked on imaging studies by lymphoma infiltrating both adrenal glands and by adrenal inflammation during the acute and subacute phases of adrenalitis. The inflammation is usually caused by granulomatous infection, and as the infection subsides the glands will atrophy and may calcify.

Notes

Adrenal: Adrenal Hemangioma

1. Chronic adrenal hemorrhage, pheochromocytoma, metastasis, adrenocortical carcinoma, and mesenchymal tumor.

2. Yes.

3. No.

4. *Dorland's Medical Dictionary* defines a phlebolith as a calculus or concretion in a vein; a vein stone.

References

Otal P, Escourrou G, Mazerolles C, et al: Imaging features of uncommon adrenal masses with histopathologic correlation, *Radiographics* 19:569–581, 1999.

Sabanegh E Jr, Harris MJ, Grider D: Cavernous adrenal hemangioma, *Urology* 42:327–330, 1993.

Cross-Reference

Zagoria RJ, *Genitourinary Radiology: THE REQUISITES,* 2nd ed, pp 368–373.

Comment

Hemangiomas can occur in almost any organ; there have been roughly 30 reported cases of these benign, mesenchymal tumors arising from the adrenal gland. Adrenal hemangiomas are usually seen in patients 50–70 years of age and have a female:male ratio of 2:1. Because they are usually nonhyperfunctional and asymptomatic, hemangiomas are usually large (more than 10 cm in diameter) at the time of incidental discovery. Hemangiomas usually involve the adrenal cortex and are encapsulated. Calcifications have been reported in two thirds of cases and can appear as dystrophic clumps or crescents, can be more characteristic phleboliths, or can be both: the question about phleboliths was intended to be a clue. When large, hemangiomas can be complicated by areas of fibrosis, necrosis, thrombosis, or hemorrhage. The sonographic appearance is nonspecific. Peripheral, nodular enhancement can be evident on CT and may be an important clue to diagnosis. MRI may be useful in the diagnostic evaluation: adrenal hemangiomas are often T2 hyperintense and contain focal hemorrhage.

Given its size and heterogeneous appearance on urography and enhanced CT, this tumor was removed. The intent of the second and third questions was to caution the radiologist about the risks of biopsy or surgery on an unsuspected pheochromocytoma.

Notes

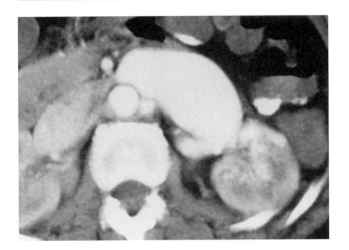 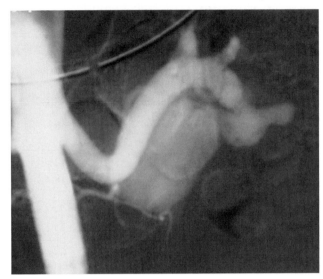

1. In this patient with gross hematuria, what is the most likely diagnosis?

2. What features on the CT scan indicate an abnormal connection between the arterial and venous systems?

3. What symptoms may result from this type of abnormality?

4. What are the common causes of this type of abnormality?

Vascular and Interventional: Renal Arteriovenous Malformation

1. Arteriovenous malformation.

2. Marked left renal vein enlargement and renal vein opacification to the same degree as in the aorta and superior mesenteric artery.

3. Gross hematuria and high output heart failure.

4. Congenital malformation and arteriovenous malformation in association with other syndromes, such as congenital telangiectasias (Osler-Weber-Rendu syndrome).

Reference

Tarkington MA, Matsumoto AH, Dejter SW, Regan JB: Spectrum of renal vascular malformation, *Urology* 4:297–300, 1991.

Cross-Reference

Zagoria RJ, *Genitourinary Radiology: THE REQUISITES,* 2nd ed, p 409.

Comment

Most arteriovenous malformations (AVMs) of the kidney are congenital. They usually come to light as a result of gross hematuria, but when there is massive shunting of blood, evidence of heart failure may develop. These abnormalities are usually diagnosed in young patients. Because of the low-resistance pathway of the AVM, the normal kidney may be underperfused, as in this case. Massive enlargement of the draining left renal vein was detected by CT scanning and led to the diagnosis of renal AVM. Selective embolization of the malformation is possible in some cases. However, when the arteriovenous connection is of large caliber with very high flow, embolic occlusion of the AVM, with maintenance of perfusion to the kidney, may be impossible.

Notes

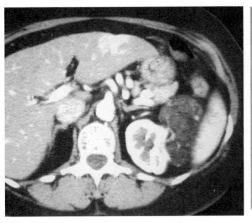 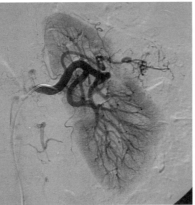 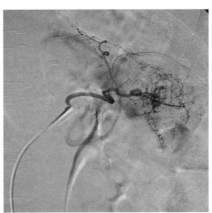

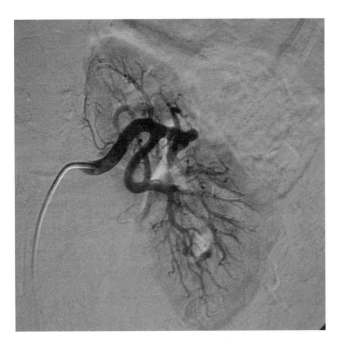

1. What is the abnormality on the CT image in the first image?

2. What risks are associated with this mass?

3. What is appropriate management for this mass?

4. If embolization is indicated, what embolization agent should be used?

Vascular and Interventional: Renal Angiomyolipoma Embolization

1. An exophytic left renal mass. Fat within the mass is diagnostic of a renal angiomyolipoma (AML).

2. AMLs contain abnormal arteries, which can lead to spontaneous hemorrhage.

3. AMLs larger than 4 cm can be treated with embolization or surgical removal.

4. Ethanol or small particles.

References

Kothary N, Soulen MC, Clark TWI, et al: Renal angiomyolipoma: long-term results after arterial embolization, *J Vasc Interv Radiol* 16:45–50, 2005.

Soulen MC, Faykus MH Jr, Shlansky-Goldberg RD, et al: Elective embolization for prevention of hemorrhage from renal angiomyolipomas, *J Vasc Interv Radiol* 5:587–591, 1994.

Cross-Reference

Zagoria RJ, *Genitourinary Radiology: THE REQUISITES*, 2nd ed, pp 106–108, 396–399.

Comment

Renal angiomyolipoma (AML) is a common benign renal tumor that is composed of thick-walled blood vessels, smooth muscle, and mature adipose tissue. Eighty percent of AMLs are sporadic and 20% are syndrome associated (tuberous sclerosis and pulmonary lymphangiomyomatosis). On CT, renal AMLs appear as well-marginated cortical masses, with mixed fatty and soft tissue density. Demonstration of macroscopic fat on CT (attenuation value under −20 Hounsfield units) is diagnostic.

Although benign, AMLs contain abnormal arteries that are prone to spontaneous hemorrhage. Hemorrhage is considered unlikely in AMLs smaller than 4 cm, and these small AMLs can be followed with imaging examinations. Once larger than 4 cm, the risk for hemorrhage is considered sufficient to warrant preventative treatment. Treatment options include embolization or partial nephrectomy. The goal of embolization in this case is necrosis of the tumor and prevention of further hemorrhage. Embolization is performed with subselective catheterization to maintain as much normal kidney as possible. Small particles 250 to 500 µm in diameter or absolute ethanol are used as the embolic agent. The second image depicts a left renal arterial selective injection showing the eccentric renal mass with mild hyperemia, a dominant feeding vessel, and parenchymal staining. Subselective catheterization of the dominant feeding vessel prior to embolization confirms the atypical nature of vessels feeding the AML in the second part of the second image. Following embolization with polyvinyl alcohol particles, there is no residual flow to the mass and excellent preservation of all major renal arterial branches (third image).

Notes

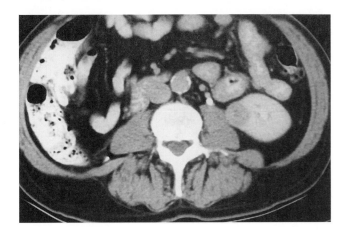

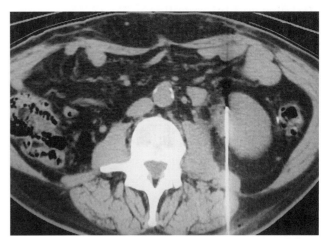

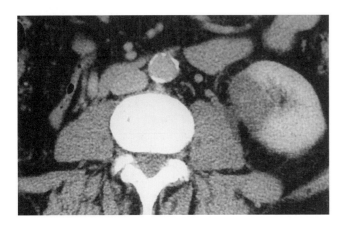

1. What are the important findings in the first image?

2. The patient had a right total nephrectomy to treat renal cell carcinoma. How does this impact treatment options?

3. Name two treatment options for this patient.

4. What is the mechanism of action of radiofrequency ablation?

Vascular and Interventional: Radiofrequency Ablation of a Renal Cell Carcinoma

1. Solid mass in the left kidney and right nephrectomy.

2. Left nephrectomy would necessitate long-term dialysis because patients with a history of cancer are not usually considered for renal transplantation.

3. Partial nephrectomy and percutaneous tumor ablation using cryotherapy or radiofrequency (RF) therapy.

4. Deposition of radiofrequency energy into a tissue causes local heating of the tissue and cell death.

References

Gervais DA, McGovern FJ, Arellano RS, et al: Radiofrequency ablation of renal cell carcinoma: part 1, indications, results, and role in patient management over a 6-year period and ablation of 100 tumors, *Am J Roentgenol* 185:64–71, 2005.

Zagoria RJ: Imaging-guided radiofrequency ablation of renal masses, *Radiographics* 24(Suppl):59–71, 2004.

Cross-Reference

Zagoria RJ, *Genitourinary Radiology: THE REQUISITES,* 2nd ed, pp 402–403.

Comment

The second image shows an RF probe positioned in a small, solid left renal tumor. The third image, obtained 12 weeks later, shows local tissue necrosis with no evidence of residual viable tumor and normal enhancement of untreated renal parenchyma.

Nephrectomy is the first-line treatment for patients with localized renal cell carcinoma. Partial nephrectomy or nephron-sparing surgery has been shown to have equivalent results in properly selected patients. However, these operations are technically difficult and, as with total nephrectomy, are associated with some morbidity.

New percutaneous techniques have been developed to treat patients with either primary or metastatic abdominal neoplastic disease. These techniques include cryoablation and radiofrequency ablation. Alternating current in the RF range causes local ionic agitation and frictional heat. As a result, interstitial temperatures in excess of 50°C produce coagulative necrosis. Shielded probes and electrodes of various sizes have been designed to concentrate the RF energy in different tissue volumes. Early studies have shown high rates of complete eradication of renal tumors with RF ablation.

Notes

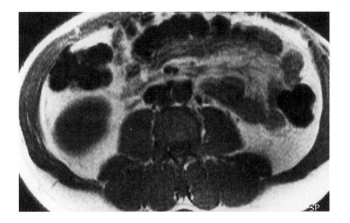

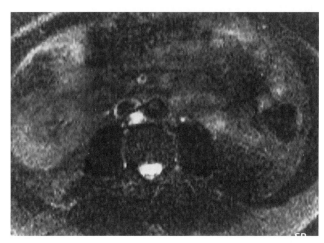

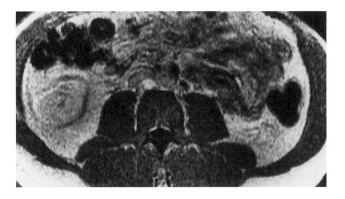

1. Describe the MRIs shown.

2. Identify the location of the abnormal tissue on these images.

3. What are the organs of Zuckerkandl? Where are they found?

4. Why is pheochromocytoma sometimes referred to as the 10% tumor?

Retroperitoneum: Recurrent Extraadrenal Pheochromocytoma

1. The first image is an axial T1W image, the second image is a T2W image with fat saturation, and the third image is an enhanced T1W image.

2. There is a small mass located between the aorta and the inferior vena cava. The mass is T1 hypointense, T2 hyperintense, and enhances after administration of intravenous gadolinium chelate.

3. A collection of sympathetic ganglia found from the origin of the inferior mesenteric artery to the aortic bifurcation.

4. Approximately 10% are extraadrenal, 10% are found in both adrenal glands, and 10% are malignant. About 10% of patients with von Hippel-Lindau disease have pheochromocytomas, and 10% of pheochromocytomas are inherited (the majority as autosomal dominant).

References

Blake MA, Kalra MK, Maher MM, et al: Pheochromocytoma: an imaging chameleon, *Radiographics* 24(Suppl): 87–99, 2004.

Mayo-Smith WW, Boland GW, Noto RB, Lee MJ: State-of-the-art adrenal imaging, *Radiographics* 21:995–1012, 2001.

Cross-Reference

Zagoria RJ, *Genitourinary Radiology: THE REQUISITES,* 2nd ed, pp 358–365, 374.

Comment

Arising from chromaffin cells of the sympathetic nervous system, pheochromocytomas may retain the capacity to produce and secrete catecholamines. Release of norepinephrine and epinephrine may lead to classic symptoms of a "crisis," or the five P's: *p*ain (head, chest, or abdomen), high blood *p*ressure, *p*alpitations, *p*erspiration, and *p*anic. Measurement of unconjugated catecholamines (norepinephrine is more sensitive than epinephrine) or their metabolites (vanillylmandelic acid) in 24-hour urine samples is the most common screening test.

Pheochromocytomas can arise in sympathetic paraganglia cells from the skull base to the urinary bladder, but 98% are discovered in the abdomen or pelvis. CT is the modality most commonly used for localizing these tumors. On CT, pheochromocytomas are most often single, solid adrenal masses that are more than 2 cm in diameter. However, adrenal pheochromocytomas can be predominantly cystic or complicated by hemorrhage. MRI can be used to confirm a suspected pheochromocytoma; on high-field MRI a pheochromocytoma is isointense to hypointense on T1W images, and approximately 50% are hyperintense on T2W images. Because pheochromocytomas are hypervascular tumors, rapid and prolonged contrast enhancement is typical on MRI. Extraadrenal pheochromocytomas are more correctly termed *extraadrenal paragangliomas*. Scintigraphy with either or both metaiodobenzylguanidine iodine 123 (a guanethidine derivative) and octreotide indium 111 (a somatostatin receptor agonist) has been used successfully to localize the tumor. PET imaging may play a role in imaging for suspected or recurrent pheochromocytoma, but the precise role of this modality is yet to be determined.

This patient had a prior resection of an adrenal pheochromocytoma but had recurrence of symptoms 1 year later. This MRI examination demonstrated recurrence of the disease (a metastasis) to the retroperitoneal nodes. The patient's symptoms resolved after resection of the metastasis.

Notes

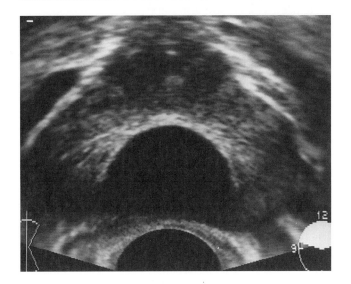 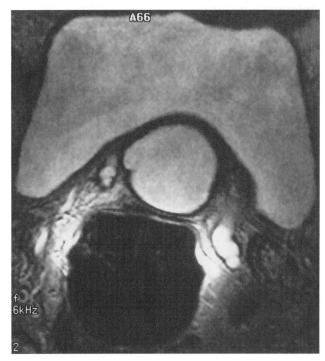

1. An axial transrectal prostatic ultrasound image and a T2W MRI from two patients with the same diagnosis are shown. What are the causes for a midline prostatic cyst?

2. What is the most common cause of a prostatic cyst?

3. Which type of prostatic cyst is associated with hypospadias and undescended testis?

4. True or false: Cysts derived from müllerian duct remnants may contain sperm.

C A S E   2 3 4

Prostate and Seminal Vesicles: Midline Prostatic Cyst

1. Most commonly, utricular cyst and müllerian cyst.

2. Benign prostatic hyperplasia.

3. Utricular cyst.

4. True.

Reference

McDermott VG, Meakem TJ III, Stolpen AH, Schnall MD: Prostatic and periprostatic cysts: findings on MR imaging, *Am J Roentgenol* 164:123–127, 1995.

Cross-Reference

Zagoria RJ, *Genitourinary Radiology: THE REQUISITES,* 2nd ed, pp 335–336.

Comment

The different causes of prostatic cysts have been classified by embryologic derivation and by location. For the radiologist, the latter classification as midline, paramedian, and lateral prostatic cysts may be more useful. Midline cysts include utricular and müllerian cysts. Paramedian cysts include both benign prostatic hypertrophy–associated cysts and ejaculatory duct cysts. Congenital prostatic and retention cysts are usually located laterally in the prostate gland, and the seminal vesicle cyst is a lateral extraprostatic cyst. Other causes of a cystic prostate mass include pyogenic abscess, parasitic cyst, and rarely carcinoma.

The most common midline prostatic cysts, the utricular and müllerian duct cysts, are derived from remnants of the paramesonephric (müllerian) duct system. In men the only derivatives of this duct system are the müllerian tubercle, which gives rise to the prostatic utricle, and the appendix testis. In addition to embryologic development and location, other similarities between these two types of cysts include a rare association with renal agenesis and prostatic carcinoma. Notably, up to 3% of these cysts may be associated with endometrial, clear cell, or squamous cell carcinomas of prostate. There are several important differences. The utricular cyst maintains a connection with the posterior urethra and may be associated with other genital tract anomalies. The müllerian duct cyst can be large and sometimes extends cephalad to the prostate, whereas the utricular cyst is intraprostatic. Stones may be found in müllerian duct cysts but not in utricular cysts. Finally, utricular cyst fluid may contain sperm, but fluid aspirated from the müllerian duct does not.

Notes

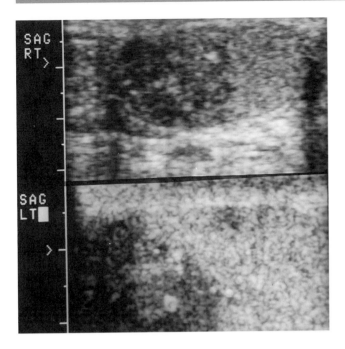 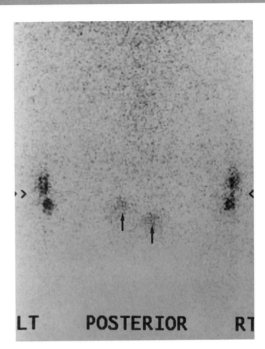

1. Images from scrotal sonography and adrenocortical scintigraphy are shown. *Arrows* indicate activity in the testes. What radiopharmaceutical is used in adrenocortical scintigraphy?

2. What is the most likely diagnosis for these testicular lesions?

3. Elevated levels of which hormone cause these lesions?

4. What is the most common disease associated with these testicular masses?

Scrotum: Testicular Adrenal Rests Associated with Congenital Adrenal Hyperplasia

1. NP-59 (131I-6β-iodomethyl-19-norcholesterol).

2. Adrenal rests.

3. Adrenocorticotropic hormone or corticotropin.

4. Congenital adrenal hyperplasia (adrenogenital syndrome).

References

Avila NA, Premkumar A, Shawker TH, et al: Testicular adrenal rest tissue in congenital adrenal hyperplasia: findings at gray-scale and color Doppler US, *Radiology* 198:99–104, 1996.

Avila NA, Shawker TS, Jones JV, et al: Testicular adrenal rest tissue in congenital adrenal hyperplasia: serial sonographic and clinical findings, *Am J Roentgenol* 172:1235–1238, 1999.

Cross-Reference

Zagoria RJ, *Genitourinary Radiology: THE REQUISITES*, 2nd ed, pp 322–325.

Comment

Elevated serum levels of corticotropin may result in the growth of rests of adrenal tissue in the testes, celiac plexus region, broad ligaments, or fetal ovarian tissue. Adrenal rests most often occur in association with congenital adrenal hyperplasia (CAH) but also have been reported in patients with Addison's disease or Cushing's syndrome. CAH is caused by an autosomal-recessive defect in the production of an adrenocortical enzyme, most often 21-hydroxylase. Elevated levels of adrenocorticotropic hormone cause rests, which are identical to hyperplastic adrenal cortex, to grow in adrenal tissue. In patients with CAH, adrenal rest tissue may hypertrophy when there is inadequate glucocorticoid replacement and may atrophy when high doses of glucocorticoid are administered. Most adrenal rests are detected in patients with CAH, but in as many as 18% of patients, adrenogenital syndrome is not discovered until testicular enlargement develops.

Adrenal rests are bilateral in 75% of cases and may be mistaken for testicular lymphoma, leukemia, or metastases. Unilateral rests may be difficult to distinguish from primary tumors of the testicle. On ultrasonography, rests are often visible in the periphery of the testicle and do not distort the outer contour of the gonad. Testicular adrenal rests differ from other intratesticular mass lesions in that the echogenic line of the testicular mediastinum or parenchymal vessels on Doppler may course through an adrenal rest undisturbed. In most cases testicular adrenal rests are hypoechoic, but they may have a hyperechoic rim or a focus of calcification, as in the case presented. Large hypoechoic rests may be associated with marked attenuation on ultrasonography. When the diagnosis is in doubt, the existence of functional adrenal tissue may be established by adrenocortical scintigraphy or testicular venous sampling.

Notes

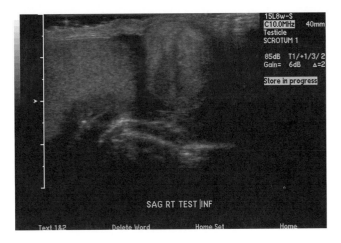

1. Where is the scrotal mass located?

2. What is the most likely organ of origin?

3. Is this entity benign or malignant?

4. What is the differential diagnosis, assuming this is a neoplasm?

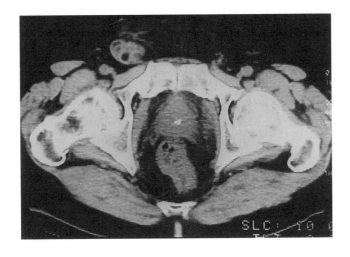 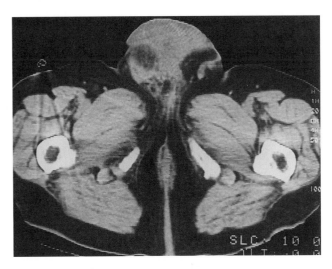

1. Given a palpable scrotal mass, what is the primary role of scrotal sonography? Why is this distinction important?

2. What is the most common tumor of the epididymis?

3. True or false: The most common extratesticular malignant tumor is a peritoneal metastasis.

4. What is the most common tumor that arises from an undescended testicle?

Scrotum: Adenomatoid Tumor of the Epididymis

1. Inferior to the testis, in the extratesticular space.

2. The tail of the epididymis.

3. Adenomatoid tumor of the epididymis is a benign tumor.

4. Leiomyoma and fibroma of the tunica vaginalis.

Reference

Woodward PF, Schwab CM, Seserhenn IA: Extratesticular scrotal masses, *Radiographics* 23:215–240, 2003.

Cross-Reference

Zagoria RJ, *Genitourinary Radiology: THE REQUISITES,* 2nd ed, p 319.

Comment

Adenomatoid tumor is the most common benign tumor arising in the extratesticular space and from the epididymis, accounting for the majority of paratesticular neoplasms. Men present between the ages of 20 and 50 years with a painless scrotal mass. At palpation, the mass is smooth, round, and usually separate from the testis. Adenomatoid tumors range in size from a few millimeters to 5 cm. They most commonly arise from the epididymal tail but can occur anywhere along the course of the epididymis, in the spermatic cord, and from the tunica albuginea. If this tumor arises from the tunica, intratesticular extension is possible. Differential diagnosis is a fibroma, usually arising from the tunica vaginalis or a leiomyoma arising from the epididymis.

Ultrasound findings include a well-defined spherical solid mass with echogenicity similar to or slightly greater than the adjacent testis. Images in multiple planes must be performed to determine with certainty that the mass is located in an extratesticular location. Doppler images reveal blood flow similar to the testis. Management is usually conservative.

Notes

Scrotum: Liposarcoma of the Spermatic Cord

1. To distinguish an intratesticular mass from an extratesticular one. Solid intratesticular masses are often malignant neoplasms; solid extratesticular masses are rarely malignant.

2. Adenomatoid tumor.

3. False.

4. Seminoma.

Reference

Frates MC, Benson CB, DiSalvo DN, et al: Solid extratesticular masses evaluated with sonography: pathologic correlation, *Radiology* 204:43–46, 1997.

Cross-Reference

Zagoria RJ, *Genitourinary Radiology: THE REQUISITES,* 2nd ed, pp. 327–329.

Comment

Malignant tumors account for only 3% of all solid extratesticular lesions, whereas 90% to 95% of solid intratesticular lesions are malignant. Ultrasonography accurately distinguishes intratesticular from extratesticular solid masses in 95% to 100% of cases and therefore is usually performed early in the evaluation of a palpable scrotal mass. However, no sonographic features reliably permit the distinction between a benign and malignant extratesticular mass. In the series of 19 solid extratesticular masses reported by Frates and colleagues, 16 were benign and included adenomatoid tumor of the epididymis, lipoma, sarcoidosis (bilateral), sperm granuloma, leiomyoma, benign inflammatory nodule, and fibroma; two of the three malignant tumors arose from the spermatic cord.

The spermatic cord originates at the internal inguinal ring and descends to the testis through the inguinal canal. It contains the testicular artery and vein, the cremasteric and deferential vessels, and the lymphatics. In addition, components of the ventral abdominal wall are incorporated in the spermatic cord and include the internal and external spermatic fascia and cremasteric layer. The predominance of mesodermal elements explains the prevalence of sarcomas among malignant tumors that arise from the spermatic cord.

Spermatic cord sarcoma is a rare cause of a solid extratesticular mass. In adults, liposarcoma, leiomyosarcoma, and malignant fibrous histiocytoma have been reported, and in infants and children, rhabdomyosarcoma is the most common type of tumor. Lymphatic spread (paraaortic lymphadenopathy) has been reported in up to one third of patients with poorly differentiated tumors.

Notes

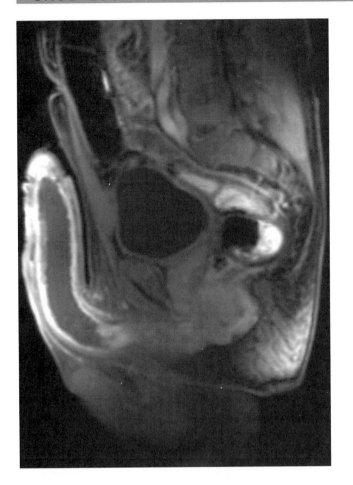

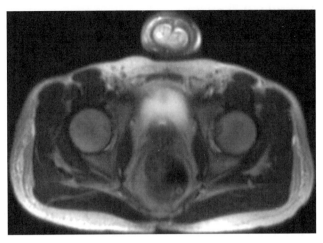

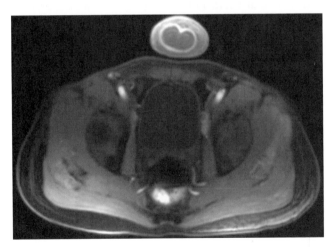

1. What are the high signal structures within the penis on the T2-weighted image?

2. What does the low signal on the contrast-enhanced sagittal and axial images imply about blood flow?

3. What are predisposing clinical factors for this disorder?

4. How should the penis be positioned for optimal MRI?

Penis: Low-Flow Priapism

1. Paired corpora cavernosa.

2. Thrombosis of the corpora cavernosa.

3. Sickle cell disease, leukemia, and tumors.

4. Abutting the anterior abdominal wall.

References

Engin G, Tunaci M, Acunas B: High-flow priapism due to cavernous artery pseudoaneurysm: color Doppler sonography and magnetic resonance imaging findings, *Eur Radiol* 9:1698–1699, 1999.

Vossough A, Pretorius ES, Siegelman ES, et al: Magnetic resonance imaging of the penis, *Abdom Imaging* 27:640–659, 2002.

Cross-Reference

Zagoria RJ, *Genitourinary Radiology: THE REQUISITES,* 2nd ed, p 346.

Comment

The male urethra is composed of the two erectile bodies, the corpora cavernosa and the central corpora spongiosum, which contains the urethra. The corpora are surrounded by three layers of tissue: the tunica albuginea, the deep penile fascia (Buck's fascia), and the superficial fascia (Colle's fascia). Blood and nerve supply is from the pudendal trunk. Venous drainage is mainly via the dorsal vein of the penis. MRI sequences should be obtained with the penis abutting the anterior abdominal wall and consist primarily of T2-weighted and contrast-enhanced images in the long and short axis.

Priapism is defined as persistent erection despite the absence of any type of sexual stimulation. There are two main types, low-flow and high-flow. Low-flow priapism occurs due to thrombosis of the dorsal vein of the penis or corpora cavernosa. The corpora will show no enhancement following contrast administration. Predisposing conditions include sickle cell disease, pelvic tumors, leukemia, and infection. High-flow priapism is usually due to a rupture of the corpora cavernosa leading to a persistent penile hematoma. In general, the two types of priapism can be distinguished clinically. When a hematoma is suspected, MRI can demonstrate both the site of the high T2 signal hematoma and associated pseudoaneurysm. Low-flow priapism is usually treated using angiography and thrombolytic therapy.

Notes

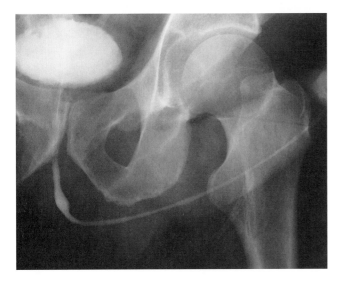

1. What type of study was performed?

2. What is the abnormal finding?

3. What is the differential diagnosis?

4. True or false: One cause of this lesion has been linked to urethral sarcoma.

Penis: Balanitis Xerotica Obliterans

1. Cystourethrogram.

2. Diffuse narrowing of the penile urethra.

3. Postinfectious urethritis, long-term urethral catheterization, chemical urethritis (rare), and balanitis xerotica obliterans (rare).

4. False (squamous cell carcinoma of the penis).

Reference

Staff WG: Urethral involvement in balanitis xerotica obliterans, *Br J Urol* 47:234–237, 1970.

Cross-Reference

Zagoria RJ, *Genitourinary Radiology: THE REQUISITES,* 2nd ed, pp 243–255.

Comment

Don't worry about making the correct diagnosis of balanitis xerotica obliterans (BXO) in this case; it is truly the "spotted zebra" of urethral inflammatory diseases. BXO is a localized variant of lichen sclerosis et atrophicus, a skin disease of unknown etiology that causes white, thickened plaques on the glans, penis, prepuce, and urethral meatus. It may result in phimosis or meatal stenosis. Uncommonly the fossa navicularis and the anterior urethra may be involved, and in these cases urethrography may reveal smooth narrowing of the anterior urethra of varying lengths.

The significance of BXO is that it is a premalignant lesion. Penile squamous cell carcinoma may be discovered long after BXO has been treated with topical steroid cream or, if this treatment is not successful, local excision. An interesting aside is that phimosis is found in as many as 75% of patients with squamous cell penile carcinoma and is the most common coexisting abnormality in patients with this malady. It is believed that the closed preputial cavity promotes the development of penile cancer by a carcinogen in smegma (the debris of desquamated cells on the inner surface of the prepuce).

The more common (and therefore more likely) diagnosis for this appearance is a postinfectious urethritis. Postinfectious (either gonococcal or nongonococcal urethritis) strictures may be multiple and may involve several centimeters of the urethra. Rarely the entire anterior urethra may narrow as a result of long-standing inflammation and fibrosis.

Notes

A